高职高专**国际护理专业**双语教材

妇产科护理学

Obstetric and Gynecological Nursing

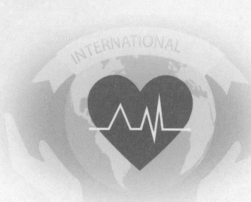

主编　任　美

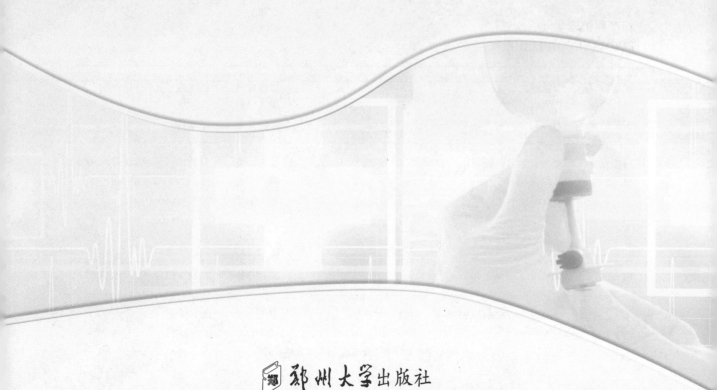

郑州大学出版社

图书在版编目（CIP）数据

妇产科护理学 = Obstetric and Gynecological Nursing：汉英对照／任美主编. -- 郑州：郑州大学出版社，2024.1

高职高专国际护理专业双语教材

ISBN 978-7-5645-9330-8

Ⅰ．①妇… Ⅱ．①任… Ⅲ．①妇产科学－护理学－高等职业教育－教材－汉、英 Ⅳ．①R473.71

中国国家版本馆 CIP 数据核字（2023）第 005017 号

妇产科护理学

FUCHANKE HULIXUE

策划编辑	李龙传		封面设计	苏永生　王深可
责任编辑	吕笑娟		版式设计	苏永生
责任校对	刘 莉		责任监制	李瑞卿

出版发行	郑州大学出版社		地　址	郑州市大学路 40 号（450052）
出版人	孙保营		网　址	http://www.zzup.cn
经　销	全国新华书店		发行电话	0371-66966070
印　刷	辉县市伟业印务有限公司			
开　本	850 mm×1 168 mm　1/16			
印　张	22.5		字　数	723 千字
版　次	2024 年 1 月第 1 版		印　次	2024 年 1 月第 1 次印刷

书　号	ISBN 978-7-5645-9330-8		定　价	69.00 元

本书如有印装质量问题，请与本社联系调换。

高职高专国际护理专业双语教材

编写委员会

主　任　许　琰

副主任　马玉霞　李福胜　倪　居

委　员　（按姓氏笔画排序）

邢华燕　何　敏　张全英　林爱琴

秦元梅　黄贺梅　梁明亮

作者名单

主　编　任　美

副主编　王珏辉　张艳亭

编　委　（按姓氏笔画排序）

王珏辉　郑州铁路职业技术学院

史利锋　河南护理职业学院

任　美　郑州铁路职业技术学院

刘淑霞　漯河医学高等专科学校

李文勤　郑州大学第五附属医院

李海燕　河南省人民医院

张　爽　郑州大学第三附属医院

张艳亭　郑州铁路职业技术学院

序

"十四五"期间,我国经济社会发展以推动高质量发展为主题,加快构建国内大循环为主体、国内国际双循环相互促进的新发展格局。职业教育是我国高等教育的重要组成部分,肩负着服务国家战略、促进高质量发展的重任。伴随着"一带一路"倡议背景下的国际产能合作,职业教育迎来了前所未有的发展机遇。2019 年《国家职业教育改革实施方案》《中国教育现代化 2035》和《关于实施中国特色高水平高职学校和专业建设计划的意见》相继出台,建设一批引领改革、支撑发展、中国特色、世界水平的高等职业院校和骨干专业群,培养具有国际视野、通晓国际规则、能够参与国际事务和国际竞争的高素质技能人才成为未来一段时期指引我国职业教育改革发展的纲领性目标。

新目标开启新征程。在新的历史机遇期,职业院校应全面对标时代发展新要求,主动承担职业教育历史使命,积极扩大对外交流合作,吸收借鉴国际先进理念,开发建设一批原创性的国际化教学标准和教学资源,为打造技能人才培养高地、开创高质量发展新局面做出重要贡献。在此背景下,郑州铁路职业技术学院联合河南中医药大学、新乡医学院第一附属医院、郑州大学第一附属医院、河南省人民医院、郑州市第三人民医院、郑州市第九人民医院、郑州市第七人民医院、河南护理职业学院,汇集骨干力量,面向国内护理专业中外合作办学项目,开发了一系列中英双语教材。

本系列教材在编写过程中紧扣创新性的编写理念,充分反映了近年来职业院校在"三教改革"方面取得的丰硕成果,在内容和形式方面具有以下鲜明特征。

1. 在深化医教协同背景下,教材内容重吸收护理学发展的新知识、新技术、新方法,全面反映了岗位实际需求和课程建设成果,充分体现了产教融合的教学特点。

2. 教材编写过程中坚持以学生为本,以人的健康为中心,更加突出医德教育,注重人文实践。

3. 教材内容取材广泛,视野宽阔,吸收融合了国外优质教学资源,为学生将来从事跨国就业奠定坚实的基础。

4. 本套教材除了纸质版外,还配套了大量数字教学资源,可供学生自主学习。

本系列教材在编写和审定过程中,得到了加拿大诺奎斯特学院、郑州大学出版社的大力支持和帮助,在此深表感谢! 编写期间相关人员参考了大量国内外专业书籍和教材,在此一并向有关作者致以谢意!

在本系列教材的编写过程中,全体编写人员本着高度负责的态度,克服了许多困难,几经修改,但因经验不足,时间仓促,书中可能有不足及错漏之处,恳请广大师生提出宝贵意见和建议,以冀再版时加以改进与完善。

许琰

2022 年 12 月

Introduction

During the 14th Five–Year Plan period, Chinese economic and social development will focus on promoting high–quality development and accelerate the establishment of a dual circulation development pattern in which domestic economic cycle plays a leading role while international economic cycle remains its extension and supplement. Vocational education, as an important component of higher education in our country, bears the responsibility of serving national strategies and promoting high–quality development. With the international production capacity cooperation under the background of the Belt and Road Initiative, vocational education has ushered in unprecedented development opportunities. In 2019, the *National Vocational Education Reform Implementation Plan*, *China's Education Modernization* 2035 and *Opinions on the Implementation of the Construction Plan of High–level Vocational Schools and Majors with Chinese Characteristics* were successively issued. These documents aim to "establish a number of world–class vocational schools and key specialty groups with Chinese characteristics that lead reform and support development" and "cultivate highly skilled technical professionals with an international perspective, understanding of international rules, and the ability to participate in international affairs and competitions". These goals serve as the guiding principles for the future period of vocational education reform and development in China.

New goals start a new journey. In this new era of historical opportunities, vocational colleges should fully align themselves with the new requirements of development, actively assume the historical mission of vocational education, and proactively expand international exchanges and cooperation. They should absorb and learn from advanced international concepts, develop and establish a set of original internationalized teaching standards and teaching resources. By doing so, they will make significant contributions to the creation of a high–level talent training hub for technical skills and the establishment of a new phase of high–quality development. Against this backdrop, in 2021, Zhengzhou Railway Vocational & Technical College, in collaboration with Henan University of Chinese Medicine, the First Affiliated Hospital of Xinxiang Medical University, the First Affiliated Hospital of Zhengzhou University, Henan Provincial People's Hospital, the Third People's Hospital of Zhengzhou, the Ninth People's Hospital of Zhengzhou, the Seventh People's Hospital of Zhengzhou, and Henan Vocational College of Nursing, has gathered key resources to develop a series of bilingual (Chinese–English) teaching materials for domestic nursing cooperative education programs.

During the development of this teaching material series, the guiding principle of "innovation" was adhered to, reflecting the fruitful achievements of vocational colleges in the "reforms in teachers, teaching materials and teaching methods" in recent years. The materials exhibit the following distinct characteristics in terms of content and format.

1. In the context of deepening the collaboration between medical and educational institutions, the teaching materials emphasize the absorption of new knowledge, technologies, and methods in nursing development. They comprehensively reflect the actual demands of the profession and the achievements in curriculum development, fully embodying the teaching characteristics of industry-education integration.

2. Throughout the process of developing the teaching materials, a student-centered approach has been maintained, with a focus on the well-being of individuals. Emphasis has been placed on medical ethics education, and significant attention has been given to incorporate humanistic practices into the materials.

3. The teaching materials draw from a wide range of sources and have a broad perspective. They incorporate and integrate high-quality teaching resources from abroad, laying a solid foundation for students' future employment in multinational settings.

4. In addition to the printed version, this set of teaching materials is accompanied by a wealth of digital teaching resources, which can be used by students for self-directed learning.

We would like to express our deep gratitude for the strong support and assistance provided by NorQuest College in Canada and Zhengzhou University Press throughout the writing and approval process of this teaching material series. We also extend our thanks to the authors of the numerous domestic and international professional books and textbooks that were referenced during the writing process.

During the writing process of this teaching material series, all the authors approached their responsibilities with a high level of dedication. They overcame numerous challenges and made multiple revisions. However, due to limited experience and time constraints, there may be some shortcomings and errors. If any teachers or students encounter issues while using these materials, we sincerely request that you provide valuable feedback and suggestions. This will allow us to make improvements and enhancements in future editions.

December, 2022

前　言

《妇产科护理学》双语教材的编写是为了适应专业建设发展的需要,为了给学习者提供清晰、准确、实用的妇产科护理学知识,促进中英文双语交流与提高,培养学习者在临床实践中解决问题的能力。本书的编写团队中吸纳了来自临床一线的专家,使所编教材更能体现行业发展现状,对接职业标准及岗位需求。本教材主要供高职护理专业学生使用。

妇产科护理学课程是高职护理专业的必修专业核心课程,也是护理专业执业资格考试的一门必考课程。本教材内容包括女性生殖系统解剖与生理、病史采集与检查、妊娠期妇女的护理、分娩期妇女的护理、产褥期管理、妊娠期并发症妇女的护理、胎儿及附属物异常的护理、妊娠合并症妇女的护理、异常分娩妇女的护理、分娩期并发症妇女的护理、产褥期疾病妇女的护理、女性生殖系统炎症患者的护理、妇产科手术患者的护理、女性生殖系统肿瘤患者的护理、妊娠滋养细胞疾病患者的护理、女性生殖内分泌疾病患者的护理、妇科其他疾病患者的护理、计划生育妇女的护理。

本教材是“理实一体”的项目任务式教材,以项目为模块组织教材内容,打破了原有教材体系的章节框架局限。教材内容上按照工作情景、任务内容、任务目标、任务实施的结构编写,符合学生认知规律,实现理论与实践的有机结合。本教材严格参照专业培养目标编写教学内容,强化理论知识的同时注重对实践应用的思考,培养学生应用知识、分析问题、解决问题的能力,注重批判性思维的培养,以利于学生更好地适应临床护理工作。

为适应互联网+教育的发展,本教材采取新形态一体化教材编写模式,实现了纸质教材和数字资源的有机结合。本教材提供了微课、课件等丰富的数字资源,学生通过扫描二维码获取,便于其深入学习和研究;每一项目后面都附有测试题,均按照护士执业资格考试的知识点进行编写和设计,通过扫描二维码进行检测;正文穿插拓展知识二维码链接,拓宽教材知识的深度和广度。

本教材的编写耗费了各位编者大量的时间和精力,在此对她们的付出深表感谢!由于编者能力有限,内容编排难免有不妥之处,欢迎广大师生批评指正!

任　美

2023 年 9 月

Preface

The development of the bilingual textbook *Obstetric and Gynecological Nursing* is aimed at meeting the needs of professional construction and providing learners with clear, accurate, practical knowledge in obstetric and gynecological nursing. It aims to promote bilingual communication and proficiency, as well as cultivate learners' ability to solve problems in clinical practice. The writing team of this book includes experts from the frontlines of clinical practice, ensuring that the content reflects the current industry development status and aligns with professional standards and job requirements. This textbook is primarily intended for use by students majoring in nursing at higher vocational institutions.

The course on obstetric and gynecological nursing is a compulsory core subject for nursing majors at higher vocational institutions, as well as an essential examinable course for obtaining a nursing professional qualification. The content of this textbook includes anatomy and physiology of the female reproductive system, medical history collection and examination, care for pregnant women during pregnancy, care for women during childbirth, postpartum management, care for women with complications during pregnancy, abnormalities in fetuses and their appendages, care for women with pregnancy-related complications or abnormal deliveries, care for women with postpartum diseases or reproductive system inflammations, care for patients undergoing obstetric-gynecological surgeries, care for patients with reproductive system tumors, care for patients suffering from trophoblastic diseases, care for patients suffering from endocrine disorders related to female reproduction, care for other gynecological disease patients, and family planning.

This textbook is a project-task-based textbook with "theory and practice as one", which organizes the content of the textbook with projects as modules, breaking the limitations of the original chapter framework of the textbook system. The textbook content is compiled according to the structure of work scenarios, task content, task objectives and task implementation, which conforms to the cognitive laws of students and realizes the organic combination of theory and practice. This textbook strictly refers to the professional training objectives to compile the teaching content, strengthens the theoretical knowledge while paying attention to the thinking of practical application, cultivates students' ability to apply knowledge, analyze problems and solve problems, and pays attention to the cultivation of critical thinking, so as to help students better adapt to clinical nursing work.

In order to adapt to the development of Internet+ education, this textbook adopts a new form of integrated textbook compilation mode, realizing the organic combination of paper textbooks and digital resources. This textbook provides rich digital resources such as micro lessons, courseware and animation, which can be obtained by students by scanning two-dimensional code, facilitating their in-depth study and research; each project is followed by a test question, which is compiled and designed according to the knowledge points of the nurse practice qualification examination, and can be detected by scanning two-dimensional code; and there are two-dimensional code links to expand knowledge, broadening the depth and breadth of the textbook knowledge.

The compilation of this textbook has taken the editors a lot of time and energy, and we would like to express our deep appreciation for their efforts! Due to limited ability, there may be some inappropriate content in the editing. Welcome the criticism and correction of teachers and students!

Ren Mei

September, 2023

目 录

绪论
（Introduction）

一 妇产科护理的历史与发展

近代以前,护理学一直作为医学领域的一个组成部分。随着社会和医学实践的发展,为适应新时期人类健康和临床医疗的需要,护理学逐渐发展并成为医学领域中一门独立的学科,妇产科护理作为护理学的亚学科,逐渐形成独立的护理专科,其护理理论和模式反映了当代妇产科护理发展的新趋势。

1. 早期妇产科护理 妇产科护理最早源于产科。人类自有繁衍以来,就有专人参与照顾妇女的生育过程,他们一般是产妇的家人或宗教及神学人员,他们照顾产妇的经验使他们成了集医、药、护为一身的原始产科医生,这就是早期的产科学及产科护理学的雏形。大约在公元前 1500 年,古埃及就有关于妇产科学的专著,描述了分娩、流产、月经及一些妇科病的处理方法。至公元前460 年,古希腊著名"医学之父"希波克拉底,在他的医学巨著中记录了阴道检查和妇科疾病的治疗经验及反对堕胎的誓言。1576 年,P. Franco 创立了三叶产钳助产术;1625 年后,H. Van Roonhyze 著有《现代妇科和产科学》,记录了为子宫破裂和异位妊娠患者实施的剖宫产术和剖腹探查术。此后,剖腹探查术开始兴起。随着无菌手术概念和麻醉学的创立,妇产科学和外科学的发展达到了新的阶段。

祖国医学发展历史悠久。公元前 1300—公元前 1200 年,甲骨文上就有王妃分娩时染疾的记载。2000 多年前的中医古典巨著《黄帝内经》里有对女子成长、发育、月经疾患、妊娠诊断及相关疾病的诊治认识。在晋朝至隋朝,太医令王叔和、巢元方所著《脉经》和《诸病源候论》里也有不少关于妇科疾病、产科疾病的病因和诊断的描述。唐代妇产科专家孙思邈在《千金要方》的《妇人方》中描述有妊娠、胎产、调经和妇科杂病。宋代和清代医学家都有对妇产科临床及护理的论述。

2. 现代妇产科护理 随着社会的进步、医学的发展,妇女生育逐渐摆脱了宗教和神学的阴影,妇女患病、生育时开始求助于专业人员或专业机构,分娩的场所也从家庭转向医院。对参与产科照顾人员的结构和学识有了更高的要求,即需要一批受过专业训练和具备产科技能的护理人员。妇产科医学的发展,如围生医学的兴起、围生监护技术的应用、产前诊断技术的提供、助孕技术(试管婴儿)的发明及妇科内分泌学的完善,为妇产科护理的发展提供了有利条件。1860 年,南丁格尔在英国圣托马斯医院创建了世界上第一所正规护士学校,着手助产士及济贫院护士的培训工作。它的出现标志着现代护理学的诞生。南丁格尔是现代护理教育的奠基人、现代护理学的创始人,也是现代妇产科护理学的创始人。

3. 当代妇产科护理发展趋势 妇产科护理与护理学发展趋势一致,也经历了由"以疾病为中心的护理"向"以患者为中心的护理"的变革,并向"以整体人的健康为中心的护理"目标进军。护士的工作场所逐渐由医院扩大到家庭、社区,工作内容也从传统、被动地执行医嘱,扩大到提供整体化护理。国内现代妇产科护理也处于迅速发展的过程中,正逐渐与世界妇产科护理接轨。

二 妇产科护理的主要内容及任务

妇产科护理是通过诊断并处理女性对现存和潜在健康问题的反应,为妇女健康提供服务的学科。它以妇产科学为理论基础,是现代护理学的重要组成部分。

1. 研究对象　生命中各阶段不同健康状况的女性,以及相关的家庭成员和社会成员。

2. 主要内容　研究女性在生命周期的妊娠、分娩、产褥期及非妊娠阶段和计划生育中的生理、病理、心理及社会等方面的问题,并对其进行护理评估,做出护理诊断,制订护理措施,最终达到护理目标。因此,妇产科护理包括孕产妇的护理、妇科疾病患者的护理、计划生育指导及妇女保健等内容。

3. 主要任务　保障妇女在整个生命周期的不同生理阶段健康、安全、幸福,保证胎儿、新生儿健康成长。

三 妇产科护理对护士的素质要求

妇产科护理作为一门独特的整体护理专业,要求妇产科护士在不断加强自身护理技能的同时,更应注重综合素质的提升。

1. 要有高尚的职业道德及进取精神　要求护士有高度的事业心和责任感,热爱本职工作,尊重生命;富有同情心和爱心,能热忱、周到地为患者服务;要有终身学习的理念,刻苦学习,不断进取。

2. 要有良好的专业素质和职业技能　广博的知识、精湛的技术、较强的理论水平和业务操作能力是保障母婴安全的基础。

3. 要有独立的护理思维与判断能力　要求护士对待工作心中有数,忙而不乱,井井有条,具有较强的应变能力和处理能力。

4. 要有健康的身体和乐观的心态　要求护士能应对繁忙、紧张的工作;善于与人合作共事,情绪稳定。妇产科工作特点既需要合作者的支持、协助,又需要护理对象的理解、配合,医护合作、护患协作尤为重要,工作中应该注意态度,控制情绪,营造和谐气氛。

妇产科护理要求护士必须具备较强的综合素质,加之飞速发展的医学科学,要求护士树立终身学习的意识,持之以恒地钻研业务,熟练掌握实践技能。妇产科护理质量关乎人口与社会的可持续发展,妇产科护士任重而道远。

Obstetric and gynecological nursing is one of the important major stem curriculums in clinical nursing. This subject explores the specific physiological and pathological phenomenon of women, ascertains the nursing problems in women's disease rehabilitation and health promotion and provides appropriate measurements to improve the holistic health level of women. Gynecological nursing science and obstetric nursing science are included in obstetric and gynecological nursing. In gynecological nursing, the existed and potential nursing problems and the interventions of women in nonpregnant period are introduced. The obstetrical nursing is mainly related to the women's problems and interventions in pregnancy, delivery and puerperium. In addition, family planning is also introduced with the development of medical science, the obstetric and gynecological nursing develops greatly in many sides, such as obstetric and gynecological nursing philosophy, the education model, psychological nursing, nursing research, especially in maternal and neonatal nursing.

"Safety motherhood, Priority childhood" is the philosophy of maternal and child healthcare. Reproduction has been given prime importance. Legislation and policy efforts have focused attention on protecting the rights of women and children. The complexity of current societal trends imposes a challenge on the providers of maternal–child healthcare. Professionals from the social science and health science, policy makers, and providers of healthcare services are combining their efforts to develop useful strategies.

Birth is a family affair, and the reproductive health of the total family is the cornerstone of a healthy society. Thus, the study of obstetrics and nursing care of women and their families during childbearing includes the study of anatomic and physiologic adaptations to human reproduction, human growth and development, interdependent relationships to society. Knowledge of the anatomy and physiology of the reproductive organs and of the development of the fetus from conception to birth is required by everyone who participates in maternity care. The health, well–being, and safety of each mother, father, and newborn must be protected, and the highest level of wellness possible for every childbearing family must be achieved in the broadest sense of physical, emotional, and social well–being.

Obstetric Nursing

Obstetrics is defined as the branch of medicine that deals with parturition, its antecedents, and its sequelae. Thus, obstetrics is concerned principally with the phenomena and management of pregnancy, labor, and the puerperium under normal and abnormal circumstances. In England and the United States, this branch of medicine was called midwifery until the latter part of the 19th century when the term obstetrics came to the forefront. Obstetric nursing is related to pregnancy, delivery and puerperium. After World War II, the terminology changed to maternity care as the focus came to be on the recipient of care rather than on the provider of care. Maternity care implies a broader meaning of care to mother, newborn, and other members of the family. It emphasizes the importance of interpersonal relationships that are significant in the family.

Perinatal Care

During the last decade, as knowledge and technology have continued to burgeon, an effort has been made to provide a conceptual umbrella to encompass maternal–fetal healthcare as a unit. Consequently, the term perinatal care has evolved. By definition, the word perinatal means from 28 gestation week to 7 days after birth. All of the definitions imply that an obstetric and pediatric orientation is involved. Hence, perinatal care is a method of healthcare delivery that decreases the segmentation and fragmentation of care for the mother and newborn. Perinatal care also has become associated with the high–risk mother and newborn in hospitals designated as tertiary care, or level III hospitals. These hospitals have the resources and expertise to manage any complication of pregnancy or that the newborn may experience. The personnel in level III institutions provide care for normal clients and for all types of maternal–fetal and neonatal illnesses and abnormalities. By contrast, level I hospitals provide for management of uncomplicated maternal and neonatal clients. In these institutions, there should be a strong component of preventive services and early detection of existing or potential problems, which then may be referred to the level III institutions. Level II hospitals provide the same services as level I hospitals; however, they can provide for some high–risk obstetric problems and certain types of neonatal illnesses that do not require the wide array of expertise and technology found in the level III hospitals.

Nurse's Responsibility

The nurse working in maternal and perinatal care has a responsibility to the woman and fetus or newborn. An understanding of one's own values and beliefs together with knowledge of the standards of care, scope of practice, and legal regulations aids in effective decision making.

The nurse has certain obligations to the woman. He or she must have the knowledge and expertise to use the equipment necessary for the woman's care, particularly fetal monitors.

The importance of the nurse recording promptly and accurately his or her observations, treatments, procedures, medicines, and any other appropriate information cannot be stressed enough. Many weak malpractice cases come to court because of errors or omissions in charting and recording.

Another important area of responsibility is to observe the newborn and mother carefully after delivery and report and record any signs of a complication or problem. Nurses can be held liable in the event of maternal or newborn complications. It is extremely important that they are knowledgeable regarding their appropriate responsibilities and care.

（任　美）

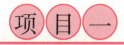

女性生殖系统解剖与生理（Anatomy and Physiology of Female Reproductive System）

项目描述

女性生殖系统与月经产生、女性性征的维持、受精、胎儿的生长发育及娩出等诸多方面关系密切。女性生殖系统的结构和功能正常是维持上述功能的基础。掌握女性生殖系统解剖与生理的基础知识是处理女性生殖系统问题的基础。

The female reproductive system functions to produce menstruation; to maintain the female characteristics; to provide a physiologic environment that allows conception, pregnancy, and birth to progress normally, and is also related to some other aspects. The normal structure and function of reproductive system provide the prerequisites. This chapter presents the normal anatomy and physiology of the female reproductive system to help the students obtain the basic knowledge and confidence in dealing with issues surrounding reproduction. Understanding the knowledge also provides the students opportunity to further study on the related knowledge and skill in obstetric and gynecological nursing.

任务一　女性生殖系统解剖（Anatomy of Female Reproductive System）

工作情景

李女士，25岁，已婚未孕，现备孕，故来妇科门诊进行常规体检。请为其做相应的检查，判断其内、外生殖器是否正常。

任务内容

女性生殖系统包括内、外生殖器，相关组织及邻近器官。骨盆为生殖器官的所在地，为生殖器官及其他盆腔脏器提供支持和保护，且与分娩关系密切。

◆能描述女性内、外生殖器的构成及解剖特点。

◆能叙述女性内生殖器的邻近器官及其临床意义。

◆能分析女性骨盆及骨盆底的结构特点及其临床意义。

一 女性外生殖器

女性外生殖器是指生殖器官的外露部分,位于两股内侧之间,前为耻骨联合,后为会阴,包括阴阜、大阴唇、小阴唇、阴蒂和阴道前庭,统称外阴(图1-1)。

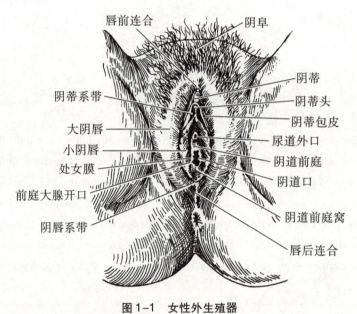

图1-1 女性外生殖器

1. 阴阜　阴阜为耻骨联合上方的脂肪垫。青春期此部位开始生长阴毛,呈倒三角形分布,并扩展至大阴唇外侧。阴毛疏密、粗细、色泽存在种族和个体差异。

2. 大阴唇　大阴唇为两股内侧的一对纵行隆起的皮肤皱襞,起自阴阜,止于会阴。大阴唇外侧面为皮肤,有色素沉着和阴毛,内含皮脂腺和汗腺;其内侧面湿润似黏膜。大阴唇皮下为疏松结缔组织和脂肪组织,内含丰富的血管、淋巴管和神经,外伤后易出血形成血肿。

3. 小阴唇　小阴唇为位于大阴唇内侧的一对薄皮肤皱襞。其表面色褐、湿润、无阴毛分布,但富含神经末梢,故极为敏感。

4. 阴蒂　阴蒂位于两侧小阴唇顶端下方,与男性阴茎海绵体组织相似,神经末梢丰富,为性反应器官。

5. 阴道前庭　阴道前庭为两侧小阴唇之间的菱形区域,前至阴蒂,后至阴唇系带。

(1)尿道外口　位于阴道前庭的前部,略呈圆形,边缘折叠而合拢。其后壁有一对尿道旁腺,其分泌物有润滑尿道口的作用,但此腺体开口小,容易有细菌潜伏。

(2)阴道口和处女膜　阴道口位于尿道外口下方、前庭的后部,其大小、形状常不规则。阴道口周围覆有一层较薄黏膜称处女膜,其中央有一孔,圆形或新月形,月经血经此排出。处女膜因初次性交撕裂或剧烈运动破裂,可有少量流血,阴道分娩时进一步破损,仅留下处女膜痕。

（3）前庭球　又称球海绵体,位于前庭两侧,由具有勃起性的静脉丛组成。

（4）前庭大腺　又称巴多林腺,位于两侧大阴唇后部及深部,被球海绵体肌覆盖,如黄豆大小,左右各一。其腺管细长（1～2 cm）,开口于小阴唇与处女膜之间的沟内中下 1/3 处,性兴奋时分泌黄白色黏液起润滑作用。正常情况检查时不能触及此腺,若腺管口闭塞,可形成前庭大腺囊肿或脓肿。

The external genitalia is also called pudenda or vulva. It consists of the mons pubis, the labia majora, the labia minora, the clitoris, the vaginal vestibule. These are all visible on external examination. It is therefore bounded anteriorly by the mons pubis, laterally by the labia majora and posteriorly by the perineum.

女性内生殖器

女性内生殖器由外向内依次包括阴道、子宫、输卵管和卵巢,其中输卵管和卵巢又合称为子宫附件（图1-2）。

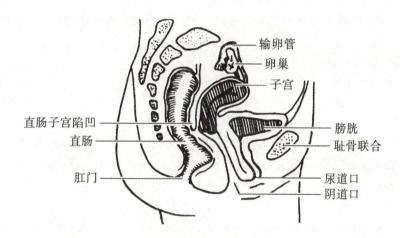

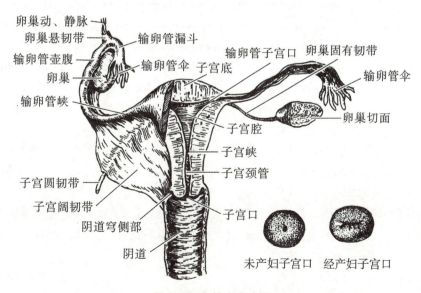

图1-2　女性内生殖器

The internal genital organs in female include the vagina, the uterus, the fallopian tubes and the ovaries. These organs are placed internally and require special instruments for inspection. And the fallopian tubes and the ovaries are also called the uterine adnexa.

1. 阴道 阴道是性交器官,也是月经血排出及胎儿娩出的通道。

(1)位置和形态 位于真骨盆下部的中央,呈上宽下窄的腔道,前壁长 7～9 cm,与膀胱和尿道相邻;后壁长 10～12 cm,与直肠贴近。正常阴道前后壁紧贴,可以防止外界的污染。阴道上端包绕子宫颈,下端开口于阴道前庭的后部。子宫颈与阴道间的圆周状隐窝称阴道穹隆,按位置可分为前、后、左、右 4 部分,其中以后穹隆位置最深,其顶端与盆腔最低点(直肠子宫陷凹)紧密相邻,临床上具有十分重要的意义,经此处穿刺或引流,是某些疾病诊断或实施手术的重要途径。

(2)组织结构 阴道壁由内而外由黏膜层、肌层和纤维组织膜组成。阴道黏膜为复层鳞状上皮细胞,无腺体,其上端 1/3 在性激素作用下发生周期性变化。阴道壁有很多横行皱襞及弹力纤维,有较大的伸展性。幼女和绝经后妇女阴道上皮较薄,皱襞少,伸展性小,容易受损而感染。阴道黏膜渗出的少量液体与脱落细胞、子宫颈黏液混合形成白带。阴道壁富含静脉丛,损伤后易出血或形成血肿。

The vagina serves three important functions: representing the excretory duct of the uterus through which secretion and menstrual flow escape; being the female organ of copulation; forming part of the birth canal during labor.

Position and Configuration

The vagina lies in the center of the lower part of the true pelvis. It is a dilatable, mucous membrane-lined passage between the bladder and the rectum. Commonly, the anterior and posterior vaginal walls are, respectively, 7-9 cm and 10-12 cm in length. At its terminal end the vaginal circumstance is attached to the uterine cervix. As a consequence, a small, pouchlike area called the posterior fornix is formed beneath the cervix. The posterior fornix is adjacent to recto-uterine and usually provides ready surgical access to the peritoneal cavity.

Structures

The vagina is composed of mucosa, muscular layer, fibrous coat. The walls of the vagina are pinkish and lined by stratified squamous epithelium. The vagina has many rugae, ridgelike structures caused by folding of the mucous membranes. These are capable of stretching to allow marked distention of the passage in the process of childbirth. The vaginal mucosa changes periodically under the effect of sex hormones. In postmenopausal women, the walls may be thin with fewer rugae and easy to be hurt and infected. The fibrous coat out of the muscular layer is highly vascular and amiable to bleeding or forming haematoma. The vaginal pH, from puberty to menopause, is acidic.

2. 子宫 子宫是孕育胚胎、胎儿和产生月经的器官。

(1)位置和形态 子宫位于盆腔中央,形状如倒置梨形。成年女性子宫重 50～70 g,长 7～8 cm,宽 4～5 cm,厚 2～3 cm,容量约 5 mL。子宫上部较宽,称为子宫体,子宫体顶部称为子宫底。子宫两侧为子宫角,与输卵管相通。子宫下部较窄呈圆柱状,称为子宫颈。子宫体与子宫颈的比例随年龄变化而不同,婴儿期为 1∶2,成年女性为 2∶1,老年人为 1∶1。子宫体与子宫颈之间形成最狭窄部分称为子宫峡部,在非孕期长约 1 cm,其上端解剖上较狭窄,称为解剖学内口;下端黏膜由子宫内膜转为子宫颈黏膜,故称为组织学内口(图 1-3)。

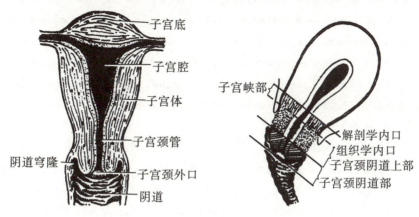

图1-3 正常子宫

（2）组织结构

1）子宫体：由内向外分为子宫内膜层、肌层和浆膜层。子宫内膜为一层粉红色黏膜组织，分为致密层、海绵层和基底层。致密层和海绵层统称为功能层，在卵巢性激素作用下发生周期性变化。基底层靠近子宫肌层，无周期性变化。子宫肌层是子宫壁最厚的一层，非孕时约0.8 cm，分为3层：外层多纵行，内层环行，中层围绕血管交织排列，有利于子宫收缩时止血。子宫浆膜层是覆盖宫底部及前后壁的盆腔腹膜，与肌层紧贴。在子宫前面向前反折，形成膀胱子宫陷凹。在子宫后面，折向直肠，形成直肠子宫陷凹，又称道格拉斯陷凹。

2）子宫颈：主要由结缔组织构成。子宫颈内腔呈梭形，称为子宫颈管，未生育的成年女性的子宫颈管长2.5～3.0 cm，其下端为子宫颈外口，开口于阴道。未经阴道分娩的妇女子宫颈外口呈圆形，经阴道分娩的妇女子宫颈外口受分娩的影响呈横裂，将子宫颈分为前后唇。子宫颈管内黏膜为单层高柱状上皮细胞，受性激素影响有周期性变化。黏膜层腺体分泌碱性黏液，形成黏液栓，堵塞子宫颈管。子宫颈外口柱状上皮与鳞状上皮交界处，是子宫颈癌的好发部位。

（3）子宫韧带 共有4对（图1-4），以维持子宫的正常位置。

1）子宫圆韧带：呈圆索状，维持子宫前倾。

2）子宫阔韧带：为一对翼形的腹膜皱襞，维持子宫在盆腔的正中位置。

3）子宫主韧带：又称子宫颈横韧带，是固定子宫颈正常位置的重要组织。

4）子宫骶韧带：间接保持子宫于前倾的位置。

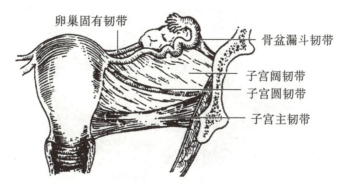

图1-4 子宫的韧带

The uterus has several functions: Proliferation of endometrium once in each menstrual cycle after puberty in anticipation of conception and shedding its lining through the process of menstruation when conception does not occur; Provision of a passage for sperm to fallopian tube after intercourse; Provision of a proliferated endometrium for the implantation of a fertilized ovum; Nurturing and enhancement of development of a placenta that will provide the means to nourish and support the developing fetus during pregnancy; Protection of the fetus and contraction during labor to expel the neonate.

Position and Configuration

The uterus, or womb, is a hollow, thick-walled, muscular organ located centrally in the female pelvis between the bladder anterior and the rectum posterior. The uterus is an inverted, flattened pear-shaped organ. In adult nulliparous woman it is approximately 7-8 cm long, 4-5 cm at its widest point, and 2-3 cm thick and weighs 50-70 g. The volume of uterine cavity is about 5 mL. It is divided into 2 main portions, the larger portion or body above and the smaller cervix below, connected by a transverse constriction, the isthmus. The body is further divided into the fundus and the cornua. Uterine isthmus is the constricted area that lies between the body and the cervix. This portion of the uterus is approximately 1 cm in length in nonpregnant state. Its upper limit marks the lower boundary of the corpus which is called the anatomical internal os. At its lower limit, the isthmus marks the transition from its own mucosa to the mucous membrane of the endocervical canal which is called the histological internal os. Cervix is cylindrical in shape and measures 2.5-3.0 cm. It extends from the isthmus and ends at the external cervical os. The exterior portion of the cervix protruding into the vagina is called the portio vaginalis cervicis, or the ectocervix. The portion lying above the vagina is called supravaginal cervix. The external orifice of uterus is round or oval before parturition but takes the form of a transverse slit in women who have borne children.

Structures

The structures are different between the uterus body and the cervix.

Uterine Ligaments

There are four pairs of ligaments of uterus: the round ligaments, the broad ligaments, the cardinal ligaments and uterosacral ligaments. In addition to the static support of these ligaments, the pelvic diaphragm provides an indirect and dynamic support.

3. 输卵管　为卵子与精子的结合场所，也是运送受精卵的管道（图1-5）。

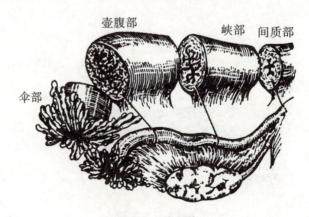

图1-5　输卵管

（1）位置和形态 输卵管为一对细长而弯曲的管道,内侧与子宫角相连,外端游离,全长8～14 cm。根据输卵管的形态由内向外可分为4部分:间质部(最狭窄处)、峡部、壶腹部(正常受精部位)和伞部(拾卵)。

（2）组织结构 输卵管壁由内向外分3层:黏膜层、平滑肌层和浆膜层。平滑肌层有节奏收缩引起输卵管由远端向近端蠕动;黏膜层由单层高柱状上皮组成,其中有分泌细胞及纤毛细胞,纤毛向宫腔方向摆动,协助受精卵的运行。输卵管黏膜层受性激素的影响有周期性变化。

The fallopian tubes are also called the uterine tubes or oviducts. They serve to convey the ova to the uterus, and also is the place the ovum meets the spermatozoon. The fallopian tubes extend from the superior angles of the uterus to the region of the ovaries, running in the superior border of the broad ligament. Each tube is 8–14 cm long and can be divided into 4 portions: uterine intramural, isthmus, ampulla and infundibulum.

The wall of the tube has 3 layers: The outer coat is serous (peritoneal), the middle coat is the muscular portion and the inner one the mucous portion.

4.卵巢 卵巢是产生与排出卵子,并分泌甾体激素的性器官。

（1）位置和形态 为一对扁椭圆形腺体,位于输卵管的后下方。成年女子的卵巢大小约为4 cm×3 cm×1 cm,重5～6 g,呈灰白色。青春期开始排卵,卵巢表面逐渐变得凹凸不平;绝经后,卵巢萎缩,变小、变硬。

（2）组织结构 卵巢表面无腹膜覆盖,表层为单层立方上皮即生发上皮,其下为致密纤维组织,称卵巢白膜。白膜下的卵巢组织分为外层的皮质与内层的髓质。皮质是卵巢的主体,由大小不等的各级发育卵泡、黄体和它们退化后形成的残余结构及间质组成;髓质与卵巢门相连,含有疏松的结缔组织及丰富的血管、神经、淋巴管及少量的平滑肌纤维(图1-6)。

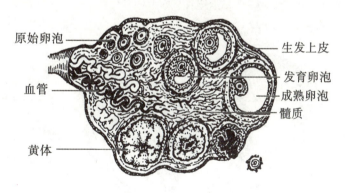

图1-6 卵巢的结构

The ovaries are two almond-shaped glandular organs. They develop and produce ova and secrete steroid sex hormones. The surface of the ovary of a girl before puberty is smooth, but in adult woman is scarred from previous ovulations. Each organ weighs approximately 5–6 g and measures about 4 cm in length, 3 cm in breadth and 1 cm in width. After menopause, the ovaries become atrophy and rigid. The paired ovaries are light gray. There is no peritoneum covering on the ovaries. The ovary is covered by the germinal epithelium (a single layer of cubical cells). The substance of the gland consists of an outer cortex and an inner medulla. The cortex consists of stromal cells thickened beneath the germinal epithelium to form the tunica albuginea, serving a protective function. During the reproductive period the cortex is studded with numerous follicular structures, called the functional units of the ovary, in various phases of their development. The medulla consists of loose connective tissues, few unstriped muscles, blood vessels and nerves.

三 血管、淋巴及神经

1. **血管** 女性内、外生殖器的血液供应,主要来自卵巢动脉、子宫动脉、阴道动脉及阴部内动脉。各部位的静脉与同名动脉伴行,但在数量上比动脉多,并在相应器官及其周围形成静脉丛,互相吻合,故盆腔感染易于蔓延。

2. **淋巴** 女性生殖器官有丰富的淋巴系统,淋巴结通常沿相应的血管排列,但数目、位置变异很大。女性生殖器官淋巴主要分为外生殖器淋巴与盆腔淋巴。当内、外生殖器发生感染或肿瘤时,往往沿各部回流的淋巴管扩散或转移,导致相应部位的淋巴结肿大。

3. **神经** 女性外生殖器的神经主要由阴部神经支配,内生殖器主要由交感神经和副交感神经支配。子宫平滑肌有自主节律活动,完全切除其神经后仍能有节律收缩,还能完成分娩活动。临床上可见低位截瘫的孕妇仍能顺利自然分娩。

四 骨盆

骨盆是躯干和下肢之间的骨性连接,是支持躯干和保护盆腔脏器的重要器官,同时也是胎儿娩出的通道,其大小、形态对分娩有直接影响。通常女性骨盆比男性宽而浅,有利于分娩。

1. **骨盆的组成** 骨盆由左右2块髋骨、1块骶骨和1块尾骨组成。每块髋骨又由髂骨、坐骨和耻骨融合而成。坐骨后缘中点的突起称为坐骨棘,是分娩过程中衡量胎先露下降程度的重要标志。耻骨两降支前部相连构成耻骨弓,所形成的角度正常为90°~100°,骶骨由5~6块骶椎融合而成,其上缘向前突出,称为骶岬。尾骨由4~5块尾椎组成(图1-7)。

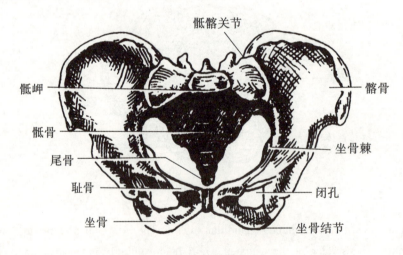

图1-7 正常女性骨盆(前上观)

关节有耻骨联合、骶髂关节及骶尾关节。以上关节和耻骨联合周围均有韧带附着,如骶骨、尾骨与坐骨结节之间的骶结节韧带,骶骨、尾骨与坐骨棘之间的骶棘韧带(图1-8)。妊娠期受激素的影响,韧带松弛,各关节的活动略有增加,尤其是骶尾关节,分娩时尾骨后移,有利于胎儿的娩出。

2. **骨盆的分界** 以耻骨联合上缘、髂耻缘、骶岬上缘的连线为界,将骨盆分为假骨盆和真骨盆两部分。

　　分界线以上部分为假骨盆,又称大骨盆,与产道无直接关系,但通过测量假骨盆某些径线可间接判断真骨盆的大小;分界线以下部分为真骨盆,又称小骨盆,是胎儿娩出的骨产道。骨盆腔为一前壁短、后壁长的弯曲管道:前壁是耻骨联合和耻骨支,两侧壁为坐骨、坐骨棘与骶棘韧带,后壁是骶骨和尾骨。

　　3.骨盆的类型　根据骨盆形状,分为4种类型(图1-9):女性型、男性型、类人猿型、扁平型。女性型骨盆最常见(占52%~58.9%),是女性正常骨盆。入口呈横椭圆形,耻骨弓较宽,坐骨棘间径≥10 cm,有利于胎儿的娩出。

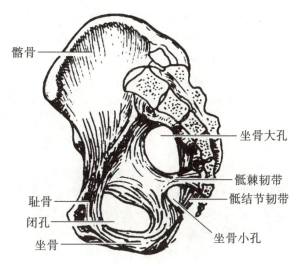

图1-8　骨盆的韧带

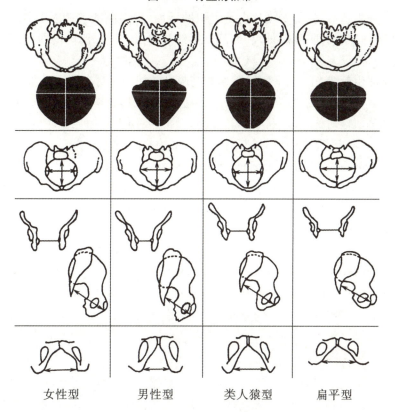

| 女性型 | 男性型 | 类人猿型 | 扁平型 |

图1-9　骨盆的类型

The pelvis is a basin-shaped ring of bones that marks the distal margin of the trunk. Its dimensions are directly related to the delivery of a neonate. For a baby to be delivered vaginally, he or she must be able to pass through the ring of pelvic bone. In general, the female pelvis is wider and shallower compared to the male pelvis. And this is helpful for the fetus to be delivered. The pelvis is composed of four united bones: the os sacrum, the os coccyx, and two os coxae (innominate bones). The pelvic joints include the pubic symphysis, the sacro-iliac joint and the sacro-coccygeal joint. There are two pairs important ligaments in the pelvis: the sacrotuberous ligaments and the sacrospinous ligaments.

The two major pelvic divisions are the pelvis major and the pelvis minor divided by the iliopectineal line or brim. The pelvis major or the false pelvis lies above the iliopectineal line, the pelvis minor or the true pelvis, located below the iliopectineal line.

There are four basic types of pelves: gynecoid type, platypelloid type, anthropoid type, and android type. The gynecoid pelvis is the normal female pelvis and also the most common one.

五 骨盆底

骨盆底是封闭骨盆出口的多层肌肉和筋膜,承托并保持盆腔脏器于正常的位置。分娩时可不同程度地损伤骨盆底组织或影响其功能。骨盆底的前面为耻骨联合下缘,后面为尾骨尖,两侧为耻骨降支、坐骨升支及坐骨结节。会阴又称会阴体,指阴道口与肛门之间的楔形软组织,厚 3 ~ 4 cm,由表及里分别为皮肤、皮下脂肪、筋膜、部分肛提肌和会阴中心腱。妊娠期会阴组织变软,伸展性很大,有利于分娩。分娩时要注意保护会阴,以免造成会阴裂伤。

骨盆底由外向内分为 3 层:外层、中层、内层。

1. 外层　位于外生殖器、会阴皮肤及皮下组织的下面,由会阴浅筋膜及其深部的 3 对肌肉(球海绵体肌、坐骨海绵体肌及会阴浅横肌)和肛门外括约肌组成。这层肌肉的肌腱汇合于阴道外口与肛门之间,形成中心腱。

2. 中层　即泌尿生殖膈,由上、下两层坚韧的筋膜及其间的一对会阴深横肌和尿道括约肌组成。

3. 内层　即盆膈,是骨盆底的最坚韧的一层,由肛提肌及其筋膜组成,自前向后依次有尿道、阴道及直肠穿过。两侧肌肉对称,合成漏斗形。肛提肌的主要作用是加强盆底的托力,其中一部分肌纤维与阴道及直肠周围密切交织,有加强肛门与阴道括约肌的作用。

The pelvic floor consists of musculofascial structures and closes the pelvic outlet. It helps to support the pelvic organs and which are placed above it. If abnormal structure and function of the pelvic floor exist, the normal position and function of pelvic organs, even the parturition can be influenced. Inappropriate management in delivery can also cause injury of pelvic floor.

The perineum is the mass of skin, muscle, and fascia between the vagina and the anus, 3 - 4 cm thick, inwards like a wedge, the termination is perineal center tendon which is in common obstetric practice referred to as the perineal body. In gestation, the perineum tissues soften to help the delivery, and they should be protected from the laceration of perineum in parturition.

六 内生殖器的邻近器官

女性生殖器官与尿道、膀胱、输尿管、直肠及阑尾相邻。当女性生殖器官出现病变时,如创伤、感染、肿瘤等,易累及邻近器官,增加诊断与治疗的难度;反之亦然。女性生殖器官的发生与泌尿系统同源,故生殖器官发育异常时也可能伴有泌尿系统的异常。

1.尿道　女性尿道长4～5 cm，短而直，开口于阴蒂下方，邻近阴道，易发生尿路感染。

2.膀胱　膀胱是一个空腔器官，位于子宫与耻骨联合之间。因覆盖膀胱顶的腹膜与子宫体浆膜层相连，充盈的膀胱可影响子宫的位置，在手术中易遭误伤，并妨碍盆腔检查，故妇科检查及术前必须排空膀胱。

3.输尿管　为一对肌性圆索状长管，长约30 cm。输尿管在腹膜后，从肾盂开始，沿腰大肌前面偏中线侧下降，在骶髂关节处，经过髂外动脉起点的前方进入骨盆腔继续下行，至阔韧带底部向前内方行，于子宫颈旁约2 cm处，在子宫动脉下方穿过，然后再经阴道侧穹隆绕向前方进入膀胱。在施行附件切除或结扎子宫动脉时，应避免损伤输尿管（图1-10）。

4.直肠　直肠上接乙状结肠，下接肛管，全长15～20 cm。前为子宫及阴道，后为骶骨，肛管长2～3 cm，在其周围有肛门内、外括约肌和肛提肌。肛门外括约肌为骨盆底浅层肌肉的一部分。妇科手术及会阴切开缝合时应注意避免损伤肛管、直肠。

5.阑尾　阑尾长7～9 cm，通常位于右髂窝内。有的阑尾下端可达右侧输卵管及卵巢部位，因此，妇女患阑尾炎时可能累及子宫附件。妊娠时阑尾的位置可随妊娠月份增加而逐渐向上外方移位。

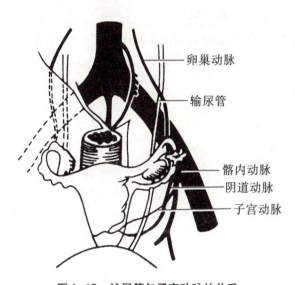

图1-10　输尿管与子宫动脉的关系

The female reproductive organs are adjacent to the urethra, bladder, ureter, rectum and appendicular appendix. When the female reproductive organs appear lesions, such as trauma, infection, tumor, easy to involve adjacent organs, increase the difficulty of diagnosis and treatment; and vice versa. The occurrence of female reproductive organs is homologous to the urinary system, so abnormal genitals development may also be accompanied by abnormal genital system.

任务实施

骨盆底功能恢复训练操作流程见表1-1。

表1-1 骨盆底功能恢复训练操作流程

项目	内容
目的	指导产妇进行盆底肌肉功能锻炼
操作前准备	1.物品准备:秒表
	2.环境准备:关闭门窗或屏风遮挡,室内温度适宜
	3.产妇准备:衣着宽松,排空膀胱,取仰卧位,尽量放松,保持平缓的呼吸
操作步骤	1.缓慢收缩:产妇吸气,然后在吸气过程中紧闭肛门,似正在制止排便。同时紧闭尿道口、阴道口,感觉像憋尿。想象电梯正在上升,一楼、二楼、三楼……当感觉到达顶层时,屏气,保持尿道口、阴道口、肛门同时紧缩。坚持数秒钟,然后缓慢放松,放松臀部和大腿。将注意力集中在尿道口,而不是肛门部。缓慢收缩动作可以锻炼盆底肌肉的耐力
	2.迅速收缩:如果通过步骤1的训练已经感到盆底肌力逐步增强,在步骤1的基础上提高收缩的速度,尽可能快地绷紧和放松耻尾肌(由小腹的耻骨部位向后到达肛门上方的尾骨),数数在1 min内可以进行多少次收缩。迅速收缩动作可以加强对盆底肌的控制能力
	3.缩肛:产妇吸气,然后在吸气过程中紧闭肛门,似正在竭力制止肛门排气,然后屏气,坚持数秒后缓慢放松。确保锻炼时松弛阴部肌肉。锻炼肛门括约肌,同时也加强整个骨盆底肌肉
	4.腹式呼吸:产妇一只手放在腹部,另一只手放在乳房下方,用腹部吸气,想象一只气球慢慢充气的过程。然后呼气,同时紧吸脐部,让脐部紧贴背脊。吸气1 s,缓缓呼气,再吸气,再呼气,循环重复4次,保持盆底肌肉松弛
整理	1.注意保护产妇隐私
	2.整理产妇衣物,整理物品
	3.注意观察产妇的反应

任务二　女性生殖系统生理(Physiology of Female Reproductive System)

工作情景

王某,13岁,月经初潮,月经持续7 d尚未结束,比较紧张,遂来医院咨询。如何对该患者进行健康指导?

任务内容

妇女一生经历不同时期,各时期具有不同的生理特征,其中生殖系统的变化最显著。女性生殖系统的生理变化与其他系统的功能息息相关,并相互影响。

任务目标

◆ 能说出卵巢激素的生理功能。
◆ 能描述卵巢的功能及周期性变化。
◆ 能描述子宫内膜的周期性变化。
◆ 能描述月经的临床表现,能进行月经期健康指导。

一 女性一生各时期的生理特点

女性从胚胎形成到衰老是一个渐进的生理过程,体现了下丘脑-垂体-卵巢轴功能发育、成熟和衰退的变化过程。女性一生根据年龄和生理特点可分为7个阶段。

1. 胎儿期 胎儿期是指从受精卵形成至胎儿娩出,一般为 266 d (从末次月经算起为 280 d)。受精卵是由父系和母系来源的23 对(46 条)染色体组成的新个体,其中 1 对染色体在性发育中起决定作用,称性染色体。性染色体 X 与 Y 决定胎儿的性别,即 XY 合子发育为男性,XX 合子发育为女性。

2. 新生儿期 新生儿期是指出生后 4 周内。女性胎儿在子宫内受到母体性腺和胎盘产生的性激素影响,其子宫内膜和乳房均有一定程度的发育,外阴较丰满。出生后数日内,由于性激素水平下降,阴道可有少量血性分泌物排出,即假月经;乳房可稍肿大,甚至分泌少量乳汁。这些都是正常生理现象,短期内会自行消失。

3. 儿童期 儿童期是指从出生后 4 周至 12 岁左右。儿童早期(8 岁以前)下丘脑-垂体-卵巢轴功能处于抑制状态,生殖器为幼稚型,子宫、卵巢及输卵管均位于腹腔内;儿童后期(约 8 岁起),下丘脑促性腺激素释放激素抑制状态解除,卵巢有少量卵泡发育,但不成熟也不排卵;子宫、卵巢及输卵管降至盆腔;乳房和内生殖器开始发育增大,脂肪分布开始出现女性特征,其他性征也开始出现。

4. 青春期 青春期是指由儿童期向性成熟期过渡的一段快速生长时期,是女性生殖器、内分泌、体格等逐渐发育成熟的过程。世界卫生组织提出青春期为 10 ~ 19 岁。此期的身体生长发育迅速,随着激素的释放,女性的第一性征进一步发育并出现第二性征,如声调较高、乳房丰满、阴毛和腋毛出现、骨盆宽大、皮下脂肪增多并出现女性分布等。月经初潮是青春期的重要标志。由于卵巢功能尚不完善,初潮后月经周期多不规律,需 5 ~ 7 年建立规律的周期性排卵后才逐渐正常。青春期女孩心理变化很大,情绪和智力发生明显的变化,容易激动,想象力和判断力明显增强。

5. 性成熟期 性成熟期是卵巢生殖功能与内分泌功能最旺盛的时期,又称生育期。一般自 18 岁左右开始,历时约 30 年。此期妇女卵巢功能成熟,有规律的周期性排卵和性激素分泌,月经周期规律,生殖器官及乳房在卵巢分泌的性激素作用下发生周期性变化。

6. 绝经过渡期 从开始出现绝经趋势至最后一次月经的时期称为绝经过渡期。一般始于 40 岁,历时短则 1 ~ 2 年,长至 10 ~ 20 年。此期卵巢功能逐渐减退,月经不规则,直至绝经,生殖器官开始逐步萎缩,丧失生育能力。此期妇女可出现潮热、出汗、情绪不稳定、头痛、失眠等症状,称为绝经综合征。

7. 绝经后期 绝经后期是指绝经后的生命时期。绝经后期的初期卵巢分泌雌激素功能停止,但卵巢间质可分泌雄激素,雄激素在外周组织转化为雌酮,成为绝经后期血液循环中的主要雌激素。一般 60 岁以后妇女机体逐渐老化进入老年期。此期卵巢功能完全衰竭,雌激素水平低落,不足以维持女性第二性征,生殖器官进一步萎缩。骨代谢失常引起骨质疏松,易发生骨折。

From embryogenesis to aging in women is a gradual physiological process, which reflects the changes in the functional development, maturation and decline of the hypothalamic – pituitary – ovarian axis. A woman's life can be divided into 7 stages according to age and physiological characteristics: fetal period, neonatal period, childhood, adolescence, latency period, menopausal transition period, and postmenopausal period.

二 月经及其临床表现

1. 月经　月经是指伴随卵巢周期性变化而出现的子宫内膜周期性脱落及出血。规律月经的建立是生殖功能成熟的重要标志。月经初潮年龄多在 13~14 岁,可以早至 11 岁,或迟至 16 岁;若 16 岁以后月经尚未来潮,应及时就医。月经初潮的早晚主要受遗传因素控制,其他因素如营养、体重也起重要作用。近年来月经初潮的年龄有提前的趋势。

2. 月经血的特征　月经血呈暗红色,除血液外,尚含有子宫内膜碎片、炎症细胞、子宫颈黏液及脱落的阴道上皮细胞。来自子宫内膜的大量纤维蛋白溶酶溶解纤维蛋白,因此,通常月经血不凝,若出血速度过快,也可形成血块。

3. 正常月经的临床表现　正常月经具有周期性和自限性。出血第 1 天为月经周期的开始,两次月经第 1 天的间隔时间,称为月经周期。一般为 21~35 d,平均 28 d。每次月经持续的时间称经期,一般为 2~8 d,平均 4~6 d。每次月经的总失血量,称为经量,正常为 20~60 mL,超过 80 mL 为月经过多。月经属生理现象,一般无特殊症状,但由于盆腔充血及前列腺素的作用,下腹及腰骶部出现下坠不适或子宫收缩痛,并可出现腹泻等胃肠功能紊乱症状。少数可有轻度神经系统不稳定症状。

4. 月经期的保健　经期由于盆腔轻度充血,子宫颈口松弛,子宫内膜剥落出血,机体抵抗力下降,若不注意经期保健,易发生妇科疾病,影响健康及生育功能。因此,经期要注意:①正确认识月经,解除思想顾虑,保持心情舒畅;②保持外阴清洁,每天清洗外阴,勤换月经垫和内裤,清洁用品专人专用;③避免吃辛辣食物和凉食,多饮温开水,保持大、小便通畅;④密切观察月经周期、经期、经量、月经性状等,如发现异常,及时就医;⑤注意休息,避免剧烈运动和重体力劳动;⑥经期禁止性生活、游泳、盆浴、坐浴、阴道冲洗和不必要的妇科检查等。

Menstruation is the periodic uterine bleeding that occurs with the shedding of the uterine mucous membrane controlled by the ovarian cycles. It is one of the marks of maturation in reproductive function. Menarche is the term applied to the first menstrual period in girls. It occurs typically at the age 13–14 years, but may occur as early as age 11 or as late as age 16 which are still be within normal limits.

Characteristic of Normal Menstrual Flow

Menstrual blood contains tissue debris, prostaglandins, mucus, and relatively large amounts of fibrinolysin from the endometrial tissue. The fibrinolysin lyses clots, so menstrual blood does not normally contain clots unless the flow excessive. It is usually scanty, viscid and dark red at first, later becoming bright red, and finally brown towards the end of the period.

Symptoms in Menstruation

The menstruation duration varies greatly in normal women. But it is consistent for a single woman. The average duration of the menstrual period is 2–7 d. 3–5 d is common, but flows as short as 1 day and as long as 8 days can occur in normal women. The average amount of blood lost is 30 mL but may range normally slight spotting to 80 mL. Loss of more than 80 mL is abnormal. There is no special symptom in menstruation. Premonitory symptoms, such as pelvic discomfort and backache, soreness of the breasts, headache and general malaise, may sometimes precede the period.

三　卵巢功能及其周期性变化

卵巢能产生卵子并排卵, 还能分泌性激素, 具有生殖和内分泌功能。

1.卵巢的周期性变化　从青春期开始到绝经前, 卵巢在形态和功能上发生周期性变化, 称为卵巢周期, 包括以下3个阶段。

(1)卵泡的发育及成熟　近青春期, 卵巢中原始卵泡开始发育, 形成生长卵泡, 每个月经周期有一批卵泡发育, 但一般只有一个优势卵泡达到完全成熟, 称为成熟卵泡或格拉夫卵泡, 直径可达18~23 mm。卵泡发育过程中分泌雌激素。

(2)排卵　随着卵泡的发育成熟, 其逐渐向卵巢表面移行并向外突出, 当接近卵巢表面时, 该处表面细胞变薄, 最后破裂, 卵细胞及其周围的透明带、放射冠及部分颗粒细胞一起被排出, 这称为排卵。排卵一般在下次月经来潮之前14 d左右, 卵子可由两侧卵巢轮流排出, 也可由　侧卵巢连续排出。

(3)黄体生成及退化　排卵后卵泡壁塌陷, 卵泡膜血管破裂, 血液流入腔内形成血体。卵泡壁的破口由纤维蛋白封闭, 在黄体生成素(LH)的刺激下, 残留的颗粒细胞变大, 胞质内出现黄色颗粒状的类脂质, 称为黄体。排卵后7~8 d黄体发育成熟, 分泌大量雌激素和孕激素。若卵子未受精, 排卵后9~10 d黄体开始退化, 周围的结缔组织及成纤维细胞侵入, 组织纤维化, 外观色白, 称为白体。正常黄体的寿命为14 d。黄体衰退后月经来潮, 卵巢中又有新的卵泡发育, 开始新的周期。若卵子受精, 则黄体在胚胎滋养细胞分泌的绒毛膜促性腺激素作用下增大, 转变为妊娠黄体, 至妊娠3个月末退化。

2.卵巢性激素的生理作用

(1)雌激素与孕激素的生理作用　见表1-2。

表1-2　雌激素与孕激素的生理作用

作用部位	雌激素	孕激素
子宫颈	使子宫颈口松弛、扩张;子宫颈黏液分泌增多且变得稀薄,富有弹性;涂片出现典型的羊齿状结晶,有利于精子穿透	使子宫颈口闭合,子宫颈黏液分泌减少且变稠,拉丝度差,易形成子宫颈管黏液栓堵塞子宫颈口,阻止精子及微生物穿过;涂片中羊齿状结晶消失,代之以椭圆体
子宫内膜	促进子宫内膜腺体、间质增生与修复,呈增生期改变	促使子宫内膜由增生期转化为分泌期,为孕卵着床做准备
子宫肌层	促进子宫发育,使子宫肌细胞增生、肥大,肌层增厚,血运增加,收缩力增强,以及对缩宫素的敏感性加强	使子宫肌纤维松弛,活动力下降,兴奋性降低,对外界刺激的反应能力下降,对缩宫素的敏感性降低
输卵管	加强输卵管节律性收缩的振幅	抑制输卵管节律性收缩的振幅
阴道上皮	使阴道上皮细胞增生、角化,使黏膜变厚,细胞内糖原含量增加,维持阴道酸性环境,增强局部抵抗力	促使阴道上皮细胞脱落加快,使阴道上皮角化现象消失,细胞呈舟状
乳腺	促进乳腺腺管增生,乳头及乳晕着色;大量雌激素抑制乳汁分泌	在雌激素影响的基础上促进乳腺腺泡发育成熟

续表1-2

作用部位	雌激素	孕激素
下丘脑	对下丘脑有正、负反馈作用	对下丘脑有负反馈作用
其他	促使阴唇发育,使其丰满、色素加深;促进其他第二性征发育;促进肝合成高密度脂蛋白,抑制低密度脂蛋白合成,降低总胆固醇水平;促进水钠潴留;维持和促进骨基质代谢	兴奋下丘脑体温调节中枢,使排卵后基础体温升高0.3~0.5 ℃;促进水钠排泄

(2)雄激素的生理作用　雄激素是维持女性生殖功能的重要激素。自青春期开始,雄激素分泌开始增加,促进阴蒂、阴唇、阴阜发育,促进阴毛和腋毛生长,维持第二性征。但雄激素过多会对雌激素产生拮抗作用。长期使用雄激素,可出现男性化表现。雄激素还与性欲有关。

The ovaries are paired sex glands or gonads in female concerned for germ cell maturation,storage and its release and steroidogenesis.

Ovarian Cycle

The ovarian cycle points to the cyclic changes in ovaries between puberty and menopause. The ovarian cycle has three phases:the follicular growth and development,ovulation,corpus luteal formation and demise.

● Follicular growth and development:The growth and development of follicle can be divided into phases as primordial follicle,preantral follicle,antral follicle,mature follicle.

● Ovulation:It is the process whereby an ovum is released from the ovary following rupture of a mature follicle and becomes available for conception. The endocrine mechanism of ovulation is the peak of LH/FSH preovulation.

● Corpus luteum formation and demise:The follicle that ruptures at the time of ovulation promptly fills with blood,forming what is sometimes called a corpus hemorrhagicum. After rupture of the follicle,capillaries and fibroblasts from the surrounding stroma proliferate and penetrate the basal lamina. The granulose and the theca cells of the follicle lining promptly begin to proliferate,and the clotted blood is rapidly replaced with yellowish,lipid-rich luteal cells,forming the corpus luteum. This is the luteal phase of the menstrual cycle,during which the luteal cells secrete estrogens and progesterone. If pregnancy occurs,the corpus luteum persists,and there are usually no more menstrual periods until after delivery. The function life span of the corpus luteum is normally within 14 days. Thereafter,the corpus luteum spontaneously degenerates. It is replaced,unless pregnancy occurs,by an avascular scar referred to as the corpus albicans.

Ovarian Steroids

The main steroids biosynthesized and secreted by ovary are estrogen,progesterone and androgen. Granulosa cells are the source of the two most important ovarian steroids,estradiol and progesterone. Although granulose cells are capable of producing progesterone independently,the biosynthesis of estrogens requires cooperation between the granulose cells and their thecal neighbors.

四 子宫内膜的周期性变化

卵巢周期使女性生殖器发生一系列周期性变化,尤以子宫内膜的周期性变化最显著。以月经

28 d 为 1 个周期,子宫内膜的周期性变化可分为 3 期。

1. 增殖期　月经周期的第 5～14 天,与卵泡期对应。在雌激素的作用下,内膜表面上皮、腺体、间质、血管均呈增殖性改变,称为增殖期。

2. 分泌期　月经周期第 15～28 天,与黄体期对应。黄体分泌的雌激素、孕激素使子宫内膜继续增厚(可达 10 mm),腺体增大并出现分泌现象,血管迅速增生、更加弯曲,间质水肿、疏松,适宜受精卵着床。

3. 月经期　月经周期第 1～4 天,是雌激素、孕激素撤退的结果。经前 24 h,内膜螺旋动脉节律性收缩及舒张,继而出现加强的血管痉挛性收缩,导致远端血管壁及组织缺血、坏死、剥脱,脱落的内膜碎片及血液一起从阴道流出,即月经来潮。

Cyclic changes in the histological structure of the endometrium are caused by the action of the ovarian hormones. For simplicity, a 28-day cycle with ovulation occurring on the 14th day will be described. Endometrial cycle has 3 phases: the proliferative phase, the secretory phase and the menstrual phase.

Proliferative Phasc

As the ovarian follicles are producing increasing amounts of estrogen, the endometrium regenerates from the deep layer and increases rapidly in thickness. It is from the 5th to 14th day of the cycle. The endometrium gradually rebuilds its substance at this phase.

Secretory Phase

After ovulation, rising levels of progesterone from the corpus luteum act on the estrogen-primed endometrium, causing the spiral arteries to elaborate and coil more tightly and converting the functional area to a secretory mucosa. The stroma becomes increasingly edematous, The uterine glands enlarge, coil, and begin secreting nutritious glycoproteins into the uterine cavity. Consequently, this phase of the cycle is called the secretory or luteal phase. The length of the secretory phase is remarkably constant, for about 14 days. In this phase, the endometrium prepares for implantation of an embryo.

Menstrual Phase

The phase is at 1-4 days a menstrual cycle. When the corpus luteum regresses, hormonal support for the endometrium is withdrawn. The endometrium becomes thinner, which adds to the coiling of the spiral arteries. Foci of necrosis appear in the endometrium, and these coalesce. Blood from the ruptured capillaries, along with mucin from the glands, fragments of endometrial tissue, and the microscopic, atrophied, and unfertilized ovum, is discharged from the uterus as the menstrual flow or menses. The cause of the vascular necrosis is associated.

五　月经周期的调节

月经周期的调节是个复杂的过程,正常月经周期的建立有赖于下丘脑-垂体-卵巢轴(HPOA)之间的神经内分泌调节,以及子宫内膜对性激素变化的周期性反应。下丘脑分泌促性腺激素释放激素(GnRH),包括卵泡刺激素释放激素和黄体生成素释放激素,作用是促进垂体合成、释放卵泡刺激素(FSH)和黄

月经周期的调节机制

体生成素(LH);垂体分泌卵泡刺激素和黄体生成素,能促进卵泡发育,刺激排卵,形成黄体,产生孕激素与雌激素;卵巢分泌雌激素和孕激素,作用于子宫内膜及其他生殖器官使其发生周期性变化,其分泌量可对下丘脑、垂体产生反馈作用(图 1-11)。

HPOA is a complete and well-balanced neuroendocrinological system. The main function of HPOA is to control the female development, maintain normal menstruation and sexual function. Thus it is also called sexual axis. Besides it involves in the modulation of the inner environment and the metabolism.

The secretion activity of HPOA is also modulated by the central nervous system. The hypothalamus occupies a key role in the control of gonadotropin secretion. Hypothalamic control is secreted by GnRH secreting into the portal hypophyseal vessels. GnRH stimulates the secretion of FSH as well as LH. FSH from the pituitary is responsible for early maturation of the ovarian follicles, and FSH and LH together are responsible for follicle maturation. A burst of LH secretion triggers ovulation and the initial formation of the corpus luteum. LH stimulates the secretion of estrogen and progesterone from the corpus luteum. The cyclic endometrium changes occur under the control of estrogen and progesterone, and this is responsible for the menstrual cycle.

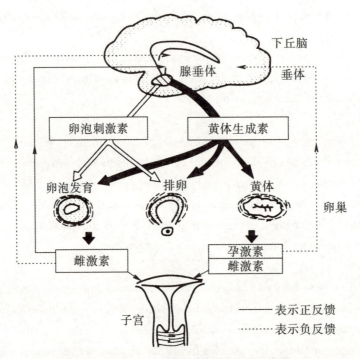

图 1-11 下丘脑-垂体-卵巢轴的相互作用

微课

课件

练习题及参考答案

（任 美）

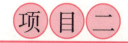

项目二

病史采集与体格检查
(Medical History Collection and Physical Examination)

项目描述

　　病史采集与体格检查是为护理对象提供护理的主要依据,也是妇产科护理临床实践的基本技能。

　　Medical history collection and physical examination are the main basis for providing nursing for nursing objects,and are also the basic skills of clinical practice in obstetric and gynecological nursing.

工作情景

　　王女士,32岁,婚后3年未孕。在家中老人的催促下,与丈夫一起来医院就诊。丈夫就诊后相关不育检查结果皆正常。妻子就诊不孕症专科。

　　①请明确采集该女性病史的方法和内容。②请明确对该女性进行体格检查的内容和方法。

任务内容

　　病史采集包括一般项目、主诉、现病史、月经史、婚育史、既往史、个人史和家族史8个方面。体格检查常常在采集病史后进行,主要包括全身检查、腹部检查和盆腔检查。

任务目标

　　◆ 能陈述妇产科病史采集方法和内容。
　　◆ 能描述妇产科体格检查的内容和方法。

一　病史采集

　　1.方法　采集病史时需要和患者进行有效的交流和充分的沟通,通过观察、会谈、阅读、身体检查、相应的实验室检查、物理学诊断、心理测试等方法获得护理对象的生理、心理、社会、精神及文化等资料。由于女性生殖系统疾病常常涉及患者的隐私和与性生活有关的内容,收集资料时会使患者感到害羞和不适,甚至不愿说出真实情况,所以在采集病史的过程中,要做到态度和蔼、语言亲切,关心体贴和尊重患者,耐心细致地询问和进行体格检查,给患者以责任感、安全感,并给予保守秘密的承诺,在可能的情况下要避免第三者在场。

2.内容

(1)一般项目 包括患者的姓名、性别、年龄、婚姻、籍贯、职业、民族、教育程度、宗教信仰、家庭住址、入院日期、入院方式、病史陈述者、可靠程度。若非患者陈述,应注明陈述者及其与患者的关系。

(2)主诉 指促使患者就诊的主要症状(或体征)与持续时间。妇科常见症状有阴道流血、白带异常、下腹疼痛、下腹部包块、外阴瘙痒、闭经及不孕等。也有无任何自觉不适,通过妇科普查而发现问题的患者。

(3)现病史 围绕主诉了解发病的时间、原因及可能的诱因、病情发展经过、就医经过、采取的护理措施及效果。可按照时间顺序进行询问。还需了解患者有无伴随症状及其出现的时间、特点和演变过程,特别是与主要症状的关系。此外,详细询问患者相应的心理反应,询问食欲、大小便、体重变化、活动能力、睡眠、自我感觉、角色关系、应激能力的变化。

(4)既往史 询问既往健康状况,曾患过何种疾病,特别是妇科疾病及与妇科疾病密切相关的病史如生殖系统炎症、肿瘤、损伤、畸形等,是否肥胖,有无肺结核、肠结核、结核性腹膜炎、肝炎、心血管疾病及腹部手术史等。为防止遗漏,可按全身各系统依次询问。同时应询问有无食物过敏史、药物过敏史,并说明对何种药物过敏。

(5)月经史 询问初潮年龄、月经周期、经期持续时间(如 13 岁初潮,月经周期 28~30 d,经期持续 4 d,可简写为 $13\frac{4}{28\sim30}$)。了解经量、经色、经质有无异常,有无经期之前或伴随月经出现的乳房胀痛、情绪异常等不适,有无痛经,历年月经的变化。常规询问末次月经日期(LMP)及经量和持续时间,若其流血情况不同于以往正常月经时,还应询问前次月经(PMP)起始日期。对于绝经后患者,应询问绝经的年龄,绝经后有无阴道流血、分泌物增多或者其他不适。

(6)婚育史 包括婚次及每次结婚年龄、男方健康情况、是否近亲结婚(直系血亲及 3 代旁系)、同居情况、双方性功能、性病史。生育史包括足月产、早产、流产次数及现存子女数,以 4 个阿拉伯数字表示,可简写为:足-早-流-存,如足月产 2 次,无早产,流产 1 次,现存子女 2 人,可记录为 2-0-1-2,也可用"孕×产×"方式表示,如孕 3 产 2(G_3P_2)。同时询问分娩方式、有无难产史、新生儿出生情况、有无产后出血或产褥感染、末次分娩或流产的时间、采用的计划生育措施及效果。

(7)个人史 患者的生活和居住情况,出生地和曾居住地区,有无烟酒嗜好,有无毒品使用史。

(8)家族史 患者的家庭成员包括父母、兄弟、姊妹及子女的健康状况。询问家族成员有无遗传性疾病(如血友病、白化病等)、可能与遗传有关的疾病(如糖尿病、高血压、癌症等)及传染病(如结核等)。

二 体格检查

体格检查应在采集病史后进行,主要包括全身检查、腹部检查和盆腔检查。盆腔检查为妇科检查所特有,又称为妇科检查。除病情危急外,应按下列先后顺序进行。

1.全身检查 测量体温、脉搏、呼吸及血压,必要时测量体重和身高。其他检查项目包括神志、精神状态、面容、体态、全身发育及毛发分布情况、皮肤、浅表淋巴结(特别是左锁骨上淋巴结和腹股沟淋巴结)、头部器官、颈(注意甲状腺是否肿大)、乳房(注意其发育、皮肤有无凹陷、有无包块、有无分泌乳汁或液体)、心、肺、脊柱及四肢。

2.腹部检查 为妇科疾病体格检查的重要组成部分,应在盆腔检查前进行。视诊观察腹部有无隆起或呈蛙腹状,腹壁有无瘢痕、静脉曲张、妊娠纹、腹壁疝、腹直肌分离等。触诊腹壁厚度,肝、脾、肾有无增大及压痛,腹部有无压痛、反跳痛和肌紧张,能否触到包块。触到包块时,应描述包块部位、大小(以厘米为单位表示或相当于妊娠月份表示,如包块相当于妊娠×个月大)、形状、质地、活动度、表面是否光滑或有高低不平隆起及有无压痛等。叩诊时注意鼓音和浊音分布范围,有无移动性浊音。必要时听诊了解肠鸣音情况。若合并妊娠,应检查腹围、子宫底高度、胎位、胎心及胎儿大小等。

3.盆腔检查 盆腔检查为妇科特有的检查,又称为妇科检查,包括外阴、阴道、子宫颈、子宫体及双侧附件检查。

(1)基本要求

1)检查者关心体贴患者,做到态度严肃,语言亲切,检查前向患者做好解释工作,检查时仔细认真,动作轻柔。同时,检查室温要适中,环境要寂静,若有其他患者在场,应注意遮挡。

2)除尿失禁患者外,检查前嘱咐患者排空膀胱,必要时导尿。大便充盈者应在排便或灌肠后进行检查。

3)为避免交叉感染,注意用具消毒,臀垫、手套、阴道扩张器(俗称阴道窥器)等检查器械均应每人次更换。

4)除尿瘘患者有时需取膝胸位外,一般盆腔检查均取膀胱截石位。不宜搬动的危重患者不能上检查台,可在病床上检查。

5)正常月经期应避免检查,若为阴道异常出血,则必须检查。检查前应先消毒外阴,以防发生感染。

6)无性生活患者禁做阴道扩张器检查和双合诊或三合诊检查,一般行直肠-腹部诊。若确有检查必要时,应先征得患者及其家属同意后,方可做阴道扩张器检查或双合诊检查。

7)怀疑有盆腔内病变而腹壁肥厚、高度紧张不合作或无性生活史患者,若妇科检查不满意,可行 B 型超声检查,必要时可在麻醉下进行盆腔检查。

8)男性医护人员对患者进行妇科检查时,应有一名女性医护人员在场。

(2)检查方法及步骤

1)外阴检查:观察外阴的发育,阴毛多少及其分布,有无畸形、炎症、溃疡、赘生物、皮肤色泽,尿道口有无红肿,前庭大腺是否肿大,阴道口及处女膜的情况等。必要时,嘱患者屏气增加腹压,以了解有无阴道前后壁膨出或子宫脱垂等。

2)阴道扩张器检查:将阴道扩张器前后两叶合拢,表面涂润滑剂以利插入,若拟做子宫颈细胞学检查或阴道分泌物涂片检查时,不宜用润滑剂,改用 0.9% 氯化钠注射液润滑,以免影响检查结果。放置阴道扩张器时,检查者用一只手拇指、示指分开小阴唇,另一只手将阴道扩张器斜行沿阴道侧后壁缓慢插入阴道内,边推进将阴道扩张器两叶转正并逐渐张开,暴露子宫颈、阴道壁及穹隆部,然后旋转阴道扩张器,充分暴露阴道各壁(图2-1、图2-2)。观察阴道时,注意阴道壁黏膜色泽,有无充血、溃疡、赘生物,观察分泌物量、色、性状及有无气味。观察子宫颈时,注意子宫颈大小、色泽、外口形状,有无糜烂、裂伤、息肉、肿物和接触性出血。必要时进行子宫颈刮片或取分泌物做涂片检查。取出阴道扩张器前,先将前后叶合拢再沿阴道侧后壁缓慢取出。

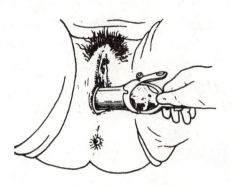

图2-1 沿阴道侧后壁放入阴道扩张器

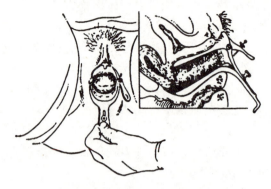

图2-2 暴露子宫颈及阴道侧壁

3）双合诊：指阴道和腹壁的联合检查，是妇科检查中最重要的项目。检查者戴无菌手套，一只手示、中两指蘸润滑剂，顺阴道后壁轻轻插入，检查阴道通畅度、深度、弹性，有无畸形、瘢痕、肿块及阴道穹隆情况。再触诊子宫颈大小、形状、硬度及外口情况，有无接触性出血。随后检查子宫体，将阴道内两指放在子宫颈后方，另一只手掌心朝下手指平放在患者腹部平脐处，当阴道内手指向上、向前方抬举子宫颈时，腹部手指往下、往后按压腹壁，并逐渐向耻骨联合部位移动，通过内、外手指分别同时抬举和按压，相互协调，即能扪清子宫位置、大小、形状、软硬度、活动度及有无压痛（图2-3）。扪清子宫后，将阴道内两指由子宫颈后方移至一侧穹隆部，尽可能往上向盆腔深部扪触；与此同时，另一只手从同侧下腹壁髂嵴水平开始，由上往下按压腹壁，与阴道内手指相互对合，以触摸该侧附件区有无肿块、增厚或压痛（图2-4）。若扪及肿块，应查清其位置、大小、形状、软硬度、活动度、与子宫的关系及有无压痛等。正常卵巢偶可扪及，触后稍有酸胀感，正常输卵管不能扪及。

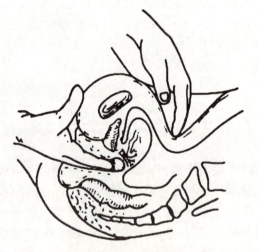

图2-3 双合诊（检查子宫）

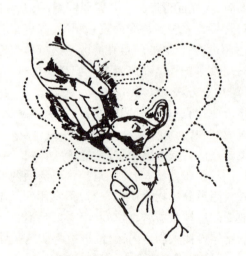

图2-4 双合诊（检查附件）

4）三合诊：指经阴道、直肠与腹壁的联合检查。方法是双合诊结束后，将一只手示指放入阴道，中指插入直肠，其余检查步骤与双合诊时相同（图2-5），是对双合诊检查不足的重要补充。对后位子宫，子宫后壁肿块，子宫骶韧带、直肠子宫陷凹及盆壁有病变者多采用。

5）直肠-腹部诊：指经直肠和腹壁的联合检查。检查者将一只手示指伸入直肠，另一只手在腹部配合检查。适用于无性生活史、阴道闭锁或月经期等其他原因，不宜行双合诊检查者。

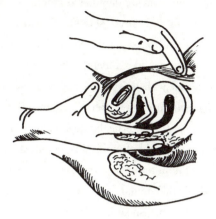

图2-5 三合诊

（3）记录 盆腔检查结束后，应将检查结果按解剖部位先后顺序记录。

1）外阴：发育情况及婚产式（如发育正常，未婚、已婚未产或经产式）。

2）阴道：是否通畅，黏膜情况，分泌物量、色、性状及有无臭味（如滑软、通畅，可见较多黄色白带，无臭味，后穹隆不饱满，无触痛）。

3）子宫颈：大小、软硬度，有无糜烂样改变、裂伤、息肉、腺囊肿，有无接触性出血和举痛（如大小正常，质中，中度单纯性子宫颈糜烂，无接触性出血，无子宫颈举痛等）。

4）宫体：位置、大小、软硬度、活动度及有无压痛（如子宫呈前倾前屈位，正常大小，质中，活动度正常，无压痛）。

5）附件：有无肿块、增厚及压痛。若扪及肿块，记录其位置、大小、形态、软硬度、活动度及与子宫的关系。左右两侧分别记录（如右侧附件可触及鸭蛋大肿块，压痛明显，左侧附件正常）。

6）实验室检查和特殊检查：摘录已有的实验室和特殊检查结果，外院检查结果应注明医院名称和检查日期。

General Physical Examination

The examination should be systematic and should include vital signs, general appearance, head and neck, breasts, heart and lungs, back, and extremities.

Abdominal Examination

Examination of the abdomen is critical in the evaluation of the gynecologic patient. The contour, whether flat, scaphoid, or protuberant, should be noted. Abdominal tenderness must be determined by placing one hand flat against the abdomen in the nonpainful areas initially, then gently and gradually exerting pressure with the fingers of the other hand. It is important to palpate any abdominal mass. The size, and whether the mass is cysticor solid, smooth or nodular, and fixed or mobile should be noted.

Pelvic Examination

The pelvic examination must be conducted systematically and with careful sensitivity. The procedure should be performed with smooth and gentle movements and accompanied by reasonable explanations.

● Vulva：The character and distribution of hair, the degree of development or atrophy of the labia, and the character of the hymen and introitus should be noted. Any clitorimegaly should be noted, as should the presence of cysts, tumors, or inflammation of Bartholin's gland. The urethra and Skene's glands should be inspected for any purulent exudates. The labia should be inspected for any inflammatory, dystrophic, or neoplastic lesions. Perineal relaxation and scarring should be noted.

● Speculum examination：The vagina and cervix should be inspected with appropriately sized bivalve speculum, which should be warmed and lubricated with warm water only, so as not to interfere with the examination of cervical cytology or any vaginal exudate. After gently spreading the labia to expose the introitus, the speculum should be inserted with the blades entering the introitus transversely, then directed posteriorly in the axis of the vagina with pressure exerted against the relatively insensitive perineum to avoid contacting the sensitive urethra. As the anterior blade reaches the cervix, the speculum is opened to bring the cervix into view. As the vaginal epithelium is inspected, it is important to rotate the speculum through 90 degrees, so that lesions on the anterior or posterior walls of the vagina ordinarily covered by the blades of the speculum are not overlooked. Vaginal wall relaxation should be evaluated using either a Sims' speculum or the posterior blade of a bivalve speculum. The cervix should be inspected to determine its size, shape, and color. Any purulent cervical discharge should be cultured. A cervical cytologic smear should be taken before the speculum is withdrawn. The exocervix is gently scraped with a wooden spatula, and the endocervical tissue is gently sampled with acytobrush.

● Bimanual examination：The bimanual pelvic examination provides information about the uterus and adnexa (fallopian tubes and ovaries). During this portion of the examination, the urinary bladder should be empty. The labia are separated, and the gloved, lubricated indexfinger is inserted into the vagina, avoiding the sensitive urethral meatus. The cervix is palpated for consistency, contour, size, and tenderness to motion. The uterus is evaluated by placing the abdominal hand flat on the abdomen with the fingers pressing gently just above the symphysis pubis. With the vaginal fingers supinated in either the anterior or the posterior vaginal fornix, the uterine corpus is pressed gently against the abdominal hand. As the uterus is felt between the examining fingers of both hands, the size, configuration, consistency, and mobility of the organ are appreciated. By shifting the abdominal hand to either side of the midline and gently elevating the lateral fornix up to the abdominal hand, it may be possible to outline a right adnexal mass. The left adnexa are best appreciated with the fingers of the left hand in the vagina. It is usually impossible to feel the normal tube, and conditions must be optimal to appreciate the normal ovary. The normal ovary has the size and consistency of a shelled oyster and may be felt with the vaginal fingers as they are passed across the undersurface of the abdominal hand.

● Rectovaginal examination：The anus should be inspected for lesions, hemorrhoids, or inflammation. Rectal sphincter tone should be recorded and any mucosal lesions should be noted. A guaiac test should be performed to determine the presence of occult blood. A rectovaginal examination is helpful in evaluating masses in the cul-de-sac, the rectovaginal septum, or adnexa. It is essential in evaluating the parametrium in patients with cervical cancer. Rectal examination may also be essential in differentiating between a rectocele and an enterocele.

● Recording：The examination result should be recorded according to the anatomy position as follows. ①External genitalia：the condition of development. ②Vagina：any obstruction and abnormal discharge. ③Cervix：size, consistency and contour (include erosion, polyps, and cyst). ④ Corpus of uterus：position, size, shape, tenderness, and mobility. ⑤ Adnexa：any mass and tenderness. ⑥ Laboratory evaluation：appropriate laboratory tests normally include a urinalysis, complete blood count, erythrocyte sedimentation rate, and blood chemistry analyses. Special tests, such as tumor marker and hormone assays, are performed when indicated.

任务实施

盆腔检查操作流程见表2-1。

表2-1 盆腔检查操作流程

项目	内容
目的	能利用妇科检查模型初步掌握盆腔检查的方法及步骤
操作前准备	1. 检查者准备:洗手、戴口罩、戴无菌手套
	2. 物品准备:一次性阴道扩张器、无菌手套、一次性臀垫、石蜡油
	3. 环境准备:温度适宜,环境安静,有遮挡保护患者隐私
	4. 受检者准备:排空膀胱,取膀胱截石位
操作步骤	1. 外阴部检查:观察外阴发育及阴毛分布情况,有无皮炎、溃疡及肿块,分开小阴唇,查看尿道口和阴道口
	2. 阴道扩张器检查:注意医患沟通 (1)放置:将阴道扩张器两叶合拢,用石蜡油或肥皂液润滑两叶前端,放置阴道扩张器前先用一只手示指和拇指分开两侧小阴唇,暴露阴道口,另一只手持预先备好的阴道扩张器,倾斜45°沿阴道侧后壁缓慢插入阴道内,边推进边将两叶转平,并逐渐张开两叶,直至完全暴露子宫颈、阴道壁及穹隆部,观察阴道黏膜、阴道分泌物及子宫颈有无异常。 (2)取出:取出阴道扩张器前应合拢两叶,再取出。在放入或取出过程中,注意避免小阴唇和阴道壁黏膜被夹入两叶侧壁间而引起剧痛或不适
	3. 双合诊:注意医患沟通。一只手示、中两指沿阴道后壁轻轻插入,检查阴道通畅度,扪及子宫颈大小、形状、硬度及外口情况,有无接触性出血。随后将阴道内两指放在子宫颈后方,另一只手的手掌心朝下,手指平放在患者腹部平脐处,检查子宫的位置、大小、形状、软硬度、活动度及有无压痛。将阴道内两指由子宫颈后方移至一侧穹隆部,尽可能往上向盆腔深部扪触,与此同时另一手从同侧下腹壁髂嵴水平开始,由上往下按压腹壁,与阴道内手指相互对合,检查附件区
整理	1. 询问患者有何不适
	2. 协助患者离开检查床
	3. 汇报检查结果

微课

课件

练习题及参考答案

(张艳亭)

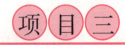

妊娠期妇女的护理
（Nursing of Gestational Women）

项目描述

　　妊娠期是女性一生中可能经历的一段特殊生理时期。女性在此时期的角色发生了重要转变,成为一名准妈妈,经历着生理和心理两方面的变化;孕妇和家庭成员都将随着妊娠的进展而进行心理和社会调适,迎接新生命的到来。护士应运用所学知识和技能,进行孕期健康教育,帮助孕妇及其家庭做好分娩前准备,促进母婴健康。

　　During the pregnancy, the woman's body undergoes many changes to accommodate the growing fetus. Besides, becoming a parent who is capable of loving and caring for a totally dependent infant is more than a biologic event. This chapter focuses first on the biophysical changes that are signs and symptoms of pregnancy and are helpful for pregnancy diagnosis. It then explores the impact of social and cultural on adjustment to pregnancy.

任务一　妊娠生理（Physiology of Pregnancy）

工作情景

　　张女士,24岁,已婚,平素月经规律,末次月经时间为2023年3月6日,现停经2个月。如果该女士确定为早孕,预产期应该是什么时间? 护士应为该女士提供哪些保健指导?

任务内容

　　妊娠是胚胎和胎儿在母体内发育成长的过程。成熟卵子受精是妊娠的开始,胎儿及其附属物自母体排出是妊娠的终止。从末次月经第1天算起,妊娠期约40周(280 d),妊娠是一个变化非常复杂而又极其协调的生理过程。

任务目标

◆ 能描述妊娠、受精、着床的定义。

◆ 能叙述胎儿附属物的组成及功能。

◆ 能解释妊娠期母体生理变化的原因及心理社会变化的特点。

一 受精与受精卵着床

1. 受精 精液射入阴道后,精子离开精液经子宫颈管进入子宫腔及输卵管腔,受生殖道分泌物中的 α 与 β 淀粉酶作用,解除了精子顶体酶上的"去获能因子",此时精子具有受精的能力,此过程称为精子获能。

成熟卵子从卵巢排出后,经输卵管伞端的拾卵作用进入输卵管内,停留在输卵管壶腹部与峡部连接处等待受精。

精子与卵子的结合过程称为受精,通常受精发生在排卵后 12 h 内,整个受精过程约为 24 h。当精子与卵子相遇后,精子顶体外膜破裂,释放出顶体酶,在酶的作用下,精子穿过放射冠、透明带,与卵子的表面接触,开始受精。精子进入卵子后,卵子透明带结构改变,阻止其他精子进入透明带,称为透明带反应。精原核与卵原核逐渐融合,核膜消失,染色体相互混合,形成二倍体的受精卵,完成受精过程。

2. 受精卵的输送与发育 受精卵进行有丝分裂的同时,借助输卵管蠕动和输卵管上皮纤毛摆动,向子宫腔方向移动,约在受精后第 3 天,分裂成 16 个细胞的实心细胞团,称为桑椹胚,随后早期囊胚形成。约在受精后第 4 天,早期囊胚进入子宫腔。受精后第 5 ~ 6 天,早期囊胚的透明带消失,在子宫腔内继续分裂发育成晚期囊胚。

3. 受精卵着床 晚期囊胚侵入子宫内膜的过程,称为孕卵植入,也称受精卵着床(图 3-1)。约在受精后第 6 ~ 7 天开始,11 ~ 12 d 结束。着床需经过定位、黏附和侵入 3 个阶段。完成着床的条件:①透明带消失;②囊胚滋养层分化出合体滋养层细胞;③囊胚和子宫内膜同步发育并相互配合;④孕妇体内有足够量的孕酮。子宫有一个极短的窗口期,允许受精卵着床。

4. 蜕膜的形成 受精卵着床后,在孕激素、雌激素的作用下,子宫内膜腺体增大,腺上皮细胞内糖原增加,结缔组织细胞肥大,血管充血,此时的子宫内膜称为蜕膜。按照蜕膜与囊胚的位置关系,将蜕膜分为三部分(图 3-2)。

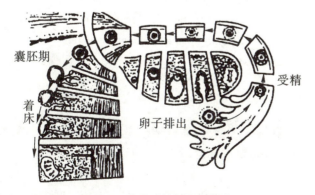

图 3-1 卵子受精与孕卵着床

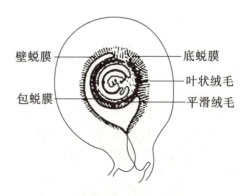

图 3-2 早期妊娠的子宫蜕膜与绒毛的关系

（1）底蜕膜　与囊胚及滋养层接触的蜕膜。将来发育成胎盘的母体部分。

（2）包蜕膜　覆盖在胚泡上面的蜕膜。随着囊胚的发育成长逐渐凸向子宫腔，约在妊娠12周左右与壁蜕膜贴近并逐渐融合，子宫腔消失，分娩时包蜕膜与壁蜕膜已无法分开。

（3）壁蜕膜　除底蜕膜、包蜕膜以外，覆盖子宫腔表面的蜕膜。

Fertilization

The mature ovum is released on the surface of the ovary, and is picked up by the fimbriated ends of the fallopian tube, and then is normally transported to the distal third of the fallopian tube (ampulla) for fertilization. After an ejaculation of enough healthy, mature, motile sperm into the vagina, thousands of spermatozoa find their way into the cavity of the uterus, and fewer reach the lumen of the fallopian tube. The spermatozoon makes its way through the cells surrounding the ovum, meanwhile, these cells become loose, and the spermatozoon finds its way through this layer to the zona pellucida. Sperm connect firmly to the surface of the zona pellucida at specific binding or "receptor" sites. The spermatozoon makes a channel through the zona pellucida as the acrosin dissolves the protein-containing zona with which it comes into contact. After the spermatozoon traverses the zona pellucida, it is in a position to penetrate the membrane of the ovum. As the spermatozoon penetrates the ovum, it brings its tail with it.

Once penetration is complete, a physiologic barrier occurs, and penetration of the ovum by other spermatozoa are prevented. Soon after penetration, the nucleus of the spermatozoon and the nucleus of the ovum undergo characteristic changes. They become pronuclei: distinct, clearly identifiable bodies of chromatin, each contained in a membrane. The male and female pronucleus fuse to form the fertilized ovum, or zygote which is called fertilization. Soon there after, the single-celled zygote undergoes first cell division through mitosis. At the 8- to 16-cell stage, the dividing ovum is delivered into the uterus. The fertilized ovum spends about 4 d in the uterine cavity developing further into a blastocyst before actual embedding takes place. Thus, a total interval is about 7 d between ovulation and implantation.

Implantation

The trophoblast is responsible for embedding the ovum, usually in the upper part of the posterior uterine wall. This process is carried out by means of enzymes. These cells not only burrow into the endometrium and eat out a nest for the ovum, but they also can digest the walls of the many small blood vessels that they encounter beneath the surface. The woman's bloodstream is tapped, and the ovum is deeply sunk in the lining epithelium of the uterus, surrounded by tiny pools of blood. Chorionic villi, develop out of the trophoblastic layer and extend into the blood-filled spaces. These chorionic villi contain blood vessels that are connected to the fetus and are extremely important because they are the sole means by which oxygen and nourishment are received from the woman. The entire ovum becomes covered with villi, which grow out radially and convert the chorion into a shaggy sac.

二 胎儿发育及生理特点

1. 胎儿发育　妊娠10周（受精后8周）内的人胚称为胚胎，为器官结构完成分化的时期。从妊娠第11周（受精第9周）起称为胎儿，为各器官进一步发育成熟的时期。胚胎及胎儿发育的特征大致如下。

8周末：胚胎初具人形，头的大小约占整个胎体的一半。可以分辨出眼、耳、口、鼻，四肢已具雏形，超声显像可见早期心脏已形成且有搏动。

12 周末:胎儿身长约 9 cm,体重约 14 g。外生殖器可初辨性别。胎儿四肢可活动。

16 周末:胎儿身长约 16 cm,体重约 110 g。从外生殖器可确定性别,头皮已长毛发,胎儿已开始有呼吸运动。部分孕妇自觉有胎动。

20 周末:胎儿身长约 25 cm,体重约 320 g。临床可听到胎心音,胎动明显增加,胎儿全身有毳毛,皮肤暗红,出生后已有心跳、呼吸、排尿及吞咽运动。自 20 周至满 28 周前娩出的胎儿,称为有生机儿。

24 周末:胎儿身长约 30 cm,体重约 630 g。各脏器均已发育,皮下脂肪开始沉积,但皮肤仍呈皱缩状。睫毛与眉毛出现。

28 周末:胎儿身长约 35 cm,体重约 1 000 g。皮下脂肪沉积不多,皮肤粉红色,可有呼吸运动,但肺泡 II 型细胞中表面活性物质含量低,此期出生者易患特发性呼吸窘迫综合征。

32 周末:胎儿身长约 40 cm,体重 1 700 g。皮肤深红,面部毳毛已脱,生活力尚可。此期出生者如注意护理,可以存活。

36 周末:胎儿身长约 45 cm,体重 2 500 g。皮下脂肪发育良好,毳毛明显减少,指(趾)甲已超过指(趾)尖,出生后能啼哭及吸吮,生活力良好。

40 周末:胎儿身长约 50 cm,体重约 3 400 g。胎儿已成熟,体形外观丰满,皮肤呈粉红色。男性睾丸已下降至阴囊内,女性大小阴唇发育良好。出生后哭声响亮,吸吮力强,能很好存活。

8 Weeks

At 8 weeks, the embryo begins to assume human form. A fetal heartbeat can be detected with real-time sonography.

12 Weeks

At 12 weeks, the fetus is about 9 cm long and weights 14 g. The sex can be distinguished because the external genitalia are beginning to show definite characteristics.

16 Weeks

At 16 weeks, the fetus is about 16 cm long and weights 110 g. The sex, as evidenced by the external genital organs, is obvious.

20 Weeks

At 20 weeks, the fetus is about 25 cm long and weights 320 g. Usually, the woman becomes conscious of slight fluttering movement. Fetal heart tones can easily be detected by auscultation at 20 weeks.

24 Weeks

At 24 weeks, the fetus is about 30 cm long and weights 630 g, and all organs have developed. The skin appears wrinkled, translucent, and is pink to red.

28 Weeks

At 28 weeks, the fetus is about 35 cm long and weights 1,000 g. A fetus often survives if born prematurely and given intensive care because the fetal lungs are capable of breathing air. But the alveolar type II cells contain low levels of surfactant, which predisposes the fetus to the idiopathic respiratory distress syndrome.

32 Weeks

At 32 weeks, the fetus is about 40 cm long and weights 1,700 g. Its skin is still red and wrinkled. The baby can survive with good care.

36 Weeks

At 36 weeks, the fetus is about 45 cm long and weights 2,500 g. After birth, the baby can cry, suck and generally survive.

40 Weeks（Full Term）

By this point,full term has been reached,and the fetus weights,about 3,400 g and is about 50 cm long. After birth,the baby cries loudly,sucks strongly and survives well.

2.胎儿生理特点

（1）循环系统

1）解剖学特点：①1 条脐静脉,带有来自胎盘氧含量较高、营养较丰富之血液进入胎体,脐静脉的末支为静脉导管。②2 条脐动脉,带有来自胎儿氧含量较低的混合血,注入胎盘与母血进行物质交换。③动脉导管,位于肺动脉与主动脉弓之间,出生后动脉导管闭锁成动脉韧带。④卵圆孔,位于左、右心房之间,多在出生后 6 个月完全闭锁。

2）血液循环特点：来自胎盘的血液经胎儿腹前壁分 3 支进入体内：一支直接入肝,一支与门静脉汇合入肝,此两支血液最后由肝静脉入下腔静脉。另一支经静脉导管直接入下腔静脉。故进入右心房的下腔静脉血是混合血,有来自脐静脉含氧较高的血,也有来自下肢及腹部盆腔脏器的静脉血,以前者为主。

卵圆孔开口处正对下腔静脉入口,下腔静脉进入右心房的血液绝大部分经卵圆孔进入左心房。上腔静脉进入右心房的血液流向右心室,随后进入肺动脉。由于肺循环阻力较大,肺动脉血液绝大部分经动脉导管流入主动脉,仅部分血液经肺静脉进入左心房。左心房含氧量较高的血液迅速进入左心室,继而入升主动脉,先直接供应心、脑及上肢,小部分左心室的血液进入降主动脉至全身,后经腹下动脉,再经脐动脉进入胎盘,与母血进行交换。可见胎儿体内无纯动脉血,而是动静脉混合血,各部分血液的含氧量不同,进入肝、心、头部及上肢的血液含氧和营养较丰富以适应需要。注入肺及身体下部的血液含氧和营养相对较少。

胎儿出生后开始自主呼吸,肺循环建立,胎盘循环停止。

（2）血液系统

1）红细胞：红细胞的生成在妊娠早期主要是来自卵黄囊,妊娠 10 周时在肝,以后在脾、骨髓,妊娠足月时至少 90% 的红细胞是由骨髓产生。红细胞总数无论是早产儿或是足月儿均较高,约为 $6.0×10^{12}$/L,胎儿期红细胞体积较大,生命周期短,约为成人的 2/3,因此需不断生成红细胞。

2）血红蛋白：胎儿血红蛋白从其结构和生理功能上可分为 3 种,即原始血红蛋白、胎儿血红蛋白和成人血红蛋白。随着妊娠的进展,血红蛋白的合成不只是数量的增加,其种类也从原始类型向成人类型过渡。

3）白细胞：妊娠 8 周后,胎儿血液循环中即出现粒细胞,12 周出现淋巴细胞,妊娠足月时白细胞计数可达（15～20）$×10^9$/L。

（3）呼吸系统　胎儿的呼吸功能是由母儿血液在胎盘进行气体交换完成的。但胎儿在出生前必须完成呼吸道（包括气管及肺泡）、肺循环及呼吸肌的发育,而且在中枢神经系统支配下能活动协调才能生存。妊娠 11 周时可观察到胎儿的胸壁运动。妊娠 16 周时可见胎儿的呼吸运动,呼吸运动次数为 30～70 次/min,时快时慢,有时也很平稳。但当发生胎儿窘迫时,正常呼吸运动可暂时停止或出现大喘息样呼吸。

（4）消化系统　妊娠 16 周,胃肠功能基本建立,胎儿能吞咽羊水,吸收水分、氨基酸、葡萄糖及其他可溶性营养物质。胎儿肝功能不太健全,肝内缺乏许多酶,不能结合因红细胞破坏产生的大量游离胆红素。胆红素经胆道排入小肠氧化成胆绿素,胆绿素的降解产物导致胎粪呈黑绿色。

（5）泌尿系统　胎儿肾在妊娠 11～14 周时有排泄功能,妊娠 14 周的胎儿膀胱内已有尿液。妊娠后半期,胎尿成为羊水的重要来源之一。

（6）内分泌系统　甲状腺是胎儿期发育的第一个内分泌腺,妊娠12周甲状腺即能合成甲状腺素。甲状腺对胎儿各组织器官发育均有作用,尤其是大脑发育。胎儿肾上腺的发育最突出,胎儿肾上腺皮质主要由胎儿带组成,能产生大量甾体激素,与胎儿肝、胎盘、母体共同完成雌三醇的合成与排泄。因此,孕妇测定血、尿雌三醇值已成为临床上了解胎儿、胎盘功能最常见的有效方法。

三　胎儿附属物的结构与功能

胎儿附属物是指胎儿以外的妊娠产物,包括胎盘、胎膜、脐带和羊水,它们对维持胎儿宫内的生命及生长发育起着重要作用。

The tissues except fetus are called the fetal appendages, which are made up of placenta, fetal membranes, umbilical cord, and amniotic fluid.

【胎盘】

1.胎盘的结构　胎盘由胎儿部分的羊膜和叶状绒毛膜及母体部分的底蜕膜构成(图3-3)。

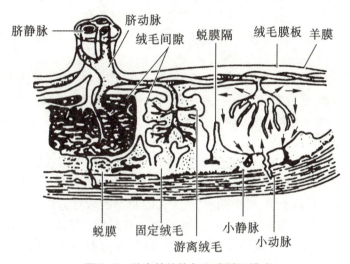

图3-3　胎盘的结构与血液循环模式

（1）羊膜　为附着在胎盘胎儿面的半透明薄膜,光滑,无血管、神经或淋巴管,有一定弹性。

（2）叶状绒毛膜　为胎盘的主要结构。晚期囊胚着床后,着床部位的滋养层细胞迅速增殖,内层为细胞滋养细胞,外层为合体滋养细胞,滋养层内面有一层胚外中胚层,与滋养层共同组成绒毛膜。在胚胎早期,整个绒毛膜表面的绒毛发育均匀,后来与底蜕膜接触的绒毛因营养丰富而高度发展,称叶状绒毛膜。胚胎表面其余部分绒毛因缺乏血液供应而萎缩退化,称为平滑绒毛膜,与羊膜共同组成胎膜。绒毛滋养层合体细胞溶解周围的蜕膜形成绒毛间隙,大部分绒毛游离其中,称为游离绒毛。少数绒毛紧紧附着于蜕膜深部起固定作用,称为固定绒毛。绒毛间隙之间有蜕膜隔将胎盘分成若干胎盘小叶,但蜕膜隔仅达绒毛间隙的2/3高度,故绒毛间隙的胎儿侧是相通的。绒毛间隙的底为底蜕膜。

（3）底蜕膜　构成胎盘的母体部分。底蜕膜的螺旋小动脉和小静脉开口于绒毛间隙,动脉因压力高把血液喷入绒毛间隙,再散向四周,经蜕膜小静脉回流入母体血液循环,故绒毛间隙充满母血。绒毛中有毛细血管,胎儿血自脐动脉入绒毛毛细血管网,再经脐静脉而入胎体内。由此可见,胎盘有母体和胎儿两套血液循环,两者的血液在各自封闭的管道内循环,互不相混,但可以通过绒毛间隙,隔着绒毛毛细血管壁、绒毛间质及绒毛表面细胞层,靠渗透、扩散及细胞的选择力进行物质交换。

妊娠足月时，胎盘为圆形或椭圆形盘状，重 450~650 g（胎盘实际质量受胎血和母血影响较大），约为足月初生儿体重的 1/6，直径为 16~20 cm，厚 1~3 cm，中间厚，边缘薄。胎盘分为胎儿面和母体面，胎儿面光滑，呈灰白色，表面为羊膜，中央或稍偏处有脐带附着。母体面粗糙，呈暗红色，由 18~20 个胎盘小叶组成。

2.胎盘的功能　胎盘具有物质交换、防御、合成等功能。

（1）物质交换功能　包括气体交换、营养物质供应、排出胎儿代谢产物等。

1）气体交换：在母体和胎儿之间，氧气（O_2）及二氧化碳（CO_2）以简单扩散的方式进行交换，替代胎儿呼吸系统的功能。子宫动脉血氧分压（PO_2）高于绒毛间隙内血 PO_2，但胎儿血红蛋白对 O_2 的亲和力强，能从母血中获得充分的 O_2。CO_2 的扩散速度比 O_2 快 20 倍，且胎儿血对 CO_2 的亲和力低于母血，故胎儿 CO_2 容易通过绒毛间隙直接向母体迅速扩散。

2）营养物质供应：葡萄糖是胎儿代谢的主要能源，以易化扩散方式通过胎盘，胎儿体内的葡萄糖均来自母体。氨基酸、钙、磷、碘和铁以主动运输方式通过胎盘。游离脂肪酸、水、钾、钠、镁，以及维生素 A、维生素 D、维生素 E、维生素 K 以简单扩散方式通过胎盘。

3）排出胎儿代谢产物：胎儿代谢产物如尿酸、尿素、肌酐、肌酸等，经胎盘进入母血，由母体排出体外。

（2）防御功能　胎盘的屏障功能很有限。各种病毒（如风疹病毒、流感病毒、巨细胞病毒等）及大部分药物均可通过胎盘，影响胎儿生长发育。细菌、弓形虫、衣原体、支原体、梅毒螺旋体等可在胎盘形成病灶，破坏绒毛结构，从而感染胎儿。母血中免疫抗体如免疫球蛋 G（IgG）能通过胎盘，使胎儿在出生后短时间内获得被动免疫力。

（3）合成功能　胎盘合体滋养细胞能合成数种激素和酶，对维持正常妊娠起重要作用。

1）人绒毛膜促性腺激素（hCG）：胚泡一经着床，合体滋养细胞即开始分泌 hCG，在受精后 10 d 左右即可用放射免疫法自母体血清、尿中测出，成为诊断早孕的敏感方法之一。至妊娠第 8~10 周时分泌达高峰，持续 1~2 周后迅速下降，至妊娠中晚期血清浓度仅为峰值的 10%，持续至分娩。正常情况下，分娩后 2 周内消失。hCG 的功能：①维持月经黄体寿命，使月经黄体增大成为妊娠黄体，增加留体激素分泌以维持妊娠；②促进雄激素芳香化转化为雌激素，同时能刺激孕酮的形成；③抑制淋巴细胞的免疫性，保护胚胎滋养层免受母体的免疫攻击；④刺激胎儿睾丸分泌睾酮，促进男胎性分化；⑤与母体甲状腺细胞促甲状腺素（TSH）受体结合，刺激甲状腺活性。

2）人胎盘催乳素：人胎盘催乳素（HPL）于妊娠 5~6 周开始分泌，至妊娠 34~36 周达高峰，直至分娩。产后 HPL 迅速下降，约产后 7 h 即不能测出。HPL 的主要功能：①促进乳腺腺泡发育，刺激乳腺上皮细胞合成乳白蛋白、乳酪蛋白、乳珠蛋白，为产后的泌乳做好准备；②促进胰岛素生成；③通过脂解作用，提高游离脂肪酸、甘油的浓度，抑制母体对葡萄糖的摄取和利用，使多余葡萄糖运转给胎儿，成为胎儿的主要能源，也是蛋白质合成的能源；④抑制母体对胎儿的排斥作用。HPL 是通过母体促进胎儿发育的"代谢调节因子"。

3）雌激素和孕激素：二者为留体激素。在妊娠早期由卵巢妊娠黄体产生，自妊娠第 8~10 周起由胎盘合成。雌激素、孕激素的主要生理作用为共同参与妊娠期母体各系统的生理变化。

4）酶：胎盘能合成多种酶，包括缩宫素酶和耐热性碱性磷酸酶，其生物学意义尚不十分明了。缩宫素酶能使缩宫素分子灭活，起到维持妊娠的作用。当胎盘功能不良时，此酶活性降低，见于死胎、子痫前期和胎儿宫内发育迟缓等。耐热性碱性磷酸酶于妊娠 16~20 周时从母血中可以测出，随着妊娠进展而逐渐增加，胎盘娩出后此值下降，产后 3~6 d 内消失。动态检测此酶的数值，可作为胎盘功能检查的一项指标。

Structures of the Placenta

The placenta is made up of amniotic membrane, chorion frondosum, and decidual basalis. By the third or fourth week of pregnancy, the chorionic villi develop blood vessels within them. These vessels are connected with the fetal bloodstream. The trophoblast cells of the chorionic villi form spaces in the decidua basalis, which fill with maternal blood to supply nourishment to the fetus. Differentiation of the chorionic villi continues, and by the third month, the placenta has formed through the union of the chorionic villi (fetal portion) and the decidua basalis (maternal portion).

During pregnancy, the placenta's weight increases in proportion to that of the fetus. The normal fetal–placental weight ratio at term is 6 : 1. The placenta grows to about 20 cm in diameter and 2 cm in thickness late in pregnancy. It appears to be a fleshy, disk–like organ that term, weight about 500 g and covers about one–quarter of the uterine wall. The structure of the placenta includes the following components.

Functions of the Placenta

- Metabolic functions: The placenta produces some nutrients needed by the embryo and for its own functions. Substances synthesized include glycogen, cholesterol, and fatty acids.

- Transfer functions: Exchange of oxygen, nutrients, and waste products across the chorionic villi occurs through several methods including simple diffusion, facilitated diffusion, active transport, and pinocytosis. Placental transfer of harmful substances also may occur. Most substances that enter the mother's bloodstream can enter the fetal circulation, and many agents enter it almost immediately.

- Gas exchange: Respiration is a key function of the placenta. Oxygen and carbon dioxide pass through the placental membrane by simple diffusion.

- Nutrient transfer: The growing fetus requires a constant supply of nutrients from the pregnant woman. Glucose, fatty acids, vitamins, and electrolytes pass readily across the placenta. Glucose is the major energy source for fetal growth and metabolic activities.

- Waste removal: In addition to carbon dioxide, urea, uric acid, and bilirubin are readily transferred from fetus to mother for disposal. Because the normal placenta removes wastes for the fetus, metabolic defects such as phenylketonuria are usually not evident until after birth.

- Antibody transfer: Many of the immunoglobulin (IgG) class of antibodies are passed from mother to fetus through the placenta. This confers passive (temporary) immunity to the fetus against diseases such as measles if the mother is immune to them. Passage of antibodies against disease is beneficial because the newborn does not produce antibodies for several months after birth.

- Endocrine functions: The placenta produces several hormones necessary for normal pregnancy. hCG causes the corpus luteum to persist for the first 6 to 8 weeks of pregnancy and secrete estrogens and progesterone. As the placenta develops further, it takes over estrogen and progesterone production and the corpus luteum regresses. When a Y chromosome is present in the male fetus, hCG also causes the fetal testes to secrete testosterone necessary for normal development of male reproductive structures. Human placental lactogen is a placental hormone that promotes normal nutrition and growth of the fetus and maternal breast development for lactation. The hormone decreases maternal insulin sensitivity and glucose use, making more glucose available for fetal nutrition. Steroid hormones secreted by the placenta include estrogens and progesterone. Estrogens cause enlargement of the woman's uterus, enlargement of the breasts, and enlargement of the external genitalia. Estriol is the most plentiful estrogen produced during pregnancy.

【胎膜】

胎膜由绒毛膜和羊膜组成。胎膜外层为绒毛膜,在发育过程中因缺乏营养供应而逐渐退化成平滑绒毛膜,妊娠晚期与羊膜紧贴,但可与羊膜完全分开。胎膜内层为羊膜,为半透明的薄膜,与覆盖胎盘、脐带的羊膜层相连接。

The fetal membranes include amnion and chorion. The shaggy chorionic villi that originally cover the ovum and invade the decidua basalis enlarge and multiply rapidly to form the chorion frondosum. This structure becomes the fetal component of the placenta. The chorionic villi covering the decidua capsularis degenerate and almost disappear leaving only a slightly roughened membrane, the chorion laeve (bald chorion). The chorion laeve lies separated from the amnion by the exocoelomic cavity until near the end of the third month, after which they establish close contact. The chorion laeve and amnion form an avascular amnio chorion, an important site of transfer and metabolic activity. The fetus is thus surrounded by two membranes, the amnion and the chorion.

【脐带】

脐带是连接胎儿与胎盘的条索状组织,胎儿借助脐带悬浮于羊水中。足月胎儿的脐带长 30～100 cm,平均 55 cm,直径为 0.8～2.0 cm。脐带的表面由羊膜覆盖,内有一条管腔大而管壁薄的脐静脉和两条管腔小而管壁厚的脐动脉,脐血管周围有保护脐血管的胚胎结缔组织,称为华通胶。胎儿通过脐带与母体进行气体、营养和代谢物质的交换。若脐带受压,可致胎儿窘迫,甚至危及胎儿生命。

The umbilical cord connects the placenta to the fetus and is usually about 30–100 cm in length and about 0.8–2.0 cm in diameter. The cord normally leaves the placenta near the center and enters the abdominal wall of the fetus at the umbilicus, just below the middle of the median line in front. However, it may insert off center or even out on the fetal membranes. It contains two arteries and one large vein, which are twisted on each other and are protected from pressure by a transparent, bluish white, gelatinous substance called Wharton's jelly.

【羊水】

羊水为充满于羊膜腔内的液体。妊娠早期的羊水是由母体血清经胎膜进入羊膜腔的透析液,妊娠中期以后,胎儿尿液成为羊水的重要来源。羊水的吸收约 50% 由胎膜完成,羊水在羊膜腔内不断进行液体交换以保持羊水量的动态平衡。母儿间的液体交换主要通过胎盘,每小时交换液体约 3 600 mL。母体与羊水的交换主要通过胎膜,每小时交换约 400 mL。羊水与胎儿的交换量较少,主要通过胎儿消化道、呼吸道、泌尿道等途径进行,故羊水通过不断更新以保持母体、胎儿、羊水三者间液体平衡。随着胚胎的发育,羊水的量逐渐增加,妊娠 38 周约 1 000 mL,此后羊水量逐渐减少,至妊娠 40 周羊水量约 800 mL。妊娠早期羊水为无色澄清液体,足月妊娠时,羊水略混浊,不透明,呈中性或弱碱性,内含有大量的上皮细胞及胎儿的一些代谢产物。

羊膜和羊水在胚胎发育中起重要的保护作用:使胚胎在羊水中自由活动;防止胎体粘连;防止胎儿受直接损伤;保持羊膜腔内恒温;有利于胎儿体液平衡;临产时,羊水直接承受宫缩压力,能使压力均匀分布,避免胎儿局部受压;羊水还可减少胎动给母体带来的不适感;临产后,前羊水囊扩张子宫颈口及阴道,破膜后羊水冲洗和润滑阴道可减少感染的发生机会。

Even before the previously noted structures become evident, a fluid-filled space develops around the embryo. This space, the amniotic cavity, is lined with a smooth, slippery, glistening membrane, the amnion. Because the amniotic cavity is filled with fluid, it is often called the bag of waters; the fetus floats and moves within this space. The amniotic fluid is composed of water（98%）and organic and inorganic solids（1% -2%）. By full term, this cavity normally contains 500 - 1,000 mL of liquor amnii, or the "waters". The amniotic fluid contains albumin, urea, uric acid, creatinine, lecithin, sphingomyelin, bilirubin, fat, fructose, leukocytes, proteins, epithelial cells, enzymes, vernix, and fetal hair. The amniotic fluid serves a number of important functions for the embryo and fetus: helping to maintain even body temperature; providing a cushion against possible injury; permitting symmetric external growth; preventing adherence of the amnion; providing space for free movement.

四 妊娠期母体变化

【生理变化】

妊娠期在胎盘产生的激素作用下,母体各系统发生了一系列生理变化,以适应胎儿生长发育的需要并为分娩做准备。

1. 生殖系统

（1）子宫 妊娠期子宫的重要功能是孕育胚胎、胎儿,同时在分娩过程中起重要作用。子宫是妊娠期及分娩后变化最大的器官。

1）子宫体:明显增大变软,至妊娠足月时子宫体积达 35 cm×25 cm×22 cm;容量约 5 000 mL,是非孕期的 500 ~ 1 000 倍;重量约 1 100 g,增加近 20 倍。子宫壁厚度非妊娠时为 1 cm,妊娠中期逐渐增厚达 2.0 ~ 2.5 cm,妊娠末期又逐渐变薄为 1.0 ~ 1.5 cm。妊娠早期子宫略呈球形且不对称,受精卵着床部位的子宫壁明显突出。妊娠 12 周时,子宫均匀增大并超出盆腔,在耻骨联合上方可触及。妊娠晚期子宫多呈不同程度的右旋,与盆腔左侧有乙状结肠占据有关。子宫增大不是由于细胞的数目增加,而主要是肌细胞的肥大,胞质内充满具有收缩活性的肌动蛋白和肌浆球蛋白,为临产后子宫收缩提供物质基础。

2）子宫峡部:是子宫体与子宫颈之间最狭窄的部分。非妊娠期长约 1 cm,随着妊娠的进展,峡部逐渐被拉长变薄,扩展成为子宫腔的一部分,临产时伸展至 7 ~ 10 cm,形成子宫下段,成为产道的一部分。

3）子宫颈:妊娠早期因充血、组织水肿,子宫颈外观肥大、着色,呈紫蓝色,质地软。子宫颈管内腺体肥大,子宫颈黏液分泌增多,形成黏稠的黏液栓,富含免疫球蛋白及细胞因子,保护宫腔不受外来感染的侵袭。

（2）卵巢 妊娠期略增大,停止排卵及新卵泡的发育。一侧卵巢可见妊娠黄体,其分泌雌激素、孕激素以维持妊娠。妊娠 10 周后,黄体功能由胎盘取代,黄体开始萎缩。

（3）输卵管 妊娠期输卵管伸长,但肌层无明显肥厚,黏膜上皮细胞变得扁平,在基质中可见蜕膜细胞。有时黏膜也可见到蜕膜样改变。

（4）阴道 妊娠期阴道黏膜水肿、充血呈紫蓝色,黏膜增厚、皱襞增多,结缔组织变松软,伸展性增加,有利于分娩时胎儿的通过。阴道脱落细胞增多,分泌物增多呈糊状。阴道上皮细胞含糖原增加,乳酸含量增加,使阴道的 pH 降低,不利于一般致病菌生长,有利于防止感染。

（5）外阴 妊娠期局部充血,皮肤增厚,大小阴唇有色素沉着。大阴唇内血管增多,结缔组织松软,伸展性增加,有利于分娩时胎儿的通过。妊娠时由于增大子宫的压迫,盆腔及下肢静脉血液回流受阻,部分孕妇可有外阴或下肢静脉曲张,产后大多自行消失。

2. 乳房 妊娠早期乳房开始增大,充血明显,孕妇自觉乳房发胀。乳头增大、着色,易勃起,乳晕着色,乳晕上的皮脂腺肥大形成散在的小隆起,称为蒙氏结节。胎盘分泌的雌激素刺激乳腺腺管的发育,孕激素刺激乳腺腺泡的发育,垂体催乳素、人胎盘催乳素等多种激素参与乳腺发育完善,为泌乳做准备。但妊娠期间并无乳汁分泌,可能与大量雌激素、孕激素抑制乳汁生成有关。在妊娠后期,尤其近分娩期,挤压乳房时可有数滴稀薄黄色液体溢出,称初乳。分娩后,随着胎盘娩出,雌激素、孕激素水平迅速下降,新生儿吸吮乳头时,乳汁正式开始分泌。

3. 血液循环系统

(1)心脏 妊娠后期,由于妊娠增大的子宫使膈肌升高,心脏向左、向上、向前移位,更贴近胸壁,心尖部左移,心浊音界稍扩大。心脏容量从妊娠早期至妊娠末期约增加10%,心率每分钟增加10~15次。由于血流量增加、血流加速及心脏移位使大血管扭曲,多数孕妇的心尖区及肺动脉区可闻及柔和的吹风样收缩期杂音,产后逐渐消失。

(2)心输出量和血容量 心输出量约自妊娠10周即开始增加,至妊娠32~34周时达高峰,维持此水平直至分娩。临产后,尤其是第二产程期间,心输出量显著增加。

血容量自妊娠6~8周开始增加,至妊娠32~34周时达高峰,增加40%~45%,平均增加约1 450 mL,维持此水平至分娩。血浆的增加多于红细胞的增加,血浆约增加1 000 mL,红细胞约增加450 mL,使血液稀释,出现生理性贫血。

(3)血压 妊娠早期及中期血压偏低,妊娠晚期血压轻度升高。一般收缩压没有变化,舒张压因外周血管扩张、血液稀释及胎盘形成动静脉短路而有轻度降低,从而脉压略增大。孕妇血压受体位影响,妊娠晚期仰卧位时增大的子宫压迫下腔静脉,回心血量减少,心输出量减少致血压下降,形成仰卧位低血压综合征,侧卧位能解除子宫压迫,改善血液回流。因此,妊娠中、晚期鼓励孕妇侧卧位休息。

(4)静脉压 妊娠期盆腔血液回流至下腔静脉的血流量增加,右旋增大的子宫又压迫下腔静脉使血液回流受阻,使孕妇下肢、外阴及直肠的静脉压增高,加之妊娠期静脉壁扩张,孕妇易发生痔、外阴及下肢静脉曲张。

(5)血液成分

1)红细胞:妊娠期骨髓造血增加,网织红细胞轻度增加。由于血液稀释,红细胞计数约为3.6×10^{12}/L(非孕妇女约为4.2×10^{12}/L),血红蛋白值约为110 g/L(非孕妇女约为130 g/L),血细胞比容从未孕时0.38~0.47降至0.31~0.34。为适应红细胞增生、胎儿生长和孕妇各器官生理变化的需要,应在妊娠中、晚期补充铁剂,以防缺铁性贫血。

2)白细胞:妊娠期白细胞计数稍增加,为$(5~12)\times10^9$/L,有时可达15×10^9/L,主要为中性粒细胞增加,淋巴细胞增加不多,单核细胞和嗜酸性粒细胞均无明显变化。

3)凝血因子:妊娠期凝血因子Ⅱ、Ⅴ、Ⅶ、Ⅷ、Ⅸ、Ⅹ均增加,仅凝血因子Ⅺ及ⅩⅢ降低,使血液处于高凝状态,产后胎盘剥离面血管内迅速形成血栓,对预防产后出血有利。血小板数无明显改变。妊娠期红细胞沉降率加快,可达100 mm/h。

4)血浆蛋白:由于血液稀释,血浆蛋白在妊娠早期即开始降低,妊娠中期时血浆蛋白值为60~65 g/L,主要是白蛋白减少,约为35 g/L,以后维持此水平至分娩。

4. 泌尿系统 由于孕妇及胎儿代谢产物增多,肾负担加重,妊娠期肾略增大。肾血流量(RPF)及肾小球滤过率(GFR)于妊娠早期均增加,并在整个妊娠期维持高水平。GFR比非妊娠时增加50%,RPF则增加35%。由于GFR增加,而肾小管对葡萄糖再吸收能力不能相应增加,故约15%的孕妇餐后可出现妊娠期生理性糖尿,应注意与糖尿病相鉴别。RPF与GFR均受体位影响,孕妇仰卧位时尿量增加,故夜尿量多于日尿量。

妊娠早期,由于增大的子宫压迫膀胱,引起尿频,妊娠12周以后子宫体高出盆腔,压迫膀胱的症状消失。妊娠晚期,由于胎先露进入盆腔,孕妇再次出现尿频,甚至腹压稍增加即出现尿液外溢现象,此现象产后可逐渐消失。右侧输尿管受右旋子宫压迫,孕妇易发生右侧肾盂肾炎,可用左侧卧位预防。

5. 呼吸系统 妊娠早期,孕妇的胸廓横径加宽,周径加大,横膈上升,呼吸时膈肌活动幅度增加。妊娠中期,肺通气量增加大于耗氧量,孕妇有过度通气现象,这有利于提供孕妇和胎儿所需的氧气。妊娠后期,因子宫增大,腹肌活动幅度减少,使孕妇以胸式呼吸为主,气体交换保持不减。呼吸次数在妊娠期变化不大,每分钟不超过 20 次,但呼吸较深。呼吸道黏膜充血、水肿,易发生上呼吸道感染。妊娠后期因横膈上升,孕妇平卧后有呼吸困难感,睡眠时稍垫高头部可减轻症状。

6. 消化系统 妊娠早期(停经 6 周左右),约有半数左右的孕妇出现晨起恶心、呕吐、食欲减退、喜食酸物或偏食,称为早孕反应。受雌激素影响,牙龈充血、水肿、增生,晨间刷牙时易有牙龈出血,孕妇常有唾液增多,有时有流涎。受孕激素影响,胃肠平滑肌张力下降,使蠕动减少、减弱,胃排空时间延长,易有上腹部饱胀感。妊娠中、晚期,由于胃部受压及幽门括约肌松弛,胃内酸性内容物可回流至食管下部,产生"灼热感"。肠蠕动减弱,易便秘,加之直肠静脉压增高,孕妇易发生痔疮或使原有痔疮加重。妊娠期增大的子宫可使胃、肠管向上及两侧移位,如发生阑尾炎时可表现为右侧腹部中或上部的疼痛。

7. 内分泌系统 妊娠期腺垂体增大 1~2 倍,嗜酸细胞肥大、增多,形成"妊娠细胞",约于产后 10 d 左右恢复。产后有出血性休克者,可使增生、肥大的垂体缺血、坏死,导致希恩综合征。由于妊娠黄体和胎盘分泌大量雌激素、孕激素对下丘脑及垂体的负反馈作用,促性腺激素分泌减少,故孕期无卵泡发育成熟,也无排卵。垂体催乳素随妊娠进展而增量,至分娩前达高峰,约为非孕妇女的 10 倍,与其他激素协同作用,促进乳腺发育,为产后泌乳做准备。促甲状腺激素(TSH)、促肾上腺皮质激素(ACTH)分泌增多,但因游离的甲状腺素及皮质醇不多,孕妇没有甲状腺、肾上腺皮质功能亢进的表现。

8. 皮肤 妊娠期垂体分泌促黑素细胞激素增加,使黑色素增加,加之雌激素明显增多,使孕妇面颊、乳头、乳晕、腹白线、外阴等处出现色素沉着。面颊呈蝶形分布的褐色斑,习称妊娠斑,于产后逐渐消退。随着妊娠子宫增大,孕妇腹壁皮肤弹力纤维过度伸展而断裂,使腹壁皮肤出现紫色或淡红色不规则平行的裂纹,称妊娠纹。产后变为银白色,持久不退。

9. 其他

(1)基础代谢率 于妊娠早期略下降,妊娠中期略增高,妊娠晚期可增高 15%~20%。

(2)体重 妊娠 12 周前无明显变化,以后体重平均每周增加 350 g,正常不应超过 500 g。至妊娠足月时,体重平均约增加 12.5 kg,增加的体重来自胎儿、胎盘、羊水、子宫、乳房、血液、组织间液、沉积脂肪等。

Reproductive Tract

● Uterus:In the nonpregnant woman,the uterus weighs approximately 70 g and is almost solid,except for a cavity of 10 mL or less. During pregnancy,the uterus is transformed into a thin-walled muscular organ of sufficient capacity to accommodate the fetus, placenta, and amnionic fluid. The total volume of the contents at term averages 5,000 mL. Thus,by the end of pregnancy,the uterus has achieved a capacity that is 500 to 1,000 times greater than the nonpregnant state. The corresponding increase in uterine weight is such that,by term,the organ weighs nearly 1,100 g. As early as 1 month after conception,the cervix begins to soften and gain bluish tones.

● Ovaries:Ovulation ceases during pregnancy,and maturation of new follicles is suspended. The single corpus luteum found in gravidas functions maximally during the first 6-7 weeks of pregnancy 4-5 weeks postovulation. Thereafter,it contributes relatively little to progesterone production. Surgical removal of the corpus luteum before 7 weeks prompts a rapid fall in maternal serum progesterone levels and spontaneous abortion. After this time, however, corpus luteum excision ordinarily does not cause abortion.

● Fallopian tubes: The fallopian tube musculature, that is, the myosalpinx, undergoes little hypertrophy during pregnancy. The epithelium of the endosalpinx somewhat flattens. Decidual cells may develop in the stroma of the endosalpinx, but a continuous decidual membrane is not formed.

● Vagina and perineum: During pregnancy, greater vascularity and hyperemia develop in the skin and muscles of the perineum and vulva, and the underlying abundant connective tissue softens. This augmented vascularity prominently affects the vagina and cervix and results in the violet color characteristic of Chadwick sign. Within the vagina, the considerably elevated volume of cervical secretions during pregnancy forms a somewhat thick, white discharge. The pH is acidic, varying from 3.5 to 6.0. This pH results from increased production of lactic acid by Lactobacillus acidophilus during metabolism of glycogen energy stores in the vaginal epithelium. Pregnancy is associated with an elevated risk of vulvovaginal candidiasis, particularly during the second and third trimesters.

The vaginal walls undergo striking changes in preparation for the distention that accompanies labor and delivery. These alterations include considerable epithelial thickening, connective tissue loosening, and smooth muscle cell hypertrophy.

Breasts

In early pregnancy, women often experience breast tenderness and paresthesias. After the second month, the breasts grow in size, and delicate veins are visible just beneath the skin. The nipples become considerably larger, more deeply pigmented, and more erectile. After the first few months, a thick, yellowish fluid—colostrum—can often be expressed from the nipples by gentle massage. During the same months, the areolae become broader and more deeply pigmented. Scattered through each areola are several small elevations, the glands of Montgomery, which are hypertrophic sebaceous glands. If breasts gain extensive size, skin striae similar to those observed in the abdomen may develop.

Cardiovascular System

● Cardiac output: Retention of sodium and water during pregnancy accounts for a total body water increase of 6 – 8 L, two thirds of which is located in the extravascular space. The total blood volume increases by about 40% above nonpregnant levels, with wide individual variations. The plasma volume rises as early as the 6th week of pregnancy and reaches a plateau by about 32 – 34 weeks' gestation. The red blood cell mass begins to increase at the start of the second trimester and continues to rise throughout pregnancy. By the time of delivery, it is 20% – 35% above nonpregnant levels. The disproportionate increase in plasma volume compared with the red cell volume results in hemodilution with a decreased hematocrit reading, sometimes referred to as physiologic anemia of pregnancy. If iron stores are adequate, the hematocrit tends to rise from the second to the third trimester.

Cardiac output rises by the 10th week of gestation; it reaches about 40% above nonpregnant levels by 20 – 24 weeks, after which there is little change. The rise in cardiac output, which peaks while blood volume is still rising, reflects increases mainly in stroke volume and, to a lesser extent, in heart rate. With twin and triplet pregnancies, the changes in cardiac output are greater than those seen with singleton pregnancies.

● Intravascular pressures: Systolic pressure falls only slightly during pregnancy, whereas diastolic pressure decreases more markedly; this reduction begins in the first trimester, reaches its nadir in mid-pregnancy, and returns toward nonpregnant levels by term.

Renal System

Renal plasma flow and the glomerular filtration rate（GFR）increase early in pregnancy, with maximumplateau elevations of 40%–50% above nonpregnant levels by mid-pregnancy, and then remain unchanged to term. The elevated GFR is reflected inlower serum levels of creatinine and urea nitrogen.

Respiratory System

As pregnancy progresses, the enlarging uterus elevates the resting position of the diaphragm. Total body oxygen consumption increases 15%–20% in pregnancy. In pregnancy, the elevationsin both cardiac output and alveolar ventilation are greater than those required to meet the increased oxygen consumption. The rise in minute ventilation reflects an approximate 40% increase in tidal volume at term; the respiratory rate does not change during pregnancy.

Gastrointestinal System

As the uterus grows, the stomach is pushed upward and the large and small bowel extend into more posterolateral regions. The appendix is displaced superiorly in the right flank area. These organs return to their normal position in the early puerperium.

Skin

Hyperpigmentation is one of the well recognized changes of pregnancy, which is manifested in linea nigra and chloasma. Chloasma is exacerbated by sun exposure, develops in 70% of pregnancies and is characterized by an uneven darkening of the skin in the centrofascial malar area. This hyperpigmentation is because of the elevated concentration of melanocytic stimulating hormone and or estrogen progesterone effect on the skin.

Weight Gain in Pregnancy

The average weight gain in pregnancy uncomplicated by generalized edema is 12.5 kg. The products of conception constitute only about 40% of the total maternal weight gain.

【心理社会调适】

在妊娠期,孕妇及家庭成员的心理会随着妊娠的进展而有不同的变化。孕妇常见的心理反应如下。

1.惊讶和震惊　在妊娠初期,不管是否计划中妊娠,几乎所有的孕妇都会产生惊讶和震惊的反应。

2.矛盾心理　在惊讶和震惊的同时,孕妇可能会出现爱恨交加的矛盾心理,尤其是未计划妊娠的孕妇。可能是因工作、学习等原因暂时不想要孩子所致;也可能是由于初为人母,既缺乏抚养孩子的知识和技能,又缺乏可以利用的社会支持系统。

3.接受　妊娠早期,孕妇对妊娠的感受仅仅是停经后的各种不适反应,并未真实感受到"孩子"的存在。随着妊娠进展,尤其是胎动的出现,孕妇真正感受到"孩子"的存在,出现了"筑巢反应",计划为孩子购买衣服、睡床等,关注孩子的喂养和生活护理等方面的知识,给未出生的孩子起名字、猜测性别等,甚至有些孕妇在计划着孩子未来的职业。

Pregnancy can be considered as the stage of family development. At this time, role of family and society will change. Expectant parents should prepare for newborn and study how to become parent. Pregnancy will also influence the relationship of couple, so they should adjust to new family.

Physiological changes of pregnancy and fear of labor can cause some psychological responses. These responses include ambivalent about the pregnancy, self as primary focus, mood swings and changes in body image. If the woman could adjust to these psychological changes, she will pass the pregnancy smoothly. Contrarily, these changes will influence the mother and fetus's health and their future life.

任务二　妊娠诊断(Diagnosis of Pregnancy)

工作情景

女性,26 岁,已婚,未避孕。平时月经规律,现月经过期已 7 d。有恶心呕吐,不能忍受炒菜的油烟味,食欲减退,有疲惫感,乳房胀痛。

①请明确该患者需做哪些检查来确诊是否妊娠。②针对该孕妇,给予孕早期饮食指导。

任务内容

根据妊娠不同时期的特点,临床上将妊娠分为 3 个时期:妊娠 13 周末以前称为早期妊娠;第 14~27 周末称为中期妊娠;第 28 周及其后称为晚期妊娠。

任务目标

◆ 能陈述早、中、晚期妊娠诊断的依据。
◆ 能复述胎产式、胎先露、胎方位的定义。

一　早期妊娠诊断

1. 症状

(1)停经　是妊娠最早的症状。月经周期正常的育龄期妇女,有性生活史,一旦月经过期10 d及以上,应首先考虑早期妊娠的可能。若停经已达8周,则妊娠的可能性更大。

(2)早孕反应　有半数左右的妇女,在停经6周左右出现晨起恶心、呕吐、食欲减退、喜食酸物或偏食,称为早孕反应。可能与体内 hCG 增多、胃酸分泌减少及胃排空时间延长有关。一般于妊娠12 周左右早孕反应自然消失。

(3)尿频　妊娠早期因增大的子宫压迫膀胱而引起,至12 周左右,增大的子宫进入腹腔,尿频症状自然消失。

2. 体征

(1)乳房变化　自妊娠8 周起,在雌激素、孕激素作用下,乳房逐渐增大。孕妇自觉乳房轻度胀痛、乳头刺痛,乳房增大,乳头及周围乳晕着色,有深褐色蒙氏结节出现。哺乳期妇女妊娠后乳汁明显减少。

(2)妇科检查　子宫增大变软,妊娠6~8 周时,阴道黏膜及子宫颈充血,呈紫蓝色,阴道检查子宫随停经月份而逐渐增大,子宫峡部极软,子宫体与子宫颈似不相连,称为黑加征。随着妊娠进展至8 周,子宫约为非妊娠子宫的2 倍,妊娠12 周时,子宫约为非妊娠子宫的3 倍,在耻骨联合上方可以触及。

3.辅助检查

（1）妊娠试验　利用孕卵着床后滋养细胞分泌 hCG，并经孕妇尿中排出的原理，用免疫学方法测定受检者血或尿中 hCG 含量，协助诊断早期妊娠。

（2）超声检查　是检查早期妊娠快速准确的方法。阴道 B 型超声较腹部超声可提前 1 周诊断早孕，最早在停经 4～5 周时，宫腔内可见圆形或椭圆形妊娠囊（图 3-4）。停经 6 周时，妊娠囊内可见胚芽和原始心管搏动。停经 14 周，测量胎儿头臀长度能较准确地估计孕周，矫正预产期，同时检测胎儿颈项透明层和胎儿鼻骨等，可作为孕早期染色体疾病筛查的指标。停经 9～14 周 B 型超声检查可以排除无脑儿等严重的胎儿畸形。

（3）子宫颈黏液检查　子宫颈黏液量少、黏稠，拉丝度差，涂片干燥后光镜下仅见排列成行的椭圆体，不见羊齿植物叶状结晶，则早期妊娠的可能性较大。

（4）基础体温测定　具有双相型体温的妇女，停经后高温相持续 18 d 不见下降者，早孕可能性大；如高温相持续 3 周以上，则早孕可能性更大。

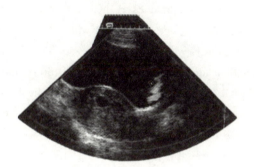

图 3-4　早孕期超声图像

Signs and Symptoms in Early Stage of Pregnancy

• Menstrual suppression：Abrupt menstrual cessation in a woman who in the past has had predictable menstrual cycles indicates the possibility of pregnancy. A woman may miss an occasional menstrual cycle for a variety of reasons, including hormonal imbalances, some chronic and systemic illnesses, psychological and emotional stress, low body fat ratio (as seen with eating disorders or in highly trained athletes), and as a side effect of some medications. In the absence of these conditions, however, and if two consecutive cycles are missed, pregnancy must be considered.

• Morning sickness：The nausea and vomiting of pregnancy are frequently called morning sickness, because these symptoms are more acute on arising. However, they may occur at any time and continue throughout the day. These symptoms are believed to be related to increased levels of hCG and estrogen. Approximately 50% of women will experience varying degrees of gastrointestinal distress in early pregnancy. Nausea and vomiting often occur at about 6 weeks of pregnancy and disappear at 12 weeks of pregnancy.

• Frequent urination：As the uterus grows, it pushes on the bladder, creating the sensation of a bladder full of urine. As the pregnancy progresses, the uterus rises out of the pelvis, and this sensation decreases.

• Breast tenderness：Many women can predict the onset of menstruation with the degree of breast tenderness they experience. The breast changes of early pregnancy may feel like an exaggeration of these changes and may be accompanied by a tingling feeling.

• Vaginal changes：After 8-10 weeks' gestation, discoloration of the vaginal mucous membrane can be observed. Elevated hormone levels thicken the vaginal mucosa, and increased vascularity, especially in the cervix, lends a blue-purple cast to the tissues. This finding, termed Chadwick's sign, is most noticeable in primigravidas (women who are pregnant for the first time) and is easily contrasted to the normal pink vagina and cervix. Vaginal secretions also increase in response to the pregnancy. Other organs in the pelvis reflect changes due to pregnancy and prepare the structures for labor and birth.

- Uterine changes: In the first 12 weeks of pregnancy, the uterus becomes more globular, enlarged, soft, and spongy. Hegar's sign describes the extreme softening of the lower uterine segment to the point where it can be compressed almost to the thinness of paper. An experienced examiner can identify this sign and support the diagnosis of pregnancy.

- Pregnancy tests: Detect human chorionic gonadotropin (hCG), which is secreted by the placenta and presents in the blood and urine of pregnant woman shortly after conception. It can be detected in as few as 8-9 days after fertilization by immunometric method. The hCG contains alpha (α) and beta (β) subunits. α-hCG is similar to the pituitary hormones; β-hCG has a unique molecular structure specific to pregnancy. Tests that identify β subunits do not cross-react with other gonadotropins. In the first trimester of normal pregnancy, the levels of β-hCG will double about every 48-72 h. In an abnormal gestation, the levels will rise to a certain point then level off or decline. Use of ultrasound plus serial mea-surements of β-hCG can identify abnormal gestations before they develop into medical emergencies.

- Visualization of the fetus: Visualizing a pregnancy through ultrasonography is increasingly the method of choice for confirming early pregnancies. An intrauterine sac is often detectable as early as 30 days after conception, and a beating fetal heart can be seen at 7-8 weeks. Sonography is invaluable for the diagnosis of spontaneous abortion and ectopic pregnancy, it can often detect extrauterine gestation before the condition becomes life-threatening. Both transabdominal and transvaginal sonography are used to diagnose pregnancy, evaluate fetal structure, and date the gestation.

二 中、晚期妊娠诊断

1. 症状　有早期妊娠的经过,孕妇感到腹部逐渐增大,自觉胎动。

2. 体征

(1)子宫增大　随着妊娠进展,子宫逐渐增大。手测子宫底高度或尺测耻上子宫高度,可以判断子宫大小与妊娠周数是否相符。子宫底高度因孕妇的脐耻间距离、胎儿发育情况、羊水量、单胎、多胎等有差异,增长过速或过缓均可能为异常(图3-5、表3-1)。

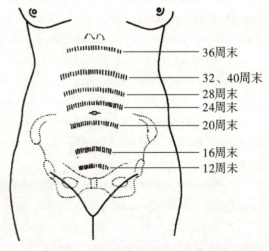

图3-5　妊娠周数与子宫底高度

表3-1　不同妊娠周数的子宫底高度

妊娠周数	妊娠月份	手测子宫底高度	尺测耻上子宫长度/cm
满12周	3个月末	耻骨联合上2~3横指	
满16周	4个月末	脐耻之间	
满20周	5个月末	脐下1横指	18(15.3~21.4)
满24周	6个月末	脐上1横指	24(22.0~25.1)
满28周	7个月末	脐上3横指	26(22.4~29.0)
满32周	8个月末	脐与剑突之间	29(25.3~32.0)
满36周	9个月末	剑突下2横指	32(29.8~34.5)
满40周	10个月末	脐与剑突之间或略高	33(30.0~35.3)

（2）胎动　指胎儿的躯体活动。孕妇于妊娠18~20周时开始自觉胎动,胎动随妊娠进展逐渐增强,至妊娠32~34周达高峰,妊娠38周后逐渐减少。胎动每小时3~5次。腹壁薄且松弛的孕妇,经腹壁可见胎动。

（3）胎心音　妊娠12周,用多普勒胎心听诊仪经孕妇腹壁能探测到胎心音,妊娠18~20周时用普通听诊仪经孕妇腹壁上能听到胎心音。胎心音呈双音,第一音与第二音相接近,如钟表的"滴答"声,速度较快,110~160次/min。注意须与子宫杂音、腹主动脉音及脐带杂音相鉴别。

（4）胎体　妊娠20周以后,经腹壁可以触及子宫内的胎体,妊娠24周以后,运用四步触诊法可以区分胎头、胎臀、胎背及胎儿四肢,从而判断胎产式、胎先露和胎方位。胎头圆而硬,用手经阴道轻触胎头并轻推,得到胎儿浮动又回弹的感觉,称为浮球感,亦称浮沉胎动感(图3-6)。

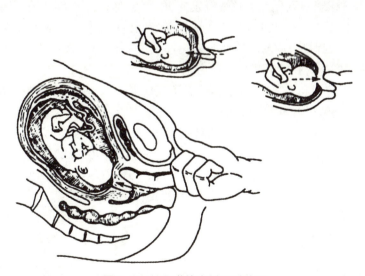

图3-6　经阴道检查浮沉胎动感

3.辅助检查　B型超声显像法不仅能显示胎儿数目、胎方位、胎心搏动、胎盘位置、羊水量、评估胎儿体重,且能测定胎头双顶径、股骨长等多条径线,了解胎儿生长发育情况。妊娠18~24周,可采用超声进行胎儿系统检查,筛查胎儿有无结构畸形。多普勒超声可探查胎心音、胎动音、脐带血流音及胎盘血流音。

Signs and Symptoms in Middle and Late Stages of Pregnancy

● Abdominal changes：The increasing size of the uterus causes a gradual increase in abdominal girth. At 12 weeks, the pregnant uterus can be palpated just above the pubic symphysis. At the end of 16 weeks, it can be found midway between the symphysis and umbilicus, and at 20 weeks, the fundus can be palpated at the level of the umbilicus. At term, the fundus can be found at the ensiform cartilage. Abdominal enlargement can be due to variety of causes, including tumor formation, edema, and body fat accumulation. These conditions usually do not cause the progressive and predictable changes in uterine size.

● Fetal movement：Fetal movement shows that the fetus is in a good condition. Quickening is an ancient term derived from the idea that life was infused into a fetus at approximately 18 – 20 weeks' gestation. It refers to the first perceptions of fetal movement as discerned by the mother. Quickening can be easily confused with intestinal gas. Women with thick abdominal walls may feel movement to a lesser degree than thinner women.

● Fetal heart sounds：Electronic Doppler monitoring allows the patient and practitioner to hear fetal heart sounds as early as the 8th week. Fetal heart sounds usually range from 110 to 160 beats/min, with an average of 130 to 140 beats/min. They are best heard over the fetal back.

● Fetal outline：At about 24 weeks' gestation, the outline of the fetus is evident to the experienced examiner. Fetal back, extremities, and head become more defined as the gestation proceeds. Uterine or other pelvic tumors usually do not have the same distinct outlines but need to be considered in diagnosis.

三 胎产式、胎先露、胎方位

妊娠28周以前,羊水较多,胎体较小,因此胎儿在子宫内的活动范围较大,胎儿在宫内的位置和姿势易于改变。妊娠32周以后,胎儿生长发育迅速,羊水相对减少,胎儿与子宫壁贴近,因此,胎儿在宫内的位置和姿势相对恒定。胎儿在子宫内的姿势,简称胎姿势。正常胎姿势为胎头俯屈,下颌贴近胸壁,脊柱略前弯,四肢屈曲交叉弯曲于胸腹部前方。整个胎体成为头端小、臀端大的椭圆形,适应妊娠晚期椭圆形子宫腔的形状。

由于胎儿在子宫内位置和姿势的不同,因此有不同的胎产式、胎先露和胎方位。尽早确定胎儿在子宫内的位置非常重要,以便及时纠正异常胎位。

1.胎产式 胎儿身体纵轴与母体身体纵轴之间的关系称为胎产式。两轴平行者称为纵产式,占妊娠足月分娩总数的99.75%。两轴垂直者称为横产式,仅占妊娠足月分娩总数的0.25%。两轴交叉者称为斜产式,属暂时的,在分娩过程中转为纵产式,偶尔转为横产式(图3-7)。

2.胎先露 最先进入骨盆入口的胎儿部分称为胎先露。纵产式有头先露、臀先露,横产式有肩先露。头先露又可因胎头屈伸程度不同分为枕先露、前囟先露、额先露、面先露(图3-8)。臀先露又可因入盆先露不同分为混合臀先露、单臀先露和足先露(图3-9)。偶见头先露或臀先露与胎手或胎足同时入盆,称为复合先露。

3.胎方位 胎儿先露部指示点与母体骨盆的关系称为胎方位,简称胎位。枕先露以枕骨、面先露以颏骨、臀先露以骶骨、肩先露以肩胛骨为指示点。根据指示点与母体骨盆左、右、前、后、横的关系而有不同的胎位(图3-10)。

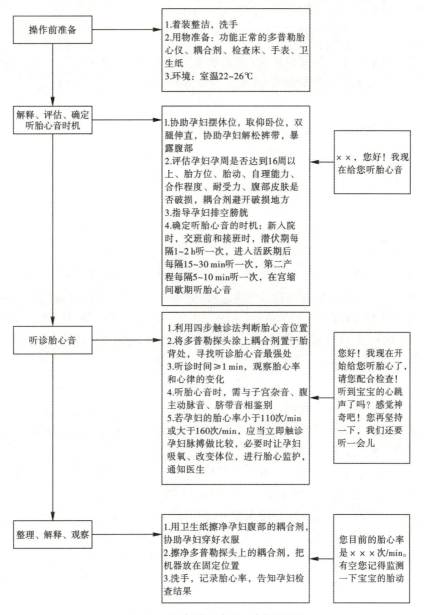

图3-11　妇产科听诊胎心音操作流程

任务三　产前检查(Prenatal Examination)

工作情景

　　孕妇,30岁,已婚,G_1P_0,妊娠36周,今日在门诊常规产检。遵医嘱为孕妇进行腹部四步触诊以判断胎产式、胎先露及胎方位,并进行骨盆外测量,了解骨产道情况。

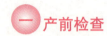 **任务内容**

产前检查包括对孕妇进行规范的检查、健康教育与指导、胎儿健康的监护与评估等,是降低孕产妇和围产儿并发症的发生率及死亡率、减少出生缺陷的重要措施。

任务目标

◆ 能叙述产前检查的目的和方法。
◆ 能描述常用的胎儿健康评估技术。

一 产前检查

规范的产前检查能够及早防治妊娠并发症或合并症和及时发现胎儿异常,评估孕妇及胎儿的安危,确定分娩时机和分娩方式,保障母儿安全。根据我国《孕前和孕期保健指南(2018)》,目前推荐的产前检查孕周分别是妊娠 6 ~ 13^{+6} 周、14 ~ 19^{+6} 周、20 ~ 24 周、25 ~ 28 周、29 ~ 32 周、33 ~ 36 周、37 ~ 41 周(每周 1 次),共 11 次。产前检查的内容包括详细询问病史、全面体格检查、产科检查、必要的辅助检查等。

【病史】

1. 年龄 < 18 岁或 ≥ 35 岁妊娠为高危因素,≥ 35 岁妊娠者为高龄孕妇。

2. 职业 从事接触有毒物质或放射线等工作的孕妇,其母儿不良结局的风险增加,建议计划妊娠前或妊娠后调换工作岗位。

3. 本次妊娠的经过 了解妊娠早期有无早孕反应、病毒感染及用药史;胎动开始时间和胎动变化;饮食、睡眠和运动情况;有无阴道流血、头痛、眼花、心悸、气短、下肢水肿等症状。

4. 推算及核对预产期 推算方法是按末次月经(LMP)第一日算起,月份减 3 或加 9,日数加 7。如为农历,月份仍减 3 或加 9,但日期加 15。实际分娩日期与推算的预产期可以相差 1 ~ 2 周。如孕妇记不清末次月经的日期,则可根据早孕反应出现时间、胎动开始时间、子宫底高度和 B 型超声检查的胎囊大小(GS)、头臀长度(CRL)、胎头双顶径(BPD)及股骨长度(FL)值推算出预产期。

5. 月经史及既往孕产史 询问初潮年龄、月经周期。经产妇应了解有无难产史、死胎死产史、分娩方式、新生儿情况及有无产后出血史,了解末次分娩或流产的时间及转归。

6. 既往史及手术史 了解有无高血压、心脏病、结核病、糖尿病、血液病、肝肾疾病等,注意其发病时间及治疗情况,并了解做过何种手术。

7. 家族史 询问家族有无结核病、高血压、糖尿病、双胎妊娠及其他与遗传相关的疾病。

8. 丈夫健康状况 着重询问健康状况,有无遗传性疾病等。

【体格检查】

观察发育、营养、精神状态、身高及步态。身材矮小者(145 cm 以下)常伴有骨盆狭窄。测量血压,正常孕妇不应超过 140/90 mmHg,超过者属病理状态。测量体重,计算体重指数(BMI),BMI = 体重(kg)/[身高(m)]^2,评估营养状况。妊娠晚期体重每周增加不应超过 500 g,超过者应注意水肿或隐性水肿的发生。检查心肺有无异常,乳房发育情况、乳头大小及有无乳头凹陷,脊柱及下肢有无畸形。

【产科检查】

产科检查包括腹部检查、骨盆测量、阴道检查等。

1.腹部检查 孕妇排尿后仰卧于检查床上,头部稍抬高,露出腹部,双腿略屈曲分开,放松腹肌。检查者站在孕妇右侧。

(1)视诊 注意腹形及大小,腹部有无妊娠纹、手术瘢痕和水肿。对腹部过大者,应考虑双胎、羊水过多、巨大儿的可能;对腹部过小、子宫底过低者,应考虑胎儿生长受限、孕周推算错误等;如孕妇腹部向前突出(尖腹,多见于初产妇)或向下悬垂(悬垂腹,多见于经产妇),应考虑有骨盆狭窄的可能。

(2)触诊 注意腹壁肌肉的紧张度,有无腹直肌分离,注意羊水量的多少及子宫肌的敏感度。用手测子宫底高度,用软尺测耻骨上方至子宫底的弧形长度及腹围值。用四步触诊法检查子宫大小、胎产式、胎先露、胎方位及先露部是否衔接(图3-12)。在做前3步手法时,检查者面向孕妇,做第4步手法时,检查者应面向孕妇足端。

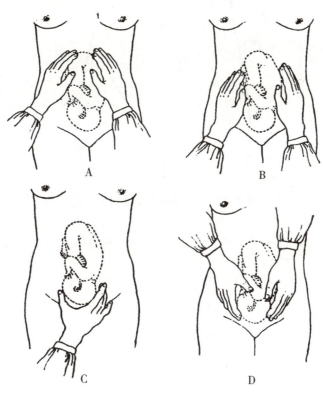

A.第一步;B.第二步;C.第三步;D.第四步。

图3-12 胎位检查的四步触诊法

1)第一步手法:检查者双手置于子宫底部,了解子宫外形并摸清子宫底高度,估计胎儿大小与妊娠月份是否相符。然后以双手指腹相对轻推,判断子宫底部的胎儿部分,如为胎头,则硬而圆且有浮球感,如为胎臀,则软而宽且形状略不规则。

2)第二步手法:检查者两只手分别置于腹部左右两侧,一只手固定,另一只手轻轻深按检查,两只手交替,分辨胎背及胎儿四肢的位置。平坦饱满者为胎背,确定胎背是向前、侧方或向后;可变形的高低不平部分是胎儿的肢体,有时可以感觉到胎儿肢体活动。

3）第三步手法：检查者右手置于耻骨联合上方，拇指与其余4指分开，握住胎先露部，进一步查清是胎头或胎臀，并左右推动以确定是否衔接。如先露部仍高浮，表示尚未入盆；如已衔接，则先露部不能被推动。

4）第四步手法：检查者两只手分别置于胎先露部的两侧，向骨盆入口方向向下深压，再次判断先露部的诊断是否正确，并确定先露部入盆的程度。

（3）听诊　胎心音在靠近胎背侧上方的孕妇腹壁上听得最清楚。枕先露时，胎心音在脐下方右或左侧；臀先露时，胎心音在脐上方右或左侧；肩先露时，胎心音在脐部下方听得最清楚（图3-13）。当腹壁紧、子宫较敏感、确定胎背方向有困难时，可借助胎心音及胎先露综合分析判断胎方位。

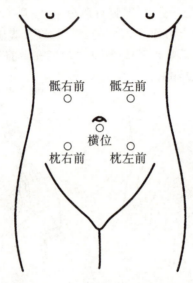

图3-13　不同胎位胎心音听诊位置

2.骨盆测量　了解骨产道情况，以判断胎儿能否经阴道分娩。骨盆测量分为骨盆外测量和骨盆内测量两种。

（1）骨盆外测量　此法常用于测量下列径线。

1）髂棘间径：孕妇取伸腿仰卧位，测量两侧髂前上棘外缘的距离（图3-14），正常值为23~26 cm。

2）髂嵴间径：孕妇取伸腿仰卧位，测量两侧髂嵴外缘最宽的距离（图3-15），正常值为25~28 cm。髂棘间径和髂嵴间径可间接推测骨盆入口横径的长度。

3）骶耻外径：孕妇取左侧卧位，右腿伸直，左腿屈曲，测量第五腰椎棘突下凹陷处（相当于腰骶部米氏菱形窝的上角）至耻骨联合上缘中点的距离（图3-16），正常值为18~20 cm。此径线可间接推测骨盆入口前后径长度，是骨盆外测量中最重要的径线。

4）坐骨结节间径：又称出口横径。孕妇取仰卧位，两腿屈曲，双手抱膝。测量两侧坐骨结节内侧缘之间的距离（图3-17），正常值为8.5~9.5 cm，平均9 cm。

5）出口后矢状径：是指坐骨结节间径中点至骶骨尖的距离，正常值为8~9 cm。出口横径与出口后矢状径之和大于15 cm者，一般足月胎儿可以娩出。

6）耻骨弓角度：用两拇指尖斜着对拢，放于耻骨联合下缘，左右两拇指平放在耻骨降支的上面，测量两拇指之间的角度即为耻骨弓角度（图3-18）。正常为90°，小于80°为异常。

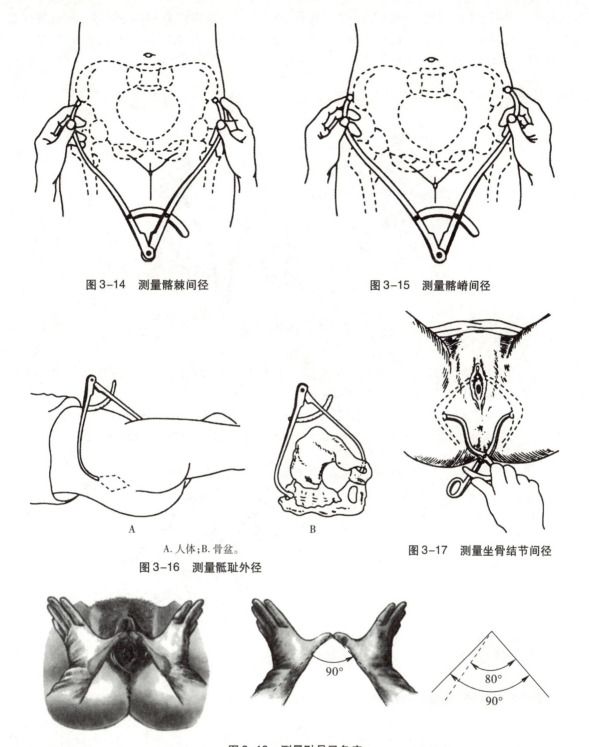

图3-14 测量髂棘间径 图3-15 测量髂嵴间径

A. 人体;B. 骨盆。

图3-16 测量骶耻外径 图3-17 测量坐骨结节间径

图3-18 测量耻骨弓角度

（2）骨盆内测量 适用于骨盆外测量有狭窄者。测量时,孕妇取膀胱截石位,消毒外阴,检查者须戴消毒手套并涂以润滑油。常用径线如下。

1）对角径:也称为骶耻内径,是自耻骨联合下缘至骶岬上缘中点的距离。检查者一只手示、中指伸入阴道,用中指尖触骶岬上缘中点,示指上缘紧贴耻骨联合下缘,并标记示指与耻骨联合下缘的接触点。中指尖至此接触点的距离，即为对角径（图3-19）。正常值为 12.5 ~ 13.0 cm，此值减去 1.5 ~ 2.0 cm，即为真结合径值，正常值为 11 cm。如触不到骶岬，说明此径线 >12.5 cm。测量时期以妊娠 24 ~ 36 周、阴道松软时进行为宜，36 周以后测量应在消毒情况下进行。

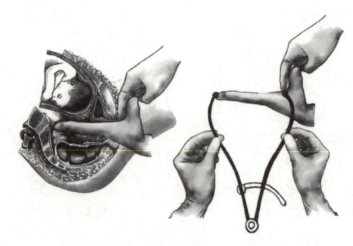

图 3-19　测量对角径

2）坐骨棘间径：测量两侧坐骨棘间的距离，正常值约 10 cm。检查者一只手的示指、中指伸入阴道内，分别触及两侧坐骨棘，估计其间的距离（图3-20）。

3）坐骨切迹宽度：为坐骨棘与骶骨下部间的距离，即骶棘韧带的宽度。检查者将伸入阴道内的示指置于韧带上，如能容纳 3 横指（5.5 ~ 6.0 cm）为正常，否则属中骨盆狭窄（图3-21）。

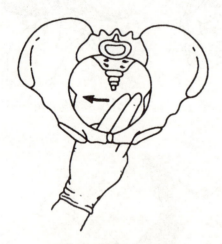

图 3-20　测量坐骨棘间径

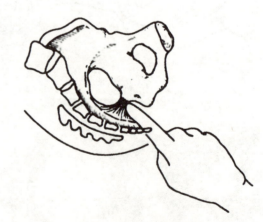

图 3-21　测量坐骨切迹宽度

3. 阴道检查　妊娠期可行阴道检查，特别是有阴道流血和阴道分泌物异常时。妊娠最后 1 个月及临产后，应避免不必要的检查，如确实需要，则需外阴消毒及戴消毒手套，以防感染。

【辅助检查】

1. 常规检查　血常规、尿常规、血型（ABO 和 Rh）、肝功能、肾功能、空腹血糖、HBsAg、梅毒螺旋体、HIV 筛查等。

2. 超声检查　妊娠 18 ~ 24 周时进行胎儿系统超声检查，筛查胎儿有无严重畸形。超声检查可以观察胎儿生长发育情况、羊水量、胎方位、胎盘位置、胎盘成熟度等。

3. 妊娠糖尿病筛查 先行 50 g 葡萄糖筛查(GCT),若 7.2 mmol/L≤血糖≤11.1 mmol/L,则进行 75 g 口服葡萄糖耐量试验(OGTT);若≥11.1 mmol/L,则测定空腹血糖。国际最近推荐的方法是可不必先行 50 g GCT,有条件者可直接行 75 g OGTT,其正常上限为空腹血糖 5.1 mmoL,1 h 血糖为 10.0 mmol/L,2 h 血糖为 8.5 mmol/L,或者将空腹血糖检测作为筛查标准。

Initial Prenatal Evaluation

The prenatal workup consists of a thorough health history, a physical examination, and laboratory tests. Prenatal forms summarize data and serve as a flow sheet for continuing visits throughout pregnancy. Advanced practice nurses (nurse practitioners or clinical specialists) often obtain the history, order diagnostic tests, conduct the physical examination, and provide complete prenatal management. Nurses usually conduct client education and orientation to prenatal services. The nurse's initial contact with the client is particularly important. By greeting the woman in a pleasant, interested, and professional manner, the nurse communicates a personalized approach to care. When the client experiences positive regard, she is more likely to keep return visits and discuss her concerns.

Diagnosis of Pregnancy and Estimating Date of Delivery

Early, accurate diagnosis of pregnancy is done by radioassay and immunologic pregnancy tests. An accurate estimated date of delivery (EDD) is important, because this allows the nurse and physician to assess the progress of gestation and evaluate term pregnancy more readily. Delivery date may be calculated by Nagele's rule based on last menstrual period (LMP), progressive measurements of the height of the fundus (McDonald's rule), and ultrasonography to measure fetal growth. Nagele's rule Count back 3 months or add 9 months from the first day of LMP and add 7 days. Correct for year if necessary. McDonald's rule for fundal height count height of fundus (cm)×8/7=gestation of pregnancy in weeks.

Physical Examination

A thorough physical examination is performed to establish a baseline for the woman's general state of health and to evaluate the pregnancy. Attention is paid to the teeth and throat, thyroid gland and lymph nodes, lungs, heart, breasts, skin, extremities, and abdomen. Characteristic changes of pregnancy are noted, and signs of infection or systemic disease are identified if present. Indications of high-risk pregnancy are identified, such as obesity, underweight for height, hypertension, severe varicosities preeclampsia, or inappropriate uterine size for dates.

Abdominal Examination

Abdominal examination is useful for providing information about the position of the fetus after the 13th week of gestation. Palpation (Leopold's maneuvers) helps to evaluate the maternal abdomen, to understand the size, fetal lie, fetal presentation, fetal position and whether the fetal presentation engaged or not. The nurse should stand at the right side of the pregnant. In the first 3 steps, the nurse faces the woman, and the last step, the nurse faces the woman's feet.

- First maneuver: While facing the woman, the nurse palpates the upper abdomen with both hands. The nurse determines the shape, size, consistency, and mobility of the form that is found. The fetal head is firm, hard, and round and moves independently of the trunk. The breech feels softer and symmetrical and has small bony prominences; it moves with the trunk.

- Second maneuver: After ascertaining whether the head or the buttocks occupies the fundus, the nurse tries to determine the location of the fetal back and notes whether it is on the right or left side of the maternal abdomen. Still facing the woman, the nurse palpates the abdomen with deep but gentle pressure, using her palms. The right hand should be steady-while the left hand explores the right side of the uterus. The Maneuver is then repeated, probing with the right hand and steadying the uterus with the left hand. The fetal back should feel firm and smooth and should connect what was found in the fundus with a mass in the inlet. Once the back is located, the nurse validates the finding by palpating the fetal extremities on the opposite side of the abdomen.

- Third maneuver: Next the nurse should determine what fetal part is lying above the inlet by gently grasping the lower portion of the abdomen just above the symphysis pubis with the thumb and fingers of the right hand. This maneuver yields the opposite information from what was found in the fundus and validates the presenting part. If the head is presenting and is not engaged, it may be gently pushed back and forth.

- Fourth maneuver: For this portion of the examination the nurse faces the woman's feet and attempts to locate the cephalic prominence or brow. Location of this landmark assists in assessing the descent of the presenting part into the pelvis. The fingers of both hands are moved gently down the sides of the uterus toward the pubis.

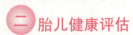

二 胎儿健康评估

评估胎儿健康包括确定是否为高危儿和监测胎儿宫内状况。

高危儿判定标准：①孕龄<37 周或≥42 周；②出生体重<2 500 g；③小于孕龄儿或大于孕龄儿；④生后 1 min 内阿普加(Apgar)评分 0~3 分；⑤产时感染；⑥高危妊娠产妇的新生儿；⑦手术产儿；⑧新生儿的兄姐有严重的新生儿病史或新生儿期死亡等。

胎儿宫内状况的监测项目如下。

1. 妊娠早期　妇科检查确定子宫大小及是否与妊娠周数相符。超声检查最早在妊娠第 6 周即可见妊娠囊和原始心管搏动。有条件时，妊娠 11~13^{+6} 周超声测量胎儿颈项透明层厚度(NT)和胎儿发育情况。

2. 妊娠中期　每次产前检查测量子宫底高度，协助判断胎儿大小及是否与妊娠周数相符。超声检查胎儿生长状况并筛查胎儿结构有无异常。每次产前检查时听取胎心率。

3. 妊娠晚期　每次产前检查测量子宫底高度并听取胎心率。超声检查不仅能判断胎儿生长状况，而且能判定胎位、胎盘位置、羊水量和胎盘成熟度。其他评估项目如下。

(1)胎动监测　胎动监测是孕妇自我评价胎儿宫内状况的简便经济的有效方法。一般孕妇妊娠 20 周开始自觉胎动，夜间和下午胎动较为活跃。胎动常在胎儿睡眠周期消失，持续 20~40 min。妊娠 28 周以后，胎动计数<10 次/2 h 或减少 50% 提示有胎儿缺氧可能。

(2)电子胎心监护　能连续观察并记录胎心率(FHR)的动态变化，同时描记子宫收缩和胎动情况，反映三者间的关系，以及时、客观地监测胎心率和评估胎儿宫内储备能力。

1)监测胎心率：胎心率基线(BFHR)是指在无胎动、无子宫收缩影响时，10 min 以上的胎心率平均值。正常的 BFHR 由交感神经和副交感神经共同调节，包括每分钟心搏次数及 FHR 变异。FHR 的正常值为 110~160 次/min，若 FHR>160 次/min 或<110 次/min，历时 10 min，称为心动过速或心动过缓。

胎心率基线变异是指 BFHR 在振幅和频率上的不规则波动或小的周期性波动，又称为基线摆动，包括胎心率的摆动幅度和摆动频率。摆动幅度是指胎心率上下摆动波的高度，振幅变动范围正常为 6~25 次/min。摆动频率是指 1 min 内波动的次数,正常为≥6 次/min。BFHR 变异表示胎儿有一定的储备能力,是胎儿健康的表现。基线波动活跃则频率增高,基线平直则频率降低或消失。BFHR 变平即变异消失,提示胎儿储备能力丧失。

2)胎心率一过性变化:受胎动、宫缩、触诊及声响等刺激,胎心率发生暂时性加快或减慢,随后又能恢复到基线水平,称为胎心率一过性变化,是判断胎儿安危的重要指标。胎心率一过性变化包括加速和减速两种情况。

加速:指宫缩时 FHR 增加≥15 次/min,持续时间≥15 s,是胎儿情况良好的表现,原因可能是胎儿躯干局部或脐静脉暂时受压。散发的、短暂的胎心率加速是无害的。但脐静脉持续受压则发展为减速。

减速:指宫缩时 FHR 减慢,包括以下 3 种情况。①早期减速:特点是 FHR 曲线下降几乎与宫缩曲线上升同时开始,FHR 曲线最低点与宫缩曲线高峰相一致,即波谷对波峰,下降幅度<50 次/min,持续时间<15 s,子宫收缩后迅速恢复正常(图 3-22)。不受孕妇体位及吸氧而改变。意义:提示胎儿有缺氧的危险。②变异减速:特点是 FHR 减速与宫缩无固定关系,下降迅速,下降幅度>70 次/min,持续时间长短不一,但恢复迅速(图 3-23)。意义:提示脐带有可能受压。可改变体位继续观察。如果存在变异减速伴有 FHR 基线变异消失,提示可能存在胎儿宫内缺氧。③晚期减速:特点是 FHR 减速多在宫缩高峰后开始出现,即波谷落后于波峰,时间差在 30~60 s,下降幅度<50 次/min,恢复所需时间较长(图 3-24)。意义:提示胎盘功能不良、胎儿有宫内缺氧。

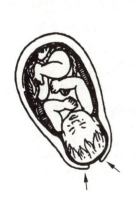

图 3-22 胎心率早期减速

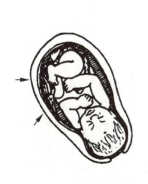
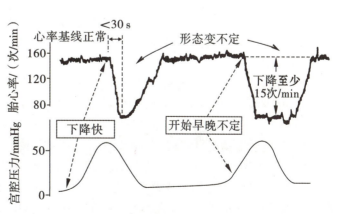

图 3-23 胎心率变异减速

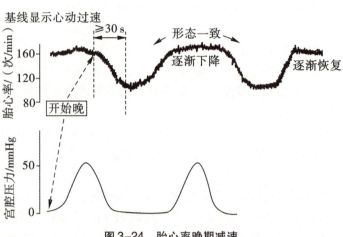

图 3-24　胎心率晚期减速

（3）预测胎儿宫内储备能力

1）无应激试验（NST）：指在无宫缩、无外界负荷刺激下，用电子胎儿监护仪进行胎心率与胎动的观察和记录，以了解胎儿储备能力。原理：在胎儿不存在酸中毒或神经受压的情况下，胎动时出现胎心率的短暂上升，预示着正常的自主神经功能。方法：孕妇取坐位或侧卧位，一般监护 20 min。由于胎儿存在睡眠周期，NST 可能需要监护 40 min 或更长时间。本试验根据 BFHR、胎动时胎心率一过性变化（变异、减速和加速）等分为 NST 反应型和无反应型。NST 反应型：指监护时间内出现 2 次或以上的胎心加速。妊娠 32 周前，加速在基线水平上 ≥10 次/min、持续时间 ≥10 s，已证明对胎儿正常宫内状态有足够的预测价值。在 BFHR 正常、变异正常且不存在减速的情况下，电子胎儿监护达到 NST 反应型即可。NST 无反应型：指超过 40 min 没有足够的胎心加速。

2）缩宫素激惹试验（OCT）：又称为宫缩应激试验（CST），其目的是观察和记录宫缩后胎心率的变化，了解宫缩时胎盘一过性缺氧的负荷变化，评估胎儿的宫内储备能力。原理：在宫缩的应激下，子宫动脉血流减少，可促发胎儿一过性缺氧表现。对已处于亚缺氧状态的胎儿，在宫缩的刺激下缺氧逐渐加重，将诱导出现晚期减速。宫缩的刺激还可引起脐带受压，从而出现变异减速。宫缩的要求：宫缩 ≥3 次/10 min，每次持续 ≥40 s。如果产妇自发的宫缩满足上述要求，无须诱导宫缩，否则可通过刺激乳头或静脉滴注子宫收缩药诱导宫缩。

OCT/CST 图形的判读主要基于是否出现晚期减速。结果阴性：无晚期减速或明显的变异减速。阳性：50% 以上的宫缩后出现晚期减速。可疑阳性：间断出现晚期减速或明显的变异减速。可疑过度刺激：宫缩>5 次/10 min 或每次宫缩持续时间>90 s 时出现胎心减速。不满意的 OCT/CST：宫缩频率<3 次/10 min 或出现无法解释的图形。

（4）胎盘功能检查

1）孕妇尿雌三醇（E_3）测定：一般测 24 h 尿 E_3 含量。24 h 尿 E_3>15 mg 为正常值，10 ~ 15 mg 为警戒值，<10 mg 为危险值。若妊娠晚期连续多次测得此值<10 mg，表示胎盘功能低下。

2）孕妇血清游离雌三醇测定：正常足月妊娠时临界值为 40 nmol/L，若每周连续测定 2 ~ 3 次，E_3 值均在正常范围，说明胎儿情况良好；若发现 E_3 值持续缓慢下降，可能为过期妊娠；下降较快者可能为重度妊娠期高血压疾病或胎儿宫内发育迟缓；急骤下降或下降>50% 时，说明胎儿有宫内死亡危险。

（5）胎儿成熟度检查　测定胎儿成熟度的方法，除计算妊娠周数、测量子宫底高度与腹围、B 型超声测量胎头双顶径外，还可经腹壁羊膜腔穿刺抽取羊水进行以下检测：①卵磷脂/鞘磷脂（L/S）比值，用于评估胎儿肺成熟度，L/S 值>2 提示胎儿肺成熟；②磷脂酰甘油（PG）测定，PG>3% 提示肺成熟；③泡沫试验或震荡试验，是一种快速而简便测定羊水中表面活性物质的试验。若两管液面均有完整的泡沫环,提示胎儿肺成熟。

（6）胎儿缺氧程度检查

1）胎儿头皮血 pH 值测定:通过采集胎儿头皮毛细血管血样测定,正常胎儿头皮血 pH 值为7.25～7.35,pH 值7.21～7.24 提示可疑酸中毒,pH 值≤7.20 提示酸中毒。

2）胎儿血氧饱和度测定:胎儿血氧饱和度（FSO₂）测定用于监测胎儿氧合状态和酸碱平衡状态,是诊断胎儿窘迫、预测新生儿酸中毒的重要指标。若 $FSO_2<30\%$,应立即采取干预措施。

（7）甲胎蛋白测定　甲胎蛋白异常增高是胎儿患有开放性神经管缺损的重要指标。多胎妊娠、死胎及胎儿上消化道闭锁等也伴有升高。

Identification of Increased Risk for Fetal Abnormalities

Women older than 35 years have increased risk for fetal abnormalities. Diagnostic procedures in early pregnancy to detect such abnormalities as Down syndrome, neural tube defect, and other chromosomal disorders are recommended. Procedures include chorionic villus sampling, which involves transcervical or transabdominal aspiration of placental samples, and amniocentesis, which involves intra-abdominal aspiration of amniotic fluid samples.

Any condition that might adversely affect the health of the woman or fetus during pregnancy, labor, or delivery places the pregnancy in a high-risk category. Various psychosocial and developmental factors can place the mother and father at high risk for parenting difficulties. The nurse assesses the family structure, communication, supports, and coping behaviors to identify strengths and stressors.

任务实施

腹部四步触诊、骨盆外测量操作流程见表3-2。

表3-2　腹部四步触诊、骨盆外测量操作流程

项目	内容
目的	能够通过腹部四步触诊判断胎产式、胎先露、胎方位及胎先露是否衔接;能够通过骨盆外测量掌握常用的骨盆外测量径线、起止点及其正常值
操作前准备	1. 操作者准备:洗手、戴口罩、手要温暖
	2. 物品准备:孕妇检查模型、骨盆测量器
	3. 环境准备:关闭门窗、屏风遮挡,做好患者隐私保护
	4. 孕妇准备:孕妇排空膀胱后仰卧于检查床上,向孕妇解释此次检查目、告知孕妇操作过程中可能出现的不适
腹部四步触诊	第一步手法:①判断宫底高度是否与孕周相符;②宫底部胎儿部分;③正确描述
	第二步手法:①检查手法;②判断腹部两侧胎儿部位;③正确描述
	第三步手法:①检查手法;②判断胎先露;③判断胎先露是否入盆
	第四步手法:①检查者站位及手法;②胎先露部胎儿部分及判断是否入盆;③正确描述
骨盆外测量	1. 垫一次性臀垫
	2. 髂棘间径(正确寻找指示点、测量外侧缘、正确读尺、记录数值)
	3. 髂嵴间径(正确寻找指示点、测量外侧缘、正确读尺、记录数值)
	4. 骶耻外径(告知体位、正确寻找指示点、正确读尺、记录数值)

续表 3-2

项目	内容
骨盆外测量	5. 坐骨结节间径(告知体位、正确寻找指示点、测量内侧缘、正确读尺、记录数值及异常值处理)
	6. 出口后矢状径(告知体位、正确寻找指示点、正确读尺、记录数值)
	7. 耻骨弓角度(正确寻找指示点、正确估值)
整理	1. 询问孕妇有何不适
	2. 协助孕妇离开检查床
	3. 汇报检查结果

任务四 妊娠期常见症状及护理(Common Symptoms and Care During Pregnancy)

工作情景

孕妇,32 岁,已婚,G_1P_0,妊娠 32^{+5} 周,自述有腰背痛、下肢痉挛,仰卧位时出现头晕、恶心、呕吐、胸闷等症状。

①请明确该患者主要的护理问题。②根据目前的情况对患者进行正确的护理。

任务内容

孕期常见症状包括恶心、呕吐、尿频、尿急、白带增多、水肿、下肢及外阴静脉曲张、便秘、腰背痛、下肢痉挛、仰卧位低血压综合征、失眠、贫血。

任务目标

◆ 能叙述孕期常见症状。
◆ 能根据孕妇症状提供对症护理措施。

孕期可出现各种与妊娠相关的症状,护理原则主要是对症护理。

1. 恶心、呕吐　半数左右妇女在妊娠 6 周左右出现早孕反应,12 周左右消失。在此期间应避免空腹,少量多餐,饮食宜清淡,避免进食油炸、难以消化或有引起不舒服气味的食物;给予精神鼓励和支持,以减少其心理的困扰和忧虑。若妊娠 12 周以后仍继续呕吐,甚至影响孕妇营养时,应考虑妊娠剧吐的可能,须住院治疗,纠正水、电解质紊乱。

2. 尿频、尿急　常发生在妊娠初 3 个月及末 3 个月。若为妊娠子宫压迫所致,且无任何感染征象,可给予解释,不必处理。孕妇无须通过减少液体摄入量的方式来缓解症状,有尿意时应及时排空。此现象产后可逐渐消失。

3. 白带增多　白带增多于妊娠初 3 个月及末 3 个月明显,是妊娠期正常的生理变化。但应排除假丝酵母菌、滴虫、淋球菌、衣原体等的感染。嘱孕妇每日清洗外阴或经常洗澡,以避免分泌物刺激外阴部,保持外阴部清洁,但严禁阴道冲洗。指导孕妇穿透气性好的棉质内裤,经常更换。分泌物过多的孕妇,可用卫生巾并经常更换,增加舒适感。

4. 水肿　孕妇在妊娠后期易发生下肢水肿,经休息后可消退,属正常。下肢有明显凹陷性水肿或经休息后不消退者,应及时诊治,警惕妊娠期高血压疾病的发生。嘱孕妇左侧卧位,解除右旋增大的子宫对下腔静脉的压迫,下肢稍垫高,避免长时间地站或坐,以免加重水肿的发生。适当限制孕妇对盐的摄入,但不必限制水分。

5. 下肢、外阴静脉曲张　孕妇应避免两腿交叉或长时间站立、行走,并注意时常抬高下肢;指导孕妇穿弹力裤或袜,避免穿妨碍血液回流的紧身衣裤,以促进血液回流;会阴部有静脉曲张者,可于臀下垫枕,抬高臀部休息。

6. 便秘　便秘是妊娠期常见的症状之一,尤其是妊娠前即有便秘者。嘱孕妇养成每日定期排便的习惯,多吃水果、蔬菜等含纤维素多的食物,同时增加每日饮水量,注意适当的活动。未经医生允许,不可随意用药。

7. 腰背痛　指导孕妇穿低跟鞋,在俯拾或抬举物品时,保持上身直立,弯曲膝部,用两下肢的力量抬起。若工作要求长时间弯腰,妊娠期间应适当给予调整。疼痛严重者,必须卧床休息(硬床垫),局部热敷。

8. 下肢痉挛　指导孕妇饮食中增加钙的摄入,若因钙磷不平衡所致,则限制牛奶(含大量的磷)的摄入量或服用氢氧化铝凝胶,以吸收体内磷质来平衡钙磷之浓度。告诫孕妇避免腿部疲劳、受凉,伸腿时避免脚趾尖伸向前,走路时脚跟先着地。发生下肢肌肉痉挛时,嘱孕妇背屈肢体或站直前倾以伸展痉挛的肌肉,或局部热敷按摩,直至痉挛消失。必要时遵医嘱口服钙剂。

9. 仰卧位低血压综合征　妊娠晚期孕妇若较长时间取仰卧姿势,由于增大的妊娠子宫压迫下腔静脉,使回心血量及心排出量减少,出现低血压。嘱左侧卧位后症状可自然消失,不必紧张。

10. 失眠　每日坚持户外活动,如散步。睡前用梳子梳头、温水洗脚、喝热牛奶等方式均有助于入眠。

11. 贫血　孕妇应适当增加含铁食物的摄入,如动物肝脏、瘦肉、蛋黄、豆类等。若需要补充铁剂,可用温水或水果汁送服,以促进铁的吸收,且应在餐后 20 min 服用,以减轻对胃肠道的刺激。向孕妇解释,服用铁剂后大便可能会变黑,或可能导致便秘或轻度腹泻,不必担心。

Nursing Care of Woman in Prenatal Period

● Rest, recreation, and sleep: Rest and sleep are essential to health. Pregnant women tire more readily and may show symptoms of fatigue, such as irritability, apprehension, worry, and restlessness. Pregnant women are advised to get as much sleep as needed; this varies by individual. Napping or resting for a half hour every morning and afternoon is beneficial.

● Exercise: Exercise during pregnancy is usually beneficial, depending on the woman's state of health, conditioning, and stage of pregnancy. Exercise provides a diversion, reduces anxiety and tension, quiets the mind, promotes sleep, helps decrease constipation, and stimulates the appetite, all of which are valuable aids to the pregnant woman. Moderate exercise involving large muscle groups, such as walking, cycling, and swimming is best. Jogging or running is acceptable for women already conditioned for this level of exercise.

● Bathing and skin care: The glands of the skin are more active during pregnancy with increased perspiration, which can result in irritation or odor. Elimination through the skin is an important method of removing body waste products. The woman should take a bath or a shower daily for cleansing; these also are refreshing and relaxing. A possible danger from tub baths during the last trimester of pregnancy is that the heavy weight of the large abdomen may affect the pregnant woman's balance, making climbing in and out of the bathtub awkward. Therefore, the likelihood of slipping or falling in the bathtub is increased.

Rubber mats or hand grips can prevent falls. Baths should not taken when there is vaginal bleeding or after rupture of the membranes to avoid infection.

● Breast care：Care of the breasts during pregnancy is an important preparation for breast－feeding. Early in pregnancy，the breasts begin to secrete colostrum and should be bathed daily with a clean washcloth and warm water. Soap，alcohol，and other drying cleansers reduce integrity of the nipple tissue，because they remove the protective skin oils and leave the ripple more prone to damage. Rubbing the nipples with a bath towel or rolling them between thumb and forefinger during the last trimester of pregnancy can help toughen them in preparation for breast－feeding. Because nipple stimulation can produce uterine activity by releasing oxytocin from the posterior pituitary，women with a history of preterm labor should consult their healthcare provider before engaging in any nipple preparation activities.

任务实施

围产期保健内容见表3-3。

表3-3 围产期保健内容

孕期检查时间	辅助检查项目	检查目的
孕 6～13^{+6} 周	基本检查项目：血、尿常规；凝血六项；血型；血糖；肝肾功能；甲功筛查；优生筛查；传染病筛查；心电图等 建议检查项目：阴道分泌物；子宫颈癌筛查；叶酸代谢；骨密度；微量元素；钙代谢等	了解孕早期孕妇健康状况及胚胎发育情况
孕 11～13^{+6} 周	NT	核实孕周，首次胚胎畸形筛查
孕 14～19^{+6} 周	唐氏筛查	筛查唐氏综合征
孕 20～24 周	血、尿常规；三维、四维彩超	早产的认识筛查和预防、胎儿畸形系统筛查
孕 24～28 周	75 g OGTT；血、尿常规	筛查妊娠糖尿病及贫血
孕 30～32 周	晚期妊娠系统彩超、血尿常规	筛查妊娠期高血压疾病及胎儿畸形
孕 33～36 周	B 族链球菌筛查、肝功能、血清胆汁酸、心电图、尿常规	筛查妊娠期肝内胆汁淤积症，了解孕妇心功能及感染情况
孕 37 周之后	产科超声检查；血尿常规；凝血功能；肝肾功能；电解质；传染病筛查	了解孕妇分娩前身体状况、胎盘功能及胎儿情况，评估分娩方式

微课　　　　　　　　课件　　　　　　练习题及参考答案

（张艳亭）

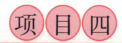

分娩期妇女的护理（Nuring of women in the Intrapartum Period）

项目描述

妊娠≥28周（≥196 d），胎儿及附属物从临产开始至全部从母体娩出的过程称为分娩。妊娠28~36⁺⁶周（196~258 d）期间分娩称为早产；妊娠37~41⁺⁶周（259~293 d）期间分娩称为足月产；妊娠≥42周（≥294 d）期间分娩称为过期产。护士应对孕妇及家属进行健康教育，使他们正确认识分娩的生理过程，做好充分的身心准备。护士协助医生正确处理产程，保证母婴安全。

Labor is a process that permits a series of extensive physiologic changes in the mother to allow for the delivery of her fetus through the birth canal. Preterm labor is defined as labor occurring after 28 weeks and before 37 weeks of gestation; partus maturus is defined as labor occurring after 37 weeks and before 42 weeks of gestation; postterm labor is defined as labor occurring after 42 weeks or more if the menstrual cycle is regular. The role of the obstetric nurse is to anticipate and assist the doctor to manage abnormalities that may occur to either the maternal or the fetal process. When a decision is made to intervene, it must be considered carefully, because each intervention carries not only potential benefits but also potential risks. In most cases, the best management may be close observation and, when necessary, cautious intervention.

任务一　影响分娩的因素（Factors Affecting Delivery）

工作情景

初孕妇，26岁，妊娠38周，阵发性腹痛8 h，子宫底高度35 cm，每2~3 min宫缩40~50 s，胎心率126次/min，宫口开大4 cm，胎头S-2，骨盆内测量对角径12 cm，坐骨棘间径9 cm，4 h后宫口开全，先露S0。胎头下降受阻，最可能的原因是什么？

影响分娩的因素包括产力、产道、胎儿及孕妇的精神心理因素,各因素均正常并能相互适应,胎儿能顺利经阴道分娩,称为正常分娩。

任务目标

◆ 能描述影响分娩的各因素。
◆ 能判断产妇影响分娩的各因素是否正常。

一 产力

将胎儿及其附属物从宫腔内逼出的力量称为产力。产力包括子宫收缩力、腹壁肌及膈肌收缩力和肛提肌收缩力。

1. 子宫收缩力 简称宫缩,是临产后的主要产力,贯穿于整个分娩过程。临产后的宫缩可使子宫颈管缩短直至消失、宫口扩张、胎先露下降、胎儿和胎盘娩出。正常子宫收缩具有以下特点。

(1)节律性 宫缩的节律性是临产的重要标志。正常宫缩是宫体肌不随意、有规律的阵发性收缩并伴有疼痛,也称阵痛。每次宫缩由弱渐强,维持一定时间,随后由强渐弱,直至消失进入间歇期(图4-1),如此反复直至分娩结束。临产开始时,宫缩间歇期为5~6 min,持续时间约30 s。随产程进展宫缩间歇期逐渐缩短,宫缩持续时间逐渐延长。当宫口开全(10 cm)后,宫缩间歇期短至1~2 min,持续时间长达60 s。

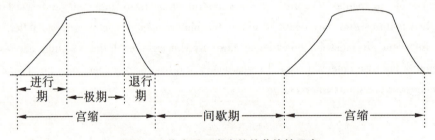

图4-1 临产后正常宫缩的节律性示意

(2)对称性和极性 正常宫缩起自两侧宫角,迅速以微波形式向子宫底中线集中,左右对称,再以每秒2 cm的速度向子宫下段扩散,约在15 s内均匀协调地扩展至整个子宫,此为子宫收缩的对称性。宫缩以宫底部最强并最持久,向下逐渐减弱,宫底部收缩力的强度几乎是子宫下段的2倍,此为宫缩的极性(图4-2)。

(3)缩复作用 宫缩时,子宫体部肌纤维短缩变宽,间歇期肌纤维不能恢复到原来的长度,经反复收缩,肌纤维越来越短,此为子宫肌纤维的缩复作用。缩复作用使宫腔内容积逐渐缩小,迫使胎先露部下降、子宫颈管逐渐缩短直至消失。

2. 腹壁肌及膈肌收缩力 腹壁肌及膈肌收缩力统称腹压,是第二产程重要的辅助力量。宫口开全后,每当宫缩时,前羊水囊或胎先露部压迫盆底组织和直肠,反射性引起排便动作。产妇主动屏气,腹壁肌及膈肌收缩使腹内压增高,促使胎儿娩出。腹压在第二产程末配合宫缩时运用最有效,过早使用腹压易使产妇疲劳、子宫颈水肿,导致产程延长。第三产程时,腹压还可促使已剥离的胎盘尽早娩出。

3.肛提肌收缩力 肛提肌收缩力可协助胎先露部在骨盆腔进行内旋转。当胎头枕部露于耻骨弓下时,能协助胎头仰伸及娩出。当胎盘娩出至阴道时,肛提肌收缩力有助于胎盘娩出。

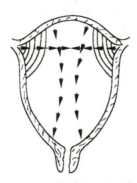

图4-2 子宫收缩的对称性和极性

The powers of labor provide the force for expulsion of the fetus and placenta from the uterus. Primary and secondary powers work together in this effort. The primary powers consist of involuntary uterine contractions that provide the force in the first stage of labor. The secondary powers are maternal pushing efforts that augment the involuntary efforts come in response to the urge to push and are generally effective only in the second stage of labor. In the first stage of labor, pushing efforts can be counter-productive to cervical dilatation.

Uterine Contractions

To expel the fetus, the uterus goes through a series of contractions (the intermittent shortening of a muscle). The key characteristics of contractions during the true labor are as following: rhythmicity, symmetry and polarity, brachystasis.

● Rhythmicity: The rhythm of uterine contraction is the important marker of labor. Each contraction includes three phases: a period when the intensity of the contraction increases (increment), a period when the contraction is at its height (acme), and a period of diminishing intensity (decrement). The duration of contractions is normally 30 s at the beginning of labor and the resting phase is 5-6 min. The contractions of the uterus during labor are intermittent, with periods of relaxation between, resembling the systole and the diastole of the heart. These periods of relaxation not only provide rest for the uterine muscles and for the mother, but also are essential to the welfare of the fetus. During the myometrial relaxation that follows the contraction in normal labor, there is a rebound phenomenon during which the uteroplacental blood flow increases above the control levels. Thus, the transfer of oxygen and other essential nutrients to the fetus is not significantly compromised.

● Symmetry and polarity: Labor contractions begin at a "pacemaker" point like cardiac contractions. This point is located in the myometrium of the uterus near the uterotubal junctions. Each contraction begins at that point and then sweeps down over the uterus as a wave known as the symmetry of uterine contractions. During labor, the uterus is differentiated into two identifiable portions, the upper and lower uterine segments. The upper segment, known as the fundus, contains the greatest concentration of myometrial cells and is the active, contractile portion of the uterus. Its function is to expel the uterine contents. The uterus displays a decreasing gradient of intensity of contractions from the fundus downward known as the polarity of uterine contractions.

- Brachystasis：As labor progresses, each individual myometrial cell as it contracts does not quite regain its normal length on relaxation. This process is known as brachystasis of the uterine muscle fibers. As this mechanism progresses, a passive lower segment is developed. With each contraction, the muscle fibers of the upper segment retract, becoming shorter as the fetus descends. The upper segment, therefore, becomes thicker. Fibers of the lower segment stretch, and consequently become thinner. The distinct boundary between the upper and lower uterine segments is called a physiologic retraction ring.

Maternal Pushing

After the cervix is dilated fully, the power most important in expulsion of the fetus is the secondary power produced by increased intra-abdominal pressure as the woman pushes or bears down. Most women experience an overwhelming urge to push when the fetal head or presenting part reaches the pelvic floor and full cervical dilatation is achieved. Increased abdominal pressure is created by deep inhalation, then purposefully contracting the abdominal muscles with the glottis closed. Bearing down efforts should coincide with uterine contractions, and the woman should be encouraged to rest between contractions. Although pushing is a necessary complement to uterine contractions in the second stage of labor, it accomplishes little in the first stage and may cause cervical edema. In the third stage of labor, spontaneous expulsion of the placenta is again aided by the woman's bearing-down efforts.

二 产道

产道是胎儿娩出的通道,分为骨产道与软产道两部分。

1. 骨产道　骨产道是指真骨盆,是产道的重要组成部分,其大小及形状与分娩关系密切。骨盆腔分为3个假想平面,即通常所称的骨盆平面:骨盆入口平面(图4-3)、中骨盆平面(图4-4)及骨盆出口平面(图4-5)。骨盆入口平面,即真假骨盆的交界面,呈横椭圆形;中骨盆平面为骨盆最小平面,是骨盆腔最狭窄的部分,呈前后径长的纵椭圆形;骨盆出口平面为骨盆腔下口,由共用底边(坐骨结节间径),但不在同一平面的两个三角形所组成。

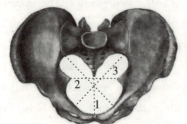 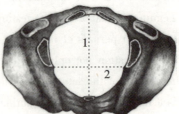 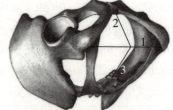

1.入口前后径11 cm; 2.入口横径13 cm; 3.入口斜径12.75 cm。 | 1.中骨盆前后径11.5 cm; 2.中骨盆横径10 cm。 | 1.出口横径9 cm; 2.出口前矢状径6 cm; 3.出口后矢状径8.5 cm。

图4-3　骨盆入口平面　　　图4-4 中骨盆平面　　　图4-5　骨盆出口平面

(1)骨盆入口平面　即真假骨盆的交界面,呈横椭圆形,共有4条径线,即入口前后径、入口横径、入口左斜径及入口右斜径。

1)入口前后径:又称真结合径,指从耻骨联合上缘中点至骶岬前缘正中的距离,平均约为11 cm,胎先露入盆与此径线关系密切。

2) 入口横径：左右髂耻缘间的最大距离，平均为 13 cm。

3) 入口斜径：左斜径为左骶髂关节至右髂耻隆突间的距离，右斜径为右骶髂关节至左髂耻隆突间的距离，平均约为 12.75 cm。

（2）中骨盆平面　为骨盆最小平面，是骨盆腔最狭窄的部分，呈前后径长的纵椭圆形。其前方为耻骨联合下缘，两侧为坐骨棘，后方为骶骨下端。有 2 条径线。

1) 中骨盆前后径：耻骨联合下缘中点通过两侧坐骨棘连线中点至骶骨下端间的距离，正常值平均为 11.5 cm。

2) 中骨盆横径：也称坐骨棘间径，是两坐骨棘间的距离，正常值平均约 10 cm，其长短与胎先露内旋转关系密切。

（3）骨盆出口平面　为骨盆腔下口，由共用底边（坐骨结节间径），但不在同一平面的两个三角形所组成。前三角顶端为耻骨联合下缘，两侧为耻骨降支；后三角顶端为骶尾关节，两侧为骶结节韧带。有 4 条径线。

1) 出口前后径：耻骨联合下缘至骶尾关节间的距离，正常值平均为 11.5 cm。

2) 出口横径：也称坐骨结节间径。两坐骨结节内侧缘的距离，正常值平均为 9 cm，此径线与分娩关系密切。

3) 出口前矢状径：耻骨联合下缘中点至坐骨结节间径中点间的距离，正常值平均为 6 cm。

4) 出口后矢状径：骶尾关节至坐骨结节间径中点间的距离，正常值平均为 8.5 cm。若出口横径稍短，而出口横径与出口后矢状径之和>15 cm 时，正常大小胎儿可以通过后三角区经阴道娩出。

连接骨盆各平面中点的假想曲线，称为骨盆轴。此轴上段向下向后，中段向下，下段向下向前（图 4-6）。分娩时，胎儿沿此轴完成一系列分娩机制，助产时也应按此轴方向协助胎儿娩出。

妇女站立时，骨盆入口平面与地平面所形成的角度，一般为 60°（图 4-7）。若骨盆倾斜度过大，可影响胎头衔接和娩出。改变体位可改变骨盆倾斜度。

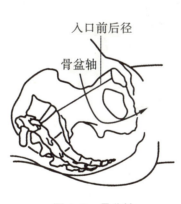

图 4-6　骨盆轴

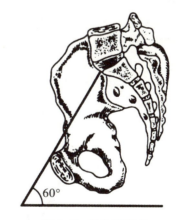

图 4-7　骨盆倾斜度

2. 软产道　软产道是由子宫下段、子宫颈、阴道及骨盆底软组织构成的弯曲管道。

（1）子宫下段的形成　由非孕时长约 1 cm 的子宫峡部伸展形成。妊娠 12 周后的子宫峡部逐渐扩展成宫腔的一部分，至妊娠末期逐渐拉长形成子宫下段。临产后的规律宫缩使子宫下段进一步拉长达 7 ～ 10 cm，成为软产道的一部分（图 4-8）。由于子宫肌纤维的缩复作用，子宫上段肌壁越来越厚，子宫下段肌壁被牵拉得越来越薄，导致子宫上下段的肌壁厚薄不同，在两者间的子宫内面形成一环状隆起，称为生理缩复环，此环在正常情况下不能从腹部见到。

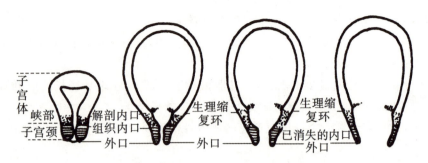

图4-8　子宫下段的形成及宫口的扩张

（2）子宫颈的变化

1）子宫颈管消失：临产前的子宫颈管长 2～3 cm，初产妇较经产妇稍长。临产后的规律宫缩牵拉子宫颈内口的子宫肌纤维及周围韧带，加之胎先露部的支撑使前羊水囊呈楔状，子宫颈内口水平的肌纤维向上牵拉，使子宫颈管形成漏斗状，随后子宫颈管逐渐变短直至消失。初产妇多是子宫颈管先缩短消失，然后宫口扩张；经产妇一般是子宫颈管缩短消失与宫口扩张同时进行（图4-9）。

2）宫口扩张：临产前，初产妇的子宫颈外口仅容一指尖，经产妇能容一指。临产后，子宫收缩及缩复、胎先露部及前羊膜囊的扩张作用，促使宫口逐渐扩张。胎膜多在宫口近开全时自然破裂，破膜后胎先露部直接压迫子宫颈，扩张宫口的作用更为显著。宫口开全（10 cm）时，足月妊娠的胎头方能通过。

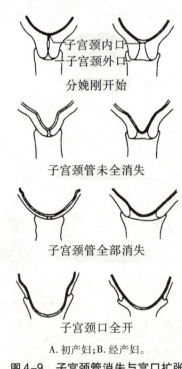

A.初产妇；B.经产妇。

图4-9　子宫颈管消失与宫口扩张

（3）骨盆底组织、阴道及会阴的变化　前羊水囊及胎先露先扩张阴道上部，破膜后的胎先露部下降直接压迫骨盆底，使软产道下段形成一个前壁短、后壁长、向前弯曲的肌性通道。阴道外口朝向前上方，阴道黏膜皱襞展平加宽腔道。会阴体由 5 cm 变成 2～4 mm，以利于胎儿通过。分娩时若保护会阴不当，易造成裂伤。

The passage is the important canal in delivery. The entire childbirth process centers on the safe passage of the fully developed fetus through the pelvis. Slight irregularities in the structure of the pelvis may delay the progress of labor, and any marked deformity may render delivery through natural passages impossible.

Bony Canal

The pelvis is divided into the false pelvis above and the true pelvis below the linea terminalis. The true pelvis forms the bony canal through which the fetus must pass during labor and birth. For convenience, the pelvis is described as having three imaginary planes.

- Pelvic inlet: Four diameters of the pelvis inlet are usually described: anteroposterior, transverse, and two obliques. Normally, the obstetrical conjugate measures 11 cm or more. The transverse diameter measures 13 cm. Each of the oblique diameters average 12.75 cm and are designated right and left, according to whether they originate at the right or left sacroiliac synchondrosis.

- Midpelvis: The midpelvis at the level of the ischial spines (midplane, or plane of least pelvic dimensions) is of particular importance following engagement of the fetal head in obstructed labor. The interspinous diameter, 10 cm or somewhat more, is usually the smallest diameter of the pelvis. The anteroposterior diameter, through the level of the ischial spines, normally measures at least 11.5 cm.

- Pelvic outlet: The outlet of the pelvis consists of two approximately triangular areas not in the same plane but having a common base, which is a line drawn between the two ischial tuberosities. The apex of the posterior triangle is at the tip of the sacrum, and the lateral boundaries are the sacrosciatic ligaments and the ischial tuberosities. The anterior triangle is formed by the area under the pubic arch. Four diameters of the pelvic outlet usually are described: the anteroposterior, transverse, anterior sa-gittal and posterior sagittal.

The anteroposterior diameter (11.5 cm) extends from the lower margin of the symphysis pubis to the tip of the sacrum. The transverse diameter (9 cm) is the distance between the inner edges of the ischial tuberosities. The anterior sagittal diameter (6 cm) extends from the lower margin of the symphysis pubis to the midpoint of the transverse diameter of pelvic outlet. The posterior sagittal diameter extends from the tip of the sacrum to a right-angle intersection with a line between diameter of the outlet usually exceeds 8.5 cm.

The pelvic cavity is the space between the inlet above, the outlet below, and the anterior, posterior, and lateral walls of the pelvis. The upper portion of the pelvic cavity is almost cylindrical, while the lower portion is curved. It is important to note the axis of the cavity as viewed from the side. During the birth process, the head must descend along the downward axis until it almost reaches the level of the ischial spines and begins to curve forward. The axis of the cavity determined the direction that the fetus takes through the pelvis in the process of birth.

Soft Birth Canal

The soft birth canal is a curved tube made from the soft tissue of the lower uterus, cervix, vagina, and pelvic floor.

- The lower segment of the uterus: The lower segment of the uterus is formed by the extension of the isthmus of the uterus which is about 1 cm long.

- Cervix change: Changes in the cervix include the disappearance of the cervical canal and dilation of the uterine orifice.

● Changes of pelvic floor tissue, vagina and perineum：The anterior amniotic fluid sac and fetal exposure expand the upper part of the vagina first, and the fetal exposure after membrane rupture descends directly to compress the pelvic floor, so that the lower part of the soft birth canal forms a muscular channel with short anterior wall and long posterior wall and curved forward.

 胎儿

胎儿能否顺利通过产道，与胎儿大小、胎方位及有无发育异常等因素有关。

1.胎儿大小 胎儿大小是决定分娩难易的重要因素，尤其是胎儿过大致胎头径线过大时，即使骨盆大小正常，也可因相对性骨盆狭窄造成难产。

（1）胎头颅骨 由顶骨、额骨、颞骨各两块及一块枕骨构成。颅骨间膜状缝隙称为颅缝，两颅缝交界处空隙较大称为囟门。胎头前方的囟门呈菱形，称为前囟（大囟门），位于胎头后方的囟门呈三角形，称为后囟（小囟）（图4-10）。在分娩过程中，颅骨轻度移位重叠使头颅变形，缩小头颅体积，有利于胎头娩出。但若胎儿过熟，颅骨较硬，胎头不易变形，可导致难产。

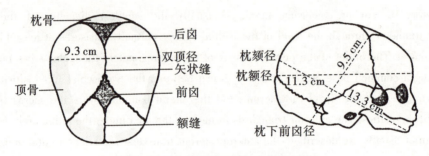

图4-10 胎头颅骨、颅缝、囟门及径线

（2）胎头径线 见表4-1。

表4-1 胎头各径线的测量方法及长度

名称	测量方法	长度/cm
双顶径（BPD）	两顶骨隆突间的距离，为胎头最大横径	9.3
枕额径	鼻根上方至枕骨隆突间的距离	11.3
枕下前囟径	前囟中央至枕骨隆突下方的距离	9.5
枕颏径	颏骨下方中央至后囟顶部的距离	13.3

2.胎方位 纵产式时，胎体纵轴与骨盆轴一致，容易通过产道。矢状缝和囟门是确定胎方位的重要标志。

3.胎儿畸形 胎儿某一部分发育异常，如脑积水、连体儿等，致胎头或胎体过大，难以顺利通过产道。

Even in an adequately sized pelvic outlet, the birth may be difficult if the fetus is too large or in a difficult position.

Fetal Size

• Fetal head：From an obstetric viewpoint, the head is the most important part of the fetus. If it can pass through the pelvic canal safely, there is usually no difficulty in delivering the rest of the body, although occasionally the shoulders may cause trouble.

The cranium, or skull, is made up of seven bones. Four of the bones lie at the base of the cranium, are closely united, and are of little obstetric interest. On the other hand, the four bones forming the upper part of the cranium—the frontal, the occipital, and two parietal bones—are of great importance. These bones are not knit closely together at the time of birth but are separated by membranous interspaces called sutures. The intersections of these sutures are known as fontanels.

• Fetal skull measurement：The most important transverse diameter of the fetal skull is the biparietal diameter, it measures, on an average, 9.3 cm. There are three important anteroposterior diameters of the fetal skull：suboccipitobregmatic diameter, occipitofrontal diameter and occipitomental diameter.

Fetal Lie

The term fetal lie refers to the relationship of the long axis (spine) of the fetus to the long axis of the mother. The longitudinal lie, in which the fetal and maternal spines are parallel, is present in more than 99% of labors at term. This is the optimal position for vaginal delivery.

四　精神心理因素

在分娩过程中产妇精神心理状态不佳可以明显影响产力,宫口扩张缓慢,胎先露部下降受阻,产程延长,产妇体力消耗过多,同时也促使产妇神经内分泌发生变化,交感神经兴奋,释放儿茶酚胺,血压升高、心率加快、呼吸急促,肺内气体交换不足,导致胎儿缺血缺氧,出现胎儿窘迫。一般来说,产妇对分娩的安全性有顾虑,并对医护人员有很大的依赖性。因此,除产妇在产前门诊接受健康宣教外,更应在分娩过程中,做好入院评估,提供必要的护理支持,讲解分娩知识,使产妇以最佳的精神心理状态顺利度过分娩全过程。

Psychological responses to the experience of labor vary widely and are influenced by a number of factors. The women's culture background is paticular important. People from diverse cultural backgrounds may differ in their beliefs about how the laboring woman should behave, the presence of support people, and the nurse's role. Preparation for childbirth often varies and may dramatically influence the coping skills of the laboring woman and her partner. In a classic study, it was found that the mate's emotional support during childbirth was a major predictor of positive perceptions of the experience. Maternal confidence in coping with labor has been found to contribute to women's perception of pain during labor. Similarly, expectations may influence psychological responses to labor. It was found that high-risk pregnant women expected more medical interventions and more difficulty coping with pain during their labor and birth than low-risk pregnant women. For both groups of women, anxiety was negatively associated with childbirth expectations. In a well-known series of classic studies, the relationship between psychological factors in pregnancy and labor.

任务实施

宫缩评估技术(表4-2)适用于对待产妇宫缩的评估,目的是准确评估宫缩的频率和强度,以判断产程的进展。

表4-2　宫缩评估技术

项目	内容
仪表	仪表端庄,衣帽整洁,洗手,剪指甲,并温暖双手,戴口罩
操作前准备	1. 评估 (1)待产妇的孕产史,本次妊娠的情况,包括孕周、妊娠合并症和并发症、相关检查结果(B型超声等)、腹痛和阴道流血的情况 (2)待产妇对宫缩检查的认知程度和心理反应 2. 环境准备:环境舒适和有效保护患者的隐私 3. 物品准备:胎心监护仪、带秒针的表、纸、笔 4. 检查用物:物品完好,将用物按使用顺序放在治疗车上
操作步骤	1. 备齐物品并检查,携带用物至床旁 2. 告知待产妇检查宫缩的目的、意义及配合方法 3. 嘱待产妇排空膀胱,仰卧于床上,露出腹部 4. 检查者将手掌放在待产妇的腹壁上感觉宫缩情况,在子宫收缩时,子宫体部隆起变硬,收缩后间歇期子宫松弛变软 5. 记录子宫收缩的持续时间、间隔时间及收缩强度 6. 观察并记录胎心监护结果,监测胎儿宫内情况 7. 协助产妇取舒适体位,整理衣裤 8. 整理用物 9. 洗手,记录
注意事项	1. 注意保护待产妇隐私 2. 操作敏捷、细心、准确 3. 动作轻柔,注意观察待产妇的反应

任务二　分娩机制（Mechanism of Labor）

任务内容

分娩机制是指胎儿先露部在通过产道时，为适应骨盆各平面的不同形态，被动地进行一系列适应性转动，以其最小径线通过产道的全过程。

任务目标

◆能描述分娩机制、步骤。
◆能用模型演示分娩的过程。

临床上以胎儿枕左前位最多见，故以枕左前位的分娩机制（图4-11）为例说明。分娩机制各动作虽分别介绍，但却是连续进行的。

1.衔接　又称入盆，指胎头双顶径进入骨盆入口平面，颅骨最低点接近或达到坐骨棘水平。胎头半俯屈状态以枕额径进入骨盆入口，由于枕额径大于骨盆入口前后径，胎头矢状缝坐落在骨盆入口右斜径上，胎头枕骨位于骨盆左前方。初产妇多在预产期前1~2周，经产妇多在分娩后开始衔接。若初产妇已临产而胎头仍未衔接，应警惕有无头盆不称。

2.下降　胎头沿骨盆轴前进的动作称为下降。下降贯穿于分娩的全过程，与其他动作相伴随。下降动作呈间歇性，宫缩时胎头下降，间歇时胎头又稍回缩。胎头下降程度可作为判断产程进展的重要标志。

3.俯屈　当胎头继续下降至骨盆底时，原来处于半俯屈状态的胎头遇肛提肌阻力，借助杠杆作用进一步俯屈，使下颌贴近胸壁，以最小的枕下前囟径取代胎头衔接时的枕额径，以适应产道形态。

4.内旋转　胎头围绕骨盆纵轴向前旋转，使矢状缝与中骨盆及骨盆出口前后径相一致，称为内旋转。内旋转动作从中骨盆平面开始至骨盆出口平面完成，一般在第一产程末完成内旋转动作。枕左前位时，盆底观胎头逆时针转45°，内旋转仅是胎头旋转，胎肩并未转动，呈头肩扭曲状态。

5.仰伸　发生在第二产程宫口开全时。完成内旋转后，俯屈的胎头下降达阴道外口时，宫缩和腹压继续迫使胎头下降，而肛提肌收缩力又将胎头向前推进，两者的合力促使胎头沿骨盆轴下段向下向前的方向转向前。当胎头枕骨达耻骨联合下缘时，以耻骨弓为支点，逐渐仰伸，胎头的顶、额、鼻、口、颏相继娩出。当胎头仰伸时，胎儿双肩径沿左斜径进入骨盆入口。

6.复位及外旋转　胎头娩出后，胎头枕部向母体左侧旋转45°，恢复胎头与胎肩的关系，称为复位。胎头娩出时，胎儿双肩径沿骨盆入口左斜径下降，为适应中骨盆及骨盆出口平面的形状，前（右）肩向前、向中线旋转45°使胎儿双肩径转成与骨盆出口前后径相一致的方向。而胎头枕部需在外继续向母体左侧旋转45°以保持胎头与胎肩的垂直关系，称为外旋转。

7.胎肩及胎儿娩出　胎头完成外旋转后，胎儿前（右）肩在耻骨弓下先娩出，随即后（左）肩从会阴前缘娩出。胎肩娩出后，胎体及下肢随之娩出，完成分娩全过程。

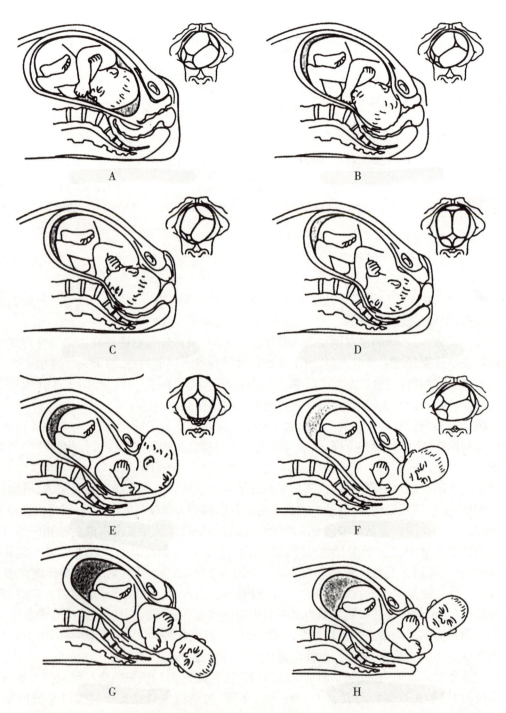

A.衔接前胎头上浮;B.衔接俯屈下降;C.继续下降与内旋转;D.内旋转已完成,开始仰伸;E.仰伸已完成;F.胎头外旋转;G.前肩娩出;H.后肩娩出。

图4-11 枕左前位分娩机制示意

The mechanism of labor consists of a combination of movements, several of which may occur at the same time. As they occur, the uterine contractions bring about important modifications in the attitude of the fetus, especially after the head has descended into the pelvis. This adaptation of the fetus to the birth canal involves the following movements: engagement, descent, flexion, internal rotation, extension, restitution, external rotation expulsion. In clinic occipito presentation is $95.55\% - 97.55\%$, the most common type of fetal position is left occipito anterior (LOA). So, we'll take LOA as an example to explain the mechanism of labor. For purposes of instruction, the various movements are described as if they occurred separately and independently.

Engagement

The mechanism by which the biparietal diameter, the greatest transverse diameter of the fetal head in occiput presentations, passes through the pelvic inlet is designated engagement. This phenomenon may take place 1-2 week before the expected period of delivery and may not occur until after the commencement of labor in many multiparous women. A normal-sized head usually does not engage with its sagittal suture directed anteroposteriorly. Instead, the fetal head usually enters the pelvic inlet either in the transverse diameter or in one of the oblique diameters.

Descent

The first requisite for the birth is descent. With primigravidas, onset of labor. This is called lightening. Because the vertex is frequently deep in the pelvis at the onset of labor, further descent does not necessarily begin until the second stage of labor. The ischial spines are used as a landmark to describe the relative position of the fetal head in the pelvis. This relationship is evaluated during each pelvic examination and recorded, along with the assessment of cervical dilatation and effacement. Descent is brought about by one or more of four forces: pressure of the amniotic fluid; direct pressure of the fundus upon the breech with contractions; bearing down efforts with the abdominal muscles; extension and straightening of the fetal body.

Flexion

Flexion occurs early in the process of descent, as the head meets resistance from the soft tissues of the pelvis, the pelvic floor, and the cervix. The head may become so flexed that the chin is in contact with the sternum. As a consequence, the smallest anteroposterior diameter (the suboccipitobregmatic plane) is substituted for the longer occipitofrontal diameter.

Internal Rotation

The head enters the pelvis in the transverse or diagonal position. When it reaches the pelvic floor, the occiput is rotated and lies beneath the symphysis pubis. In other words, with internal rotation, the sagittal suture is in the anteroposterior diameter of the outlet. Internal rotation is completed at the end of the first stage of labor.

Extension

When, after internal rotation, the sharply flexed head reaches the vulva, it undergoes extension which is essential to birth. This brings the base of the occiput into direct contact with the inferior margin of the symphysis pubis. Because the vulvar outlet is directed upward and forward, extension must occur before the head can pass through it. With progressive distention of the perineum and vaginal opening, an increasingly larger portion of the occiput gradually appears. The head is born by further extension as the occiput, bregma, forehead, nose, mouth, and finally the chin pass successively over the anterior margin of the perineum.

Restitution and External Rotation

The delivered head next undergoes restitution. If the occiput was originally directed toward the left, it rotates toward the left ischial tuberosity, if it was originally directed toward the right, the occiput rotates to the right.

Restitution of the head to the oblique position is followed by completion of external rotation to the transverse position, a movement that corresponds to rotation of the fetal body, serving to bring its bisacromial diameter into relation with the anteroposterior diameter of the pelvic outlet. Thus, one shoulder is anterior behind the symphysis and the other is posterior.

Expulsion

Almost immediately after the external rotation, the anterior shoulder appears under the symphysis pubis and becomes arrested temporarily beneath the pubic arch to act as a pivotal point for the other shoulder. As the anterior margin of the perineum becomes distended, the posterior shoulder is born, assisted by an upward lateral flexion of the newborn's body. Once the shoulders are delivered, the body is quickly extruded.

任务三　先兆临产、临产诊断及产程分期(Premonitory Signs, Diagnosis and Stages of Labor)

工作情景

孕妇,28 岁,妊娠 39 周,G_2P_0。出现宫缩 1 d,宫缩持续约 20 s,每隔 10 min 左右 1 次。孕妇认为自己已临产,遂来院就诊。

①该孕妇是否已经临产? ②如何判断临产?

任务内容

分娩发动前,孕妇出现预示不久即将临产的症状,称为先兆临产。如果出现有规律且逐渐增强的子宫收缩,持续 30 s 或以上,间歇 5~6 min,同时伴随进行性子宫颈管消失、子宫颈口扩张和胎先露下降,则为临产。

任务目标

◆ 能区分先兆临产和临产。
◆ 能描述产程分期。

一　先兆临产

分娩发动前,孕妇出现预示不久即将临产的症状,称为先兆临产。

1. 不规律宫缩　又称假临产,常在预产期前 1~2 周出现。其特点为:宫缩持续时间短(<30 s)且不恒定,间歇时间长而不规则;宫缩的强度不加强;不伴随出现子宫颈管消失和子宫颈口扩张;常在夜间出现,白天消失;给予强效镇静剂可以抑制宫缩。

2. 胎儿下降感　随着胎先露下降入骨盆,宫底随之下降,多数孕妇会感觉上腹部较前舒适,进食量也增加,呼吸轻快。由于胎先露入盆压迫了膀胱,孕妇常出现尿频症状。

3. 见红　在分娩发动前 24 ~ 48 h（少数 1 周内），因子宫颈内口附近的胎膜与该处的子宫壁分离，毛细血管破裂导致少量出血，与子宫颈管内的黏液相混排出，称为见红，是分娩即将开始的可靠征象。但若出血量超过月经量，则可能为妊娠晚期出血性疾病。

 临产

临产的标志为有规律且逐渐增强的子宫收缩，持续 30 s 或以上，间歇 5 ~ 6 min，同时伴随进行性子宫颈管消失、子宫颈口扩张和胎先露下降。用镇静剂不能抑制宫缩。

三 总产程及产程分期

总产程即分娩全过程，从临产开始至胎儿胎盘完全娩出为止。临床上分为 3 个产程。

1. 第一产程（子宫颈扩张期）　是指从开始出现规律宫缩到宫口开全。初产妇需要 11 ~ 22 h，经产妇需要 6 ~ 16 h。

2. 第二产程（胎儿娩出期）　是指从宫口开全至胎儿娩出。未实施硬膜外麻醉者，初产妇最长不应超过 3 h，经产妇不应超过 2 h；实施硬膜外麻醉镇痛者，可在此基础上延长 1 h，即初产妇最长不应超过 4 h，经产妇不应超过 3 h。

3. 第三产程（胎盘娩出期）　是指从胎儿娩出到胎盘娩出。一般 5 ~ 15 min，不超过 30 min。

Premonitory Signs of Labor

During the last few weeks of pregnancy, a number of changes indicate that labor is approaching.

- False labor：They are merely an exaggeration of the intermittent uterine contraction (Braxton Hicks) that has occurred throughout the entire gestation, but now they may be accompanied by discomfort.

- Lightening：Lightening occurs 10–14 d before birth, particularly in primigravidas. This alteration is brought about by a settling of the fetal head into the pelvis. Lightening may take place suddenly so that the woman arises one morning entirely relieved of the abdominal tightness and diaphragmatic pressure that she had experienced previously. In multigravid women, lightening is more likely to occur after labor begins.

- Show：Another sign of impending labor is the pink vaginal discharge commonly termed "show". It often occurs 24–48 h before labor. The mucous plug that has filled the cervical canal during pregnancy (and that contains accumulated cervical secretions) may be expelled when the cervix softens in the last days of pregnancy. The pressure of the descending presenting part of the fetus causes the minute capillaries in the cervix to rupture. This blood is mixed with the mucus, creating a pink tinge. The "show" must be differentiated from a substantial discharge of blood, which may indicate an obstetric complication.

Diagnosis of Labor

The onset of labor is marked by regular and increasing uterine contraction, with the duration of 30 s or more, the resting period 5–6 min, accompanied by cervical effacement, fetal presentation descent.

Stages of Labor

The process of labor is divided into three stages. It begins with the onset of regular labor contractions and ends with delivery of the placenta.

- The first stage of labor：The dilating stage, begins with the onset of regular labor contractions and ends with the complete dilatation of the cervix. This stage may be subdivided into two phases：latent and active.

● The second stage of labor: The pelvic stage, begins with the complete dilatation of the cervix and ends with the delivery or birth of the newborn.

● The third stage of labor: The placental stage, begins with the birth of the newborn and terminates with the delivery of the placenta. The average duration is 5-15 min, and no more than 30 min in the third stage.

任务实施

在分娩过程中通过阴道检查评估技术(表4-3)判断产程进展。该技术适用于子宫颈扩张或胎头下降不明;产程进展缓慢,试产6~8 h无进展;疑有脐带先露或头盆不称者。禁用于前置胎盘或怀疑前置胎盘者。

表4-3　阴道检查评估技术

项目	内容
目的	1. 评估待产妇的子宫颈情况、胎膜是否破裂、胎先露部及下降位置
	2. 初步判断待产妇是否可以进行阴道试产
操作前准备	1. 评估:待产妇的孕产史,本次妊娠的情况,包括孕周、妊娠合并症和并发症、相关检查结果(B型超声等)、腹痛和阴道流血的情况;待产妇对阴道检查的认知程度和心理反应
	2. 物品准备:无菌包1个(内装弯盘2个、卵圆钳4把)、0.5%聚维酮碘(碘伏)、纱布缸1个、无菌持物筒1个、无菌持物钳1把、一次性臀垫1块、无菌手套
	3. 助产士准备:着装整齐,洗手,剪指甲
	4. 环境准备:关闭门窗或屏风遮挡,保护产妇隐私,室内温度适宜
	5. 产妇准备:排空膀胱
操作步骤	1. 用物推至待产妇旁边,遮挡、查对,向待产妇解释检查的目的
	2. 协助待产妇取膀胱截石位,暴露会阴
	3. 按外阴消毒的程序消毒外阴
	4. 戴无菌手套,铺无菌孔巾,暴露会阴
	5. 右手示指和中指伸入阴道,了解骨产道的情况,包括骨盆的对角径、坐骨棘间径、坐骨切迹的情况。了解软产道的情况,包括宫口开大的情况、子宫颈成熟度及有无水肿,了解先露部的方位和下降程度。触诊宫口开大情况时,示指先触到胎儿的先露部,然后由中心向外摸清子宫颈的边缘,再沿边缘画圈并估计子宫颈开大的程度(以厘米为单位),如已摸不到子宫颈边缘,表明宫口已开全。触诊时摸清颅缝和囟门的位置可以确定先露部的方位,再以先露部骨质最低点与坐骨棘平面的关系来确定胎头位置高低
	6. 为待产妇穿上裤子,摆好舒适的体位,整理床单位
	7. 记录阴道检查结果,进行Bishop评分
	8. 整理产妇衣物,整理物品
	9. 洗手,记录
注意事项	1. 注意观察待产妇的反应
	2. 注意保护待产妇隐私
	3. 注意无菌操作

任务四　正常分娩妇女的护理（Nursing of Normal Delivery Women）

工作情景

李女士,25 岁,G_1P_0,孕 38^{+5} 周。昨日发现内裤上有少量血液,未在意。今天早上出现小腹阵痛,遂来医院就诊。产科检查发现宫口开大 1 指。产妇因害怕疼痛,情绪非常紧张。

①根据上述表现,李女士目前处于第几产程？②如何对其进行正确的护理？

任务内容

分娩全过程是指从临产开始至胎儿胎盘完全娩出,分为 3 个时期:第一产程、第二产程、第三产程。护理人员要识别各产程临床表现,实施恰当的护理,协助医生处理好产程,从而保障母婴安全。

任务目标

◆能进行产程观察(观察宫缩、监测胎心、了解宫口扩张情况)。
◆能完成接生准备、产程护理配合,能协助产后观察及护理。

一　第一产程妇女的护理

第一产程即子宫颈扩张期,是产程的开始。在规律宫缩的作用下,宫口扩张、胎先露下降。但第一产程时间长,可发生各种异常,需严密观察胎心、宫缩,通过阴道检查判断宫口扩张与胎先露下降及胎方位、产道等有无异常。

【护理评估】

1.健康史　了解产妇是否有不良孕产史。重点询问本次妊娠的经过,包括末次月经,预产期,有无阴道流血、腹痛、高血压等异常情况。询问宫缩开始的时间、强度及频率,有无见红、阴道流液等。

2.身体状况

(1)宫缩规律　第一产程开始时,子宫收缩力弱,持续时间较短,约 30 s,间歇期较长,为 5~6 min。随产程进展,宫缩强度增加,持续时间延长,间歇期缩短。当宫口开全时,宫缩持续时间可长达 1 min,间歇仅 1~2 min。

产程中需重视观察并记录子宫收缩的情况,包括宫缩持续时间、间歇时间及强度。临床常用触诊观察法及电子胎儿监护两种方法。

1)触诊观察法:是监测宫缩最简单的方法。观察者将手掌放于孕妇腹壁的宫体近宫底处,宫缩时宫体部隆起变硬,间歇期松弛变软。

2)电子胎儿监护:用电子胎儿监护仪描述宫缩曲线,可以直观地看出宫缩强度、频率和持续时间,是反映宫缩的客观指标。监护仪有外监护及内监护两种。外监护临床应用最广,适用于产程的任何阶段,将宫缩压力探头固定在孕妇腹壁宫体近宫底部即可。宫缩的观察不能完全依赖电子胎儿监护,对做电子胎儿监护的孕妇,护士至少要亲自评估 1 次宫缩。内监护有宫腔内感染的可能且价格昂贵,临床应用较少。

(2)胎心　胎心率是产程中极为重要的观察指标。临产后更应严密监测胎心的频率、规律性和宫缩后胎心变化。胎心监测有听诊和电子胎儿监护两种方法。

1)听诊:临床现多采用电子胎心听诊器。此方法简单,但仅获得每分钟胎心率,不能分辨胎心率变异、瞬间变化及其与宫缩、胎动的关系,需注意同时监测孕妇脉搏,与孕妇脉搏区分。

2)电子胎儿监护:多用于外监护描记胎心曲线。观察胎心率变异及其与宫缩、胎动的关系。此方法较能准确判断胎儿在宫内的状态。但是,电子胎儿监护可能出现假阳性,不能过度依赖。

(3)宫口扩张与胎头下降　宫口扩张与胎头下降的速度和程度是产程观察的两个重要指标,通过阴道检查可了解宫口扩张及胎头下降情况。

1)宫口扩张:表现为子宫颈管逐渐变软、变短、消失,子宫颈展平并逐渐扩大。开始宫口扩张速度较慢,后期速度加快。当宫口开全(10 cm)时,子宫下段、子宫颈及阴道共同形成桶状的软产道。根据宫口扩张情况第一产程又分为潜伏期和活跃期。潜伏期是宫口扩张缓慢阶段,一般初产妇不超过20 h,经产妇不超过 14 h。活跃期为宫口扩张的加速阶段,一般宫口开至 4～5 cm 即进入活跃期,最迟至 6 cm 才进入活跃期,直至宫口开全(10 cm)。此期宫口扩张速度应≥0.5 cm/h。

2)胎先露下降:是决定胎儿能否经阴道分娩的重要指标。随着产程进展,先露部逐渐下降,并在宫口开大 4～6 cm 后快速下降,直到先露部达到外阴及阴道口。临床上以胎头颅骨最低点与坐骨棘平面的关系判断胎头下降的程度。胎头颅骨最低点平坐骨棘平面时,以"0"表示;在坐骨棘平面上 1 cm 时,以"-1"表示;在坐骨棘平面下 1 cm 时,以"+1"表示,其余以此类推(图 4-12)。潜伏期胎头下降不明显,活跃期下降加快,通过肛查或阴道检查判断宫口扩张和胎头下降情况。

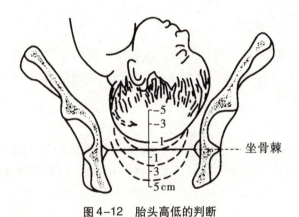

坐骨棘

图 4-12　胎头高低的判断

(4)胎膜破裂　胎儿先露部衔接后,将羊水分隔为前后两部,在胎先露部前面的羊水称为前羊水。当宫缩时羊膜腔内压力增加到一定程度时胎膜自然破裂,前羊水流出。自然分娩胎膜破裂多发生在宫口近开全时。评估胎膜是否破裂,确定破膜时间,羊水颜色、性状及量。也可用 pH 试纸检测,pH≥7.0 时破膜的可能性大。破膜后,宫缩常暂时停止,产妇略感舒适,随后宫缩重现且较前增强。

3.心理-社会状况　因产房陌生的环境和人员、对分娩结局的未知、宫缩所致的疼痛等,产妇可表现出焦虑、恐惧等。应注意评估产妇对分娩的认识、对疼痛的耐受程度、对自然分娩的信心、与医务人员的配合程度等,给予正确的护理。

4.辅助检查　用 B 型超声、胎儿监护仪、多普勒超声等检测胎儿宫内安危。

【护理诊断】

1. 分娩疼痛　与逐渐增强的宫缩有关。

2. 舒适度减弱　与子宫收缩、膀胱充盈、胎膜破裂等有关。

3. 焦虑　与知识缺乏,担心自己和胎儿的安全有关。

【护理措施】

1. 心理护理　向产妇及家属介绍分娩的基本知识,帮助产妇消除宫缩疼痛引起的恐惧,缓解其紧张情绪。耐心倾听产妇诉说,给予产妇支持和鼓励,及时提供产程进展的情况,增加产妇对自然分娩的信心。发挥产妇家庭支持系统的作用,鼓励家属在产程中多陪伴并支持产妇。

2. 一般护理

(1)监测生命体征　监测产妇生命体征并记录。宫缩时,血压会升高 5～10 mmHg,间歇期恢复。产程中应每隔 4～6 h 测量 1 次,若发现血压升高或为高危人群,应增加测量次数并给予相应的处理。

(2)饮食指导　为保证分娩的顺利进行,应鼓励孕妇在宫缩间歇期少量多次摄入无渣食物。

(3)休息与活动　宫缩不强且未破膜时可以鼓励产妇在室内适度活动,以缩短第一产程。

(4)排尿及排便　临产后,鼓励孕妇每 2～4 h 排尿 1 次,以免膀胱充盈影响宫缩及胎先露下降。

3. 产程观察及护理

(1)观察宫缩　潜伏期应每 2～4 h 观察 1 次,活跃期每 1～2 h 观察 1 次,一般需要连续观察至少 3 次宫缩。根据产程进展情况决定处理方法,若产程进展好则继续观察;若产程进展差,子宫收缩欠佳应及时处理。

(2)监测胎心　胎心听诊应在宫缩间歇期完成。潜伏期每小时听胎心 1 次,活跃期每 15～30 min 听诊胎心 1 次,每次听诊 1 min。也可用胎心监护仪连续描记。

(3)观察子宫颈扩张和胎头下降程度　通过阴道检查判断宫口扩张程度及胎头下降程度。临产后适时在宫缩时行阴道检查,一般潜伏期 2～4 h 查 1 次,活跃期 1 h 查 1 次,总产程不超过 10 次。

(4)胎膜破裂的处理　一旦胎膜破裂,应立即听胎心,判断是否出现脐带脱垂,并观察羊水性状和流出量、有无宫缩,同时记录破膜时间。若胎头尚未入盆,应卧床休息,抬高臀部,防止脐带脱垂,并保持产妇外阴清洁干燥,防止上行感染。破膜超过 12 h 尚未分娩者,应遵医嘱给予抗生素预防感染。

4. 疼痛护理　向产妇介绍分娩疼痛产生的原因,教会产妇减轻分娩疼痛的方法,必要时实施分娩镇痛。目前通常使用的分娩镇痛方法有两种:一种是非药物性的分娩镇痛,如连续的分娩陪伴、拉玛泽减痛分娩法、产程中的自由体位、音乐止痛法、穴位镇痛、水疗、催眠疗法、芳香疗法等;另一种是药物性分娩镇痛,即应用麻醉药或镇痛药来达到镇痛效果,常用的有连续硬膜外镇痛、产妇自控硬膜外镇痛、腰麻-硬膜外联合阻滞、微导管连续腰麻镇痛、产妇自控静脉瑞芬太尼镇痛、氧化亚氮吸入镇痛等。目前认为对没有分娩镇痛禁忌证的产妇,当出现规律宫缩、疼痛视觉模拟评分法(VAS)评分>3 分,至第二产程均可用药物性分娩镇痛。注意观察药物的不良反应,如恶心、呕吐、呼吸抑制等,一旦发现立即停止镇痛,遵医嘱给予对症治疗。

Nursing Assessment

Assessment during the first stage of labor includes vaginal examination and assessment of contractions, vital signs, and FHR.

- Uterine contractions: Frequency, duration, and intensity of the contractions should be monitored closely and recorded, whether or not an electronic fetal monitor is used. As labor progresses, the character of the contractions changes. They become stronger in intensity, last longer and come closer together. If the monitor is not being used, one effective method the nurse can use when timing contractions is to keep her fingers lightly on the fundus. The fingers are recommended because they are more sensitive than the palm. Assessing contractions in this manner enables the nurse to detect the beginning the contraction by the gradual tensing and rising forward of the fundus and to feel the contraction through its three phases until the uterus relaxes again. It is important to observe the frequency and duration of the contractions and to be assured that the uterine muscle relaxes completely after each contraction.

● Vital signs: Temperature, pulse, respiration and blood pressure should be evaluated on admission and every 4 h in normal labor when membranes are intact or more frequently as necessary, depending on the clinical situation and treatments used. If membranes have ruptured, it would be wise to evaluate the temperature every 2 h to screen for the development of amnionitis.

● Assessment of FHR: Assessment of FHR constitutes one of the most important responsibilities during the intrapartum period. Whether using electronic FHR monitoring or intermittent auscultation with uterine palpation, it is recommended that for low−risk clients, the nurse assesses, interprets and records FHR every 60 min after a contraction in the first stage of labor and every 15 min in the second stage of labor. With high−risk clients, the recommendations are different, but the nurse still has the choice of electronic fetal monitoring or intermittent auscultation. The electronic fetal monitor is widely used in the hospital setting to assess fetal well−being and evaluate uterine contraction during labor. As mentioned previously, the fetus must be assessed before and after ambulation, enema administration, artificial rupture of membranes, and the administration of analgesia or anesthesia. It is important to assess FHR immediately after the rupture of membranes because there is a possibility that with the gush of water, the cord may be prolapsed, and any indication of fetal distress from the pressure on the umbilical cord can be detected by a decrease in the FHR.

● Vaginal examination: The frequency with which vaginal examinations are required during labor depends on the individual case, often one or two such examinations are sufficient, whereas in some instances, more are required. In the presence of ruptured membranes, it is especially important to limit the number of vaginal examinations to protect against infection. In the presence of vaginal bleeding, placenta previa must first be ruled out before a vaginal examination can safely be done, or perforation of the placenta could be a catastrophic consequence.

Nursing Intervention

As previously emphasized, the nurse must have an empathic, nonjudgmental, and supportive attitude toward the woman to interpret the progress of labor and perform certain technical procedures skillfully. It should be pointed out that " supportive care " includes not emotional support, but also aspects of physical care that contribute to the woman's well-being and comfort and hence to her emotional equilibrium.

● Psychological support: The nurse can provide psychological support via verbal or nonverbal communication. Many of the physical care activities that nurses perform consist, in part at least, of " laying on of hands. " This type of communication can be a way of demonstrating the nurse's concern and empathy, especially when verbal communication is difficult or impossible. This contact can take the form of a back rub, stroking the client's brow, and so forth. Many of the relaxation techniques practiced in the prepared childbirth classes rely on the use of touch. The nurse must use professional judgment regarding its use, and rapport with the client helps to indicate a correct decision. It also is an effective means of incorporating the partner into the care and support of his or her significant other.

● Supportive milieu: During early labor, the client usually prefers to move around the room and frequently is more at ease sitting in a comfortable chair. She can be permitted and encouraged to do this and whatever else seems to be most relaxing and pleasant to her if there are no contraindicating conditions.

Once labor is well established, the laboring woman should not be left alone. The morale of women in labor is sometimes hopelessly shattered when they are left by themselves for long periods, regardless of whether or not they have been prepared for labor during pregnancy. During labor, most women are more sensitive to the behavior of those around them, particularly in relation to her perception of how much concern healthcare personnel show for her safety and well-being. For instance, careless remarks dropped in conversation often are misinterpreted as indicative of negligence, and lack of feeling. Comments and laughter overheard in the corridor outside the client's room may contribute to her uneasiness. Therefore, the nurse must be on guard against unfortunate happenings of this kind.

The nurse should not underestimate the usefulness of suggestion for the woman in labor. Because the woman responds readily to suggestions, especially in early labor, the nurse can use suggestibility to great advantage in her supportive care.

● Assisting with maternal birthing position: If monitors are not used and no contraindicating high-risk conditions exist, the client can be encouraged to assume any position that is comfortable for her, such as side, semi-sitting, squatting, all fours, or sitting. Generally, women should avoid laboring on their back, because the weight of the gravid uterus could theoretically compress the major maternal vessels. With vena cava occlusion, the return of blood to the heart is decreased, and this might result in a fall in maternal cardiac output, maternal hypotension, and decreased uterine blood flow. Thus for many clients, contractions become stronger and less frequent when the woman changes position from her back to her side, because the uteroplacental perfusion improves.

Position changes during labor can improve maternal comfort; the woman may find that she prefers various positions at various points in the labor, and the nurse should help her to assume whichever position seems most comfortable and safe for the woman and fetus. Frequent position changes may help with promoting fetal rotation and descent. Sometimes a position change will help to relieve mild fetal distress if the distress is caused by umbilical cord compression. If there is evidence of umbilical cord compression, monitoring FHR with various fetal positions may help provide information about which positions the woman should avoid and which are safe to assume. If the woman is experiencing backache, a change in position may help to promote fetal rotation and relieve the pressure of the presenting part on the sacrum.

For some women, the upright position while walking enhances labor. This is due to the effect of gravity on the improved application of the presenting part against the cervix, and the improved alignment of the presenting vertex into the pelvic canal.

● Management of contractions: Studies of pain have demonstrated that the anticipation of pain can raise the anxiety level significantly and lower pain tolerance. Thus, the client reacts sooner to even minimal pain stimuli. The pain is subjectively intensified and even a slight amount of pain seems great. Furthermore, other sensations may be misinterpreted as pain (e. g. , pressure, stretching).

The heightening of the anticipation of pain increases the response to pain; soon a vicious cycle is established. The nurse can help to break this cycle or prevent it from becoming established by intervening at the anticipation-anxiety junction. This is done by reminding the client that a contraction is over (and the pain is gone) and that because another contraction is not expected for several minutes, this is the time for her to rest and relax. The anxiety related to the anticipation of pain is lowered or eliminated, and the subjective intensification is diminished. It is obvious that the nurse or some other reliable person should be in continuous attendance to do this.

● Breathing techniques: The woman who has been prepared for childbirth has been schooled in breathing techniques, such as diaphragmatic breathing or rapid, shallow costal breathing. With coaching from her partner or her nurse, she is usually able to accomplish conscious relaxation.

A different situation exists with the woman who has had no childbirth preparation. It is often best to help such aclient relax by encouraging and coaching her to keep breathing slowly and evenly during the early contractions and to assume a pattern of more rapid and shallow breathing that is most comfortable during the late active phase. Women with no training in breathing techniques may need to be reminded not to hold their breath during the contractions.

● Food and fluid intake: Beliefs regarding the appropriateness of fluid and food intake during labor vary greatly in the literature and in clinical practice. If the client is admitted in the latent phase of labor, the physician may order a clear liquid diet. The client in active labor is usually not given solid or liquid foods because many women experience nausea and vomiting during labor and delivery. The other concern is the potential risk of aspiration of gastric contents. Gastric emptying is slower in pregnancy than in the nonpregnant state, and labor may contribute to a slowing in gastric contents.

Nursing interventions to combat the dry mouth and potential for dehydration are to provide mouth care and offer clear fluids. Intravenous fluid administration for all labors is common practice in hospitals. Intravenous solutions are started for the following reasons: prevention of dehydration, electrolyte imbalance, and acidosis; a "life line" for emergencies; usually required before the administration of analgesia, anesthesia; administration of oxytocin prophylactically after the delivery to prevent uterine atony.

● Bladder care: The client should be encouraged to void at least every 2-4 h. The laboring woman often attributes all of her discomfort to the intensity of uterine contractions and therefore is unaware that the pressure of a full bladder has increased her discomfort. With epidural anesthesia, she may be unable to sense bladder fullness. In addition to causing unnecessary discomfort, a full bladder may be a serious impediment to labor or the cause of urinary retention in the puerperium. If the distended bladder can be palpated above the symphysis pubis and the client is unable to void, the physician should be notified. Straight catheterization may be prescribed in such cases.

二 第二产程妇女的护理

第二产程即胎儿娩出期,从宫口开全至胎儿娩出。第二产程应密切观察产程,指导产妇正确使用腹压,做好接产前的准备,正确保护会阴并娩出胎儿。

【护理评估】

1.健康史 了解第一产程的经过与处理、有无妊娠并发症或合并症。

2.身体状况

（1）规律宫缩加强　进入第二产程后，宫缩的频率和强度达到高峰，宫缩持续约 1 min 或以上，宫缩间歇期仅 1～2 min。

（2）排便感　当胎头下降压迫盆底组织时，产妇有反射性排便感，并不自主地产生向下用力屏气的动作，会阴膨隆、变薄，肛门括约肌松弛。

（3）胎头拨露　胎头于宫缩时露出于阴道口，在宫缩间歇期又缩回阴道内（图 4-13A）。

（4）胎头着冠　当胎头双顶径越过骨盆出口，宫缩间歇期胎头不再回缩（图 4-13B）。

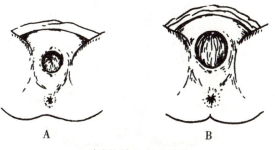

A.胎头拨露；B.胎头着冠。

图 4-13　胎头拨露及胎头着冠

（5）胎儿娩出　当胎头枕部在耻骨弓下露出时，胎头仰伸，顶、额、鼻、口、颏部相继娩出。接着胎头复位及外旋转，随后前肩和后肩相继娩出，胎体很快娩出，后羊水随之涌出。经产妇第二产程短，有时仅需几次宫缩即可完成胎头娩出。

3.心理-社会状况　进入第二产程后，宫缩强而频，产妇常因阵痛加剧和急于结束分娩而焦虑。评估产妇的心理状态、对自然分娩的信心及家属对产妇的支持情况。

4.辅助检查　胎儿监护仪监测宫缩和胎心变化，以及时发现异常情况。

【护理诊断】

1.疼痛　与子宫收缩及会阴伤口有关。

2.有受伤的危险　与可能发生的会阴裂伤、胎儿窘迫、新生儿产伤有关；与会阴保护及接生手法不当有关。

3.焦虑　与对分娩结局的不确定有关。

【护理措施】

1.一般护理　第二产程期间，助产士应陪伴在旁，以及时提供产程进展信息，给予产妇安慰、支持和鼓励，缓解其紧张和恐惧，同时进行协助其饮水、擦汗等生活护理。

2.密切监测胎心　此期宫缩频而强，应增加胎心监测频率，每次宫缩过后或每 5 min 监测1 次，听诊胎心应在宫缩间歇期且至少听诊 30 s。有条件者建议行连续电子胎心监护，每次宫缩后评估胎心率与宫缩的关系等。若发现胎心异常，应立即行阴道检查，综合评估产程进展情况，尽快结束分娩。

3.密切监测宫缩　第二产程宫缩持续时间可达 60 s，间隔时间 1～2 min。宫缩的质量与第二产程时限密切相关，必要时可给予缩宫素加强宫缩。

4.指导产妇用力　推荐产妇在有向下屏气用力的感觉后再指导用力，从而更有效地利用好腹压。方法是让产妇双足蹬在产床上，两手握住产床把手，宫缩时深吸气后屏气，然后如排便样向下用力以增加腹压。于宫缩间歇期，产妇自由呼吸并全身肌肉放松。宫缩时，再做同样的屏气动作,以加速产程进展。

5. 做好接产的准备 初产妇胎头拨露3～4 cm、经产妇宫口近开全、会阴膨隆紧张时,应做好接产的准备。让产妇仰卧于产床(有条件的医院可采取自由体位),两腿屈曲分开,露出外阴部,用温水清洁外阴部,聚维酮碘溶液消毒外阴部2～3次,顺序是大阴唇、小阴唇、阴阜、大腿内上1/3、会阴及肛门周围(图4-14)。接产者按要求洗手、戴手套、穿手术衣,准备接产。

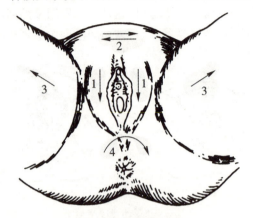

图4-14 外阴消毒顺序

6. 接产

(1)评估是否需行会阴切开术 综合评估胎儿大小、会阴体长度及弹性后,确定是否需行会阴切开术,防止发生严重会阴裂伤。

(2)接产要领 正确保护会阴,协助胎头俯屈,控制胎头娩出的速度,让胎头以最小径线(枕下前囟径)缓慢通过阴道口,减少会阴撕裂的风险。

(3)接产步骤 接产者站在产妇正面,当宫缩来临产妇有便意时指导产妇屏气用力。胎头着冠时,指导产妇何时用力和呼气。会阴水肿、过紧、炎症,耻骨弓过低,胎儿过大、娩出过快等,均易造成会阴撕裂。接产者应在接产前作初步评估,接生时个体化指导产妇用力,并用手控制胎头娩出速度,同时左手轻轻下压胎头枕部,协助胎头俯屈,使胎头双顶径缓慢娩出,此时若娩出过急则可能撕裂会阴。当胎头枕部在耻骨弓下露出时,让产妇在宫缩间歇时期稍向下屏气,左手协助胎头仰伸,使胎头缓慢娩出,清理口腔黏液。胎头娩出后,不宜急于娩出胎肩,而应等待宫缩使胎头自然完成外旋转复位,胎肩旋转至骨盆出口前后径。再次宫缩时接生者右手托住会阴,左手将胎儿颈部向下牵拉胎头,使前肩从耻骨弓下顺势娩出,继之托胎颈向上,使后肩从会阴前缘缓慢娩出。双肩娩出后,保护会阴的右手放松,双手协助胎体娩出(图4-15)。胎儿娩出后用器皿置于产妇臀下计量产后失血量。

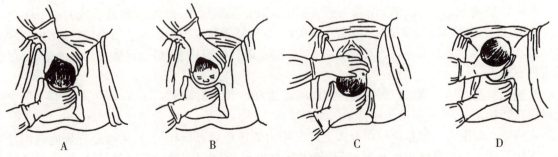

A.协助胎头俯屈;B.协助胎头仰伸;C.协助前肩娩出;D.协助后肩娩出。

图4-15 接产步骤

The second stage of labor begins with complete dilatation of the cervix and ends with the birth. The complete dilatation of the cervix can be definitely confirmed only by a vaginal examination. However, the experienced nurse is often able to suspect complete dilatation by observing changes in the clients' behavior. It has traditionally been considered prolonged if more than 2 h. However, if descent is progressive and electronic fetal monitoring used for close surveillance, a longer second stage can be a safe option and operative intervention may not be necessary. To determine if the duration of second stage is significantly increasing the risk of birth injury, the nurse must always keep in mind "who" is going through this process. Characteristics such as a large fetus, a post-term pregnancy, a smaller size woman, or a more difficult presentation increase the likelihood of cephalopelvic disproportion or fetal distress. If these conditions occur, a cesarean birth may be necessary to prevent second stage birth injuries.

Nursing Intervention

● Methods for bearing down: During the second stage of labor, the client is asked to exert her abdominal forces and bear down. The bearing down efforts were thought to be best when the client used long and sustained pushes with no audible sounds made.

The following is a description of how the nurse can assist the client during second stage in the semi-fowler position: The woman's head and shoulders can be raised to a 45° angle and supported firmly during the contraction. The client's thighs are flexed on the abdomen, with hands grasped just below the knees when a contraction begins. The client can be encouraged to work with the urge to push, she should be instructed that the action is similar to straining during a bowel movement. The long breath-holding pushes may be used if needed to hasten birth.

● Preparing the perineum: When the woman is positioned on the birthing or delivery table or bed, the nurse carries out the procedure for cleansing the vulva and the surrounding. If the birth is to be conducted with the client in the recumbent position, this may be done with the knees drawn up slightly and the legs separated. Once the birth attendant has scrubbed and donned sterile gown and gloves, the client is draped with towels and sheets appropriate for the purpose. After the client has been prepared for birth, catheterization, if needed, is carried out. Sometimes it is difficult to catheterize a client in the second stage of labor, because the fetus's head may compress the urethra. If the catheter does not pass easily, it should not be forced.

● Birth: As soon as the head distends the vaginal orifice to diameter of 6 or 8 cm (crowning) a towel may be placed over the rectum while forward pressure is exerted on the newborn's chin with one hand, at the same time that downward pressure is applied to the occiput by the other hand. This technique, called the Ritgen maneuver, provides control the head as it emerges and directs the extension phase of birth so that the head is born with the smallest diameter presenting. The head is usually delivered between contractions and as slowly as possible. At this time, the woman may complain about a "splitting" sensation caused by the extreme vaginal stretching as the head is born.

Control of the head by the Ritgen maneuver, extension, and slow delivery between contractions help to prevent lacerations. If a tear seems to be inevitable, an incision called an episiotomy may be made in the perineum. This prevents lacerations and facilitates the delivery.

Immediately after the birth of the head, the mouth and nose are routinely suctioned with the bulb syringe. After suctioning, a finger is passed along the occiput to the newborn's neck to feel whether a loop or more of umbilical cord encircles it. If such a coil is felt, it should be gently drown down and if loose enough, slipped over the newborn's head. This is done to prevent interference with the oxygen supply, which could result from pressure of the shoulder on the umbilical cord. If the cord is too tightly coiled to permit this procedure, it must be clamped and cut before the shoulders are delivered; the newborn must be extracted immediately before asphyxiation results.

The anterior shoulder is usually brought under the symphysis pubis first and then the posterior shoulder is delivered, after which the remainder of the body follows without particular mechanism. The exact time of the birth should be noted. The newborn usually cries immediately, and the lungs gradually become expanded. The pulsations in the umbilical cord begin to diminish about this time.

● Episiotomy: An episiotomy is an incision of the perineum made to facilitate delivery. The incision is made with blunt-pointed straight scissors about the time that the head distends the vulva and is visible to a diameter of several centimeters. The incision may be made in the midline of the perineum, a median episiotomy, or it may be begun in the midline and directed downward and laterally away from the rectum, a mediolateral episiotomy. In the latter instance, the incision may be directed to either the right or the left side of the woman's pelvis.

三 第三产程妇女的护理

第三产程是胎盘娩出期,护理人员需要正确处理已娩出的新生儿,做到早接触、早吸吮、早开奶;仔细检查胎盘完整性,检查软产道有无损伤,预防产后出血。

【护理评估】

1. 健康史　了解第一、第二产程的经过及其处理。

2. 身体状况

(1)子宫收缩　胎儿娩出后,宫底降至平脐,产妇感到轻松,宫缩暂停数分钟后再现,应注意评估子宫收缩情况。

(2)胎盘剥离征象　胎儿娩出后,由于宫腔容积突然明显缩小,胎盘不能相应缩小,胎盘附着面与子宫壁发生错位而剥离。剥离面出血形成胎盘后血肿,子宫继续收缩,胎盘后血肿增大,直至胎盘完全剥离而排出。胎盘剥离的征象:①子宫底变硬呈球形,胎盘剥离后降至子宫下段,下段被扩张,子宫体呈狭长形被推向上,宫底升高达脐上(图4-16);②阴道口外露的一段脐带自行延长;③少量阴道流血;④用手掌尺侧在产妇耻骨联合上方轻压子宫下段,宫体上升而外露的脐带不再回缩。

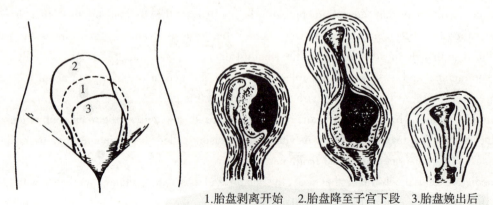

1.胎盘剥离开始　2.胎盘降至子宫下段　3.胎盘娩出后

图4-16　胎盘剥离时子宫形状

（3）胎盘排出方式　①胎儿面娩出式：多见，胎盘从中央开始剥离，而后向周围剥离，其特点是先排出胎盘，随后见少量阴道流血；②母体面娩出式：少见，胎盘边缘先开始剥离，血液沿剥离面流出，其特点是先有较多阴道流血，然后胎盘娩出。

（4）检查胎盘、胎膜的完整性　胎盘娩出后，评估胎盘、胎膜是否完整，胎盘周边有无断裂的血管，判断是否有副胎盘。

（5）仔细检查软产道　注意有无子宫颈裂伤、阴道裂伤及会阴裂伤。

3. 心理-社会状况评估　产妇情绪状态、对新生儿性别及外形等是否满意，评估亲子间互动，评估家属对分娩结局是否满意。

【护理诊断】

1. 潜在并发症　产后出血、新生儿窒息。

2. 有亲子关系无效的危险　与疲乏、会阴切口疼痛或新生儿性别不理想有关。

【护理措施】

1. 新生儿护理

（1）清理呼吸道　不建议常规使用吸球或吸痰管清理呼吸道。若咽部及鼻腔分泌物较多，可用吸球吸引，以免发生吸入性肺炎。当确认呼吸道通畅而仍未啼哭时，可用手抚摸新生儿背部或轻拍新生儿足底。新生儿大声啼哭后即可处理脐带。

（2）Apgar 评分　是快速评估新生儿出生后的一般情况的方法，以出生后 1 min 内的心率、呼吸、肌张力、喉反射及皮肤颜色 5 项体征为依据，每项为 0 ~ 2 分，满分为 10 分（表 4-4）。若评分为 8 ~ 10 分，正常；4 ~ 7 分属轻度窒息，又称青紫窒息，需采用清理呼吸道、人工呼吸、吸氧、用药等措施才能恢复；0 ~ 3 分属重度窒息，又称苍白窒息，需紧急抢救，在直视下行喉镜气管内插管并给氧。对缺氧严重的新生儿，应在出生后 5 min、10 min 时再次评分，直至连续两次评分均≥8 分。1 min 评分反映胎儿在宫内的情况；5 min Apgar 评分则反映复苏效果，与近期和远期预后关系密切。脐动脉血气代表新生儿在产程中血气变化的结局，提示有无缺氧、酸中毒及其严重程度，反映窒息的病理生理本质，较 Apgar 评分更为客观、更具有特异性。

表 4-4　新生儿 Apgar 评分法

体征	0 分	1 分	2 分
心率	0	<100 次/min	≥100 次/min
呼吸	0	浅慢，不规则	佳，哭声响亮
肌张力	松弛	四肢稍屈曲	四肢屈曲，活动好
喉反射	无反射	有些动作	咳嗽，恶心
皮肤颜色	全身苍白	身体红，四肢青紫	全身粉红

我国新生儿窒息标准：①5 min Apgar 评分≤7 分，仍未建立有效呼吸；②脐动脉血 pH 值<7.15；③排除其他引起低 Apgar 评分的病因；④产前具有可能导致窒息的高危因素。以上①~③为必要条件，④为参考指标。

（3）处理脐带　新生儿娩出后，若母儿健康，可采取延迟断脐，可在新生儿出生后 30 ~ 60 s 或脐带血管停止搏动后再结扎脐带。目前临床多用脐带夹处理脐带，助产士更换手套，用 2 把无菌止血钳分别在距离脐带根部 2 cm 和 5 cm 处夹住脐带，在距离脐带根部 2 cm 处一次断脐，应避免二次断脐。此外,也可以采用无菌棉线在脐根 0.5 cm 处结扎第一道,在结扎线外 0.5 cm 处结扎第二道,在第二道结扎线外 0.5 cm 处剪断脐带。若为早产儿,视母儿具体情况延迟 30～45 s 断脐,若新生儿发生窒息或产妇有大出血风险,应立即断脐对新生儿及产妇进行紧急处理。

(4)一般护理 新生儿体格检查;将新生儿足底印及母亲拇指印留于新生儿病历上;新生儿手腕带和包被标明性别、体重、出生时间、母亲姓名,帮助新生儿早接触、早吸吮,吸吮时间不少于 30 min;注意新生儿保暖。

2. 协助胎盘娩出 正确处理胎盘娩出可预防产后出血。在胎儿前肩娩出后将缩宫素 10～20 U 稀释于 250～500 mL 0.9%氯化钠注射液中快速静脉滴注,并控制性牵拉脐带,确认胎盘已完全剥离。以左手握住宫底,拇指置于子宫前壁,其余 4 指放于子宫后壁并按压,同时右手轻拉脐带。当胎盘娩至阴道口时,接产者双手捧起胎盘,向一个方向旋转并缓慢向外牵拉,协助胎盘、胎膜完整剥离排出(图 4-17)。若在胎膜排出过程中,发现胎膜部分断裂,可用血管钳夹住断裂上端的胎膜,再继续向原方向旋转,直至胎膜完全排出。

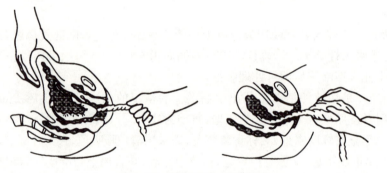

图 4-17 协助胎盘、胎膜娩出

3. 检查胎盘、胎膜 将胎盘铺平,先检查胎盘母体面胎盘小叶有无缺损。然后将胎盘提起,检查胎膜是否完整,再检查胎盘胎儿面边缘有无血管断裂,以及时发现副胎盘。若有副胎盘、部分胎盘残留或大部分胎膜残留时,应在无菌操作下伸手入宫腔取出残留组织。若确认仅有少量胎膜残留,可给予子宫收缩剂待其自然排出。

4. 检查软产道 胎盘娩出后,应仔细检查产妇会阴、小阴唇内侧、尿道口周围、阴道及子宫颈有无裂伤。若有裂伤,应立即缝合。

5. 产后 2 h 护理 胎盘娩出 2 h 内是产后出血的高危期,有时被称为第四产程。

(1)观察产后出血情况 重点观察产妇血压、脉搏、子宫收缩情况、阴道流血量,膀胱是否充盈,会阴及阴道有无血肿等,发现异常及时处理。

(2)促进舒适 为产妇擦汗更衣,及时更换床单及会阴垫,提供清淡、易消化流质食物,帮助产妇恢复体力。

(3)情感支持 帮助产妇接受新生儿,协助产妇和新生儿进行皮肤接触和早吸吮,建立母子情感。

The third stage of labor, the placental stage, begins after the birth of the newborn and terminates with the birth of the placenta. Immediately after delivery of the newborn, the height of the uterine fundus and its consistency are ascertained by palpating the uterus through a sterile towel placed on the lower abdomen. The physician places his or her hand on top of the sterile drape and holds the uterus gently, with the fingers behind the fundus and the thumb in front. So long as the uterus remains hard and there is no bleeding, the policy is ordinarily one of watchful waiting until the placenta is separated.

Nursing Assessment

• Placental separation and delivery：Because attempts to deliver the placenta before its separation from the uterine wall are not only futile but may be dangerous, it is most important that the signs of placental separation be well understood. The following signs indicate that the placenta has loosened and is ready to deliver：a lengthening of the umbilical cord, a sudden gush of vaginal blood, or a change in the shape of the uterus. When the placenta has separated and the uterus is firmly contracted？ The client is asked to bear down so that the intra-abdominal pressure helps expel the placenta. If this fails, or if it is not practical because of anesthesia, gentle pressure is exerted downward with the hand on the fundus, and the placenta is gently guided out of the vagina. This procedure, known as placental expression, must be done gently and without squeezing. Placental expression should never be attempted unless the uterus is hard；otherwise, the organ may be turned inside out. This is one of the gravest complications of obstetrics and is known as inversion of the uterus. Once the placenta is expelled, it is carefully inspected to make sure that it is intact. If a piece is left in the uterus, it may cause subsequent hemorrhage. Prolonged placental separation, known as "retained placenta", has been defined by duration of third stage longer than 30 min, because incidence of hemorrhage increases significantly after that length of time.

• Use of oxytocics：After the separation and delivery of the placenta in the third stage of labor, hemostasis along the inner uterine surface is achieved at the placental site by contraction of the myometrium, causing vasoconstriction of the uterine spiral arteries. Oxytocic agents are used widely in the normal third stage of labor. If an intravenous infusion is in place, our standard practice has been to add 20 units of oxytocin per liter of infusion.

• Lacerations of the birth canal：During the process of a normal delivery, lacerations of the perineum and vagina may be caused by rapid and sudden expulsion of the head, excessive size of the newborn, and friable maternal tissues. In other circumstances, they may be caused by difficult forceps deliveries, breech extractions, or contraction of the pelvic outlet in which the head is forced posteriorly. Some tears are unavoidable, even in the most skilled hands, but control of the head is extremely important to deter perineal lacerations.

Postpartum care begins immediately after the delivery；mother and newborn are making adjustments that need to be assessed. If problems arise, actions need to be taken promptly to ensure well-being. The first maternal assessment is to be done in the delivery room before transfer. The immediate postpartum checks, performed every 15 min for the first hour, every 30 min for the second hour, include blood pressure, pulse, respirations, massaging the fundus and observing the vaginal flow, inspecting the perineum, and assessing for bladder distention.

Meticulous assessment is essential, because the mother is at great risk at this time for postpartum he-morrhage and development of a hematoma.

During this period the fundus is massaged and its condition and position are documented. Vaginal bleeding is assessed and documented in regard to amount, color, and presence of clots or foul odor. Problems arise when amounts are not standardized and when measurement differs among nurses. A plate with scale is put under the hip to measure the quantity of vaginal bleeding duration the first two hours after birth.

Nursing Intervention

Nursing interventions at this stage focus on anticipation of potential complications and providing supportive and positive care that promotes family interaction.

● Immediate care for the newborn: Routine use of bulb syringe or suction tubes for airway clearance is not recommended. If the pharynx and nasal secretions are more, bulb syringe can be used to avoid aspiration pneumonia. The nurse notes the time of birth, the sex of the newborn and sets the 1-minute timer for the Apgar score (The Apgar system of scoring, developed in 1953 by the late Dr. Virginia Apgar, provides an index for assessing the newborn's condition at birth). If the baby appears normal and is not in obvious respiratory distress, blood and body fluids are wiped away, a warm blanket is placed over the newborn, and the cord is being clamped and cut by the birth attendant. The change in environment and sudden stimulation usually cause vigorous crying in the newborn. The nurse should assess and record the newborn's 1-minute Apgar score and reset the timer for the 5-minute score.

As long as the 1-minute Apgar score is satisfactory, the newborn can be placed on the mother's abdomen. The skin-to-skin contact helps to keep the newborn warm and promotes bonding between the mother and the newborn. The mother may want to attempt breast-feeding at this time.

A cord clamp is placed on the cord, and the excess is cut off with sterile scissors. Two completed identification bands are placed on the newborn's extremities, and one is placed on the mother's wrists. Prophylactic eye care and vitamin K injection may be performed at this time.

● Postpartum hemorrhage: If the uterus shows any tendency to relax, it is to be massaged immediately with firm but gentle circular strokes until it contracts effectively. Relaxation of the uterus is a prime cause of postpartum hemorrhage, and surveillance of the uterus and the amount of bleeding is of extreme importance at this time. The nurse has an intravenous infusion with an oxytocic for immediate administration ready in the event that the attendants suspect hemorrhage is imminent.

任务实施

母乳喂养有利于母婴健康,但有些产妇在母乳喂养过程中可能会出现一些问题,尤其是初产妇易出现哺乳困难,做好母乳喂养指导和乳房护理(表4-5),对母儿都具有重要意义。

表4-5　母乳喂养指导和乳房护理

项目	内容
目的	1. 熟练掌握母乳喂养的优点和方法
	2. 学会哺乳前后乳房的护理
	3. 具有保护产妇隐私的意识,关心、体贴母婴
操作前准备	1. 用物准备:清洁的毛巾、脸盆、热水
	2. 环境准备:环境舒适、温暖、整洁,必要时屏风遮挡
	3. 产妇准备:洗净双手,取舒适体位
	4. 护士准备:着装规范,修剪指甲,洗净双手,寒冷季节应预热双手
	5. 婴儿准备:为婴儿更换清洁的尿布

续表4-5

项目	内容
操作步骤	1.核对、解释:核对母婴床号、姓名,讲解母乳喂养的优点
	2.哺乳前准备 (1)乳房准备:先用温热毛巾洗净乳头、乳晕,再用毛巾湿热敷乳房3~5 min,轻轻按摩 (2)安置体位:协助母婴取舒适、放松的体位,例如坐于靠背椅上、侧卧于床上等
	3.指导母亲正确的哺乳姿势 (1)母亲一只手抱紧婴儿,前臂搂住婴儿身体,上臂支撑婴儿头和颈,婴儿的头和身体呈一直线 (2)母婴紧密相贴,婴儿的脸朝向乳房,鼻头对准乳头 (3)母亲另一只手拇指与其余四指分开,拇指放于与婴儿鼻子齐平的乳房上侧,其余四指并拢放于乳房下方胸壁,示指将乳房支撑至自然高度 (4)手指不要离乳头太近,轻轻挤捏,使乳房形态有利于婴儿含接
	4.帮助婴儿正确含接乳头:母亲先用乳头触碰婴儿的嘴唇,诱发觅食反射,在婴儿嘴张大,舌下压的瞬间,把乳头和大部分乳晕放入婴儿口中,此时婴儿下唇向外翻,舌呈勺状,包裹乳头,慢而深、有节律地吮吸。此时可看到婴儿吞咽的动作,并能听到吞咽的声音。母亲一只手扶住乳房,防止堵塞婴儿口鼻,影响呼吸,还要防止婴儿头后仰而影响吞咽
	5.哺乳结束后,用示指轻压婴儿下颏取出乳头,避免强行牵拉造成乳头皮肤损伤
	6.用少许乳汁涂抹于乳头和乳晕周围,防止乳头皲裂
	7.把婴儿竖着抱起,让婴儿头趴在母亲肩上,轻拍背1~2 min,排出胃内空气,以防吐奶
操作后处理	1.协助母亲放下婴儿,帮助母亲取舒适体位
	2.整理用物,清洁双手,记录
	3.交代注意事项
注意事项	1.做到按需哺乳,产后半小时开奶
	2.乳汁分泌不足的产妇,让婴儿充分吸空一侧乳房后再吮吸另一侧

微课

课件

练习题及参考答案

（任　美）

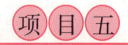

项目五

产褥期管理
（Puerperium Management）

项目描述

产褥期是指从胎盘娩出至产妇全身各器官（除乳腺外）恢复至正常未孕状态所需要的一段时期，一般为6周。产褥期是产妇各系统恢复的关键时期，因此，了解产褥期管理的相关知识，为产褥期妇女提供护理，对促进产妇的康复非常重要。

The postpartum period, or puerperium encompasses the time from the completion of placenta delivery to the organs except breast have returned to their pregnant state. It refers to 6−week period following childbirth. During this time, mothers experience numerous physiologic and psychosocial changes. The physical postpartum care a woman receives can influence her health for the rest of her life. The emotional support she receives can influence the emotional health of her child and family and can be felt into next generation.

任务一　正常产褥（Normal Puerperium）

工作情景

陈女士，28岁，G_1P_1，孕40周临产入院。入院次日晨4时行会阴侧切术，产钳助娩一女婴，体重4 000 g。产妇产后第1天，查体发现体温37.8 ℃，脉搏70次/min，呼吸18次/min，血压120/75 mmHg；子宫平脐，阴道流出血鲜红色；会阴切口缝合处水肿，无压痛。产妇自述尿量增多，且哺乳时出现下腹部疼痛；乳房胀痛，但无乳汁分泌；产妇住在母婴病房，自感焦虑。

①请明确该产妇主要的护理问题。②请根据目前的情况对产妇进行正确的护理。

任务内容

产褥期妇女全身各系统发生了较大的生理变化，其中生殖系统变化最明显。同时，伴随着新生儿的出生，产妇及其家庭也经历着心理和社会的适应过程。

◆能描述正常产褥期母体的生理变化。
◆能为产褥期妇女提供心理调适指导。

一　产褥期妇女的生理变化

1.生殖系统的变化

(1)子宫　子宫是产褥期生殖系统中变化最大的器官,其主要变化是子宫复旧。子宫复旧是指妊娠子宫自胎盘娩出后逐渐恢复至未孕状态的过程,一般为6周,主要变化为子宫体肌纤维缩复、子宫内膜再生、子宫血管变化及子宫颈和子宫下段的复原。

1)子宫体肌纤维缩复:子宫复旧不是肌细胞数目减少而是肌细胞缩小。随着肌纤维不断缩复,子宫体积和重量均发生变化。胎盘娩出后,子宫逐渐缩小,产后1周子宫缩小至妊娠12周大小,在耻骨联合上方可扪及;产后10 d子宫降至骨盆腔内,在腹部检查摸不到子宫底;产后6周子宫恢复至正常非妊娠前大小。子宫重量也逐渐减少,分娩结束时约1 000 g,产后1周约500 g,产后2周约为300 g,产后6周子宫逐渐恢复到50~70 g。

2)子宫内膜再生:胎盘胎膜娩出后,遗留在宫腔内的表层蜕膜逐渐变性、坏死、脱落,随恶露自阴道排出;接近肌层的子宫内膜基底层逐渐再生出新的功能层,将子宫内膜修复。胎盘附着部位的子宫内膜修复约需至产后6周,其余部位的子宫内膜修复大约需要3周的时间。

3)子宫血管变化:胎盘娩出后,胎盘附着面缩小为原来的一半,使螺旋动脉和静脉窦压缩变窄,数小时后形成血栓,出血量逐渐减少直到最后停止,最终被机化吸收。在新生的内膜修复期,胎盘附着面因复旧不良出现血栓脱落,可引起晚期产后出血。

4)子宫颈和子宫下段的复原:由于产后肌纤维缩复,子宫下段逐渐恢复至非孕时的子宫峡部。胎盘娩出后子宫颈外口呈环状如袖口。产后2~3 d,宫口可容纳2指;产后1周,子宫颈内口关闭,子宫颈管复原;产后4周,子宫颈完全恢复至非孕时形态。由于分娩时子宫颈外口发生轻度裂伤(多在子宫颈3点、9点处),初产妇子宫颈外口由产前的圆形(未产型)变为产后的"一"字形横裂(已产型)。

(2)阴道　分娩后的阴道腔扩大、阴道黏膜及周围组织水肿、黏膜皱襞减少甚至消失,导致阴道壁松弛、肌张力低下。阴道壁肌张力在产褥期逐渐恢复,但不能完全恢复至未孕时的张力。阴道腔逐渐缩小,阴道黏膜皱襞在产后3周重新呈现。

(3)外阴　分娩后的外阴轻度水肿,于产后2~3 d逐渐消退。因会阴部血液循环丰富,若有轻度撕裂或会阴侧切开缝合,多于产后3~4 d愈合。

(4)盆底组织　分娩过程中,由于胎先露长时间压迫,盆底组织过度伸展导致弹性降低,而且常伴有盆底肌纤维部分撕裂,因此,产褥期应避免过早进行较强的体力劳动,坚持做产后康复锻炼,有利于盆底肌的恢复。

2.乳房　妊娠期孕妇体内雌激素、孕激素、人胎盘催乳素升高,使乳腺发育、乳腺体积增大、乳晕加深,为泌乳做好准备。当胎盘剥离娩出后,产妇血中雌激素、孕激素及人胎盘催乳素水平急剧下降,抑制下丘脑分泌的催乳素抑制因子释放,在催乳素作用下,乳汁开始分泌。婴儿吸吮及不断排空乳房能够促进乳汁不断分泌,同时婴儿吸吮反射性地引起宫缩,促进子宫复旧。由于乳汁分泌量与产妇营养、睡眠、情绪和健康状况密切相关,保证产妇休息、足够睡眠和营养丰富饮食,并避免精神刺激至关重要。若此期乳汁不能正常排空，可出现乳汁淤积，导致乳房胀痛及硬结形成；若乳汁不足，可出现乳房空软。

3. 血液循环系统　由于分娩后子宫胎盘血液循环终止和子宫缩复，大量血液从子宫涌入产妇的血液循环，另外妊娠期潴留的组织液回吸收，产后 72 h 内产妇循环血量增加 15% ~ 25% ，应注意预防心力衰竭的发生。循环血量于产后 2 ~ 3 周恢复至未孕状态。

产褥早期血液仍然处于高凝状态，有利于胎盘剥离创面形成血栓，减少产后出血量。纤维蛋白原、凝血酶、凝血酶原于产后 2 ~ 4 周内降到正常。血红蛋白水平于产后 1 周左右回升。白细胞总数于产褥早期较高，可达 $(15 ~ 30) \times 10^9/L$ ，一般产后 1 ~ 2 周恢复正常。淋巴细胞稍减少，中性粒细胞增多，血小板增多。红细胞沉降率于产后 3 ~ 4 周降至正常。

4. 消化系统　妊娠期胃肠肌张力及蠕动力均减弱，胃液中盐酸分泌量减少，产后需 1 ~ 2 周逐渐恢复。产妇因分娩时能量的消耗及体液流失，产后 1 ~ 2 d 内常感口渴，喜进流质饮食或半流质饮食，但食欲差，以后逐渐好转。产妇因卧床时间长、缺少运动、腹肌及盆底肌肉松弛、肠蠕动减弱等，容易发生便秘和肠胀气。

5. 泌尿系统　妊娠期体内潴留的大量液体在产褥早期主要由肾脏排出，故产后 1 周内尿量增多。妊娠期发生的肾盂及输尿管生理性扩张，产后 2 ~ 8 周恢复正常。因分娩过程中膀胱受压，膀胱黏膜水肿、充血及肌张力降低，以及会阴伤口疼痛、不习惯卧床排尿、器械助产、区域阻滞麻醉等，均可导致尿潴留的发生。

6. 内分泌系统　产后雌激素、孕激素水平急剧下降，产后 1 周降至未孕时水平。人胎盘催乳素于产后 6 h 已测不出。催乳素水平受哺乳的影响：若产妇哺乳，催乳素水平于产后下降，但仍高于非孕时水平；若产妇不哺乳，催乳素于产后 2 周降至非孕时水平。月经复潮及排卵恢复时间受哺乳影响：不哺乳产妇一般在产后 6 ~ 10 周月经复潮，产后 10 周左右恢复排卵；哺乳期产妇月经复潮延迟，平均在产后 4 ~ 6 个月恢复排卵。产后月经复潮较晚者，复潮前多有排卵，故哺乳期妇女虽无月经来潮，仍有受孕的可能。

7. 腹壁的变化　腹部皮肤受妊娠子宫增大影响，部分弹力纤维断裂，腹直肌呈不同程度分离，使产后腹壁明显松弛，其紧张度需产后 6 ~ 8 周恢复。妊娠期出现的下腹正中线色素沉着，在产褥期逐渐消退。初产妇腹部紫红色妊娠纹变为银白色。

Reproductive System

● Uterus：Uterine involution is the process whereby the uterus returns to its nonpregnant state. The woman is in danger of hemorrhage from the uterus until involution is complete. Involution depends on three processes：contraction of muscle fibers，catabolism，and regeneration of uterine epithelium. Involution begins immediately after delivery of the placenta，when uterine muscle fibers contract firmly. The uterus decreases in size when muscle fibers contract intensively. Although the total number of cells remains unchanged，the enlarged muscle cells of the uterus undergo catabolic changes in protein cytoplasm that cause a reduction in individual cell size.

Regeneration of the uterine epithelial lining begins soon after childbirth. Within 2–3 d，the remaining decidua separates into two layers. The first layer is superficial and shed in lochia. The basal layer remains intact and is the source of new endometrium. New endometrium is generated at the site from glands and tissue that remain in the lower layer of the decidua after separation of the placenta. Regeneration of the endometrium，except at the site of placental attachment，occurs by 3 weeks. Healing at the placental site occurs more slowly and requires approximately 6 weeks.

Immediately after birth the uterus weighs about 1,000 g. At the end of the first week，it weights about

500 g. By the time involution is complete, it will weigh approximately 50 g—its prepregnant weight.

● Cervix: Immediately after childbirth, the cervix is formless, flabby, and open wide enough to admit the entire hand. Small tears or lacerations may be present, and the cervix is often edematous. Cervix is a rapid healing place. By the end of the first week the cervix feels firm. The internal os closes as before pregnancy, but the shape of the external os is permanently changed. It remains slightly open and appears slit-like rather than round, as in the nulliparous woman.

Vagina: Soon after childbirth, the vaginal walls appear edematous, and very few vaginal rugae (folds). Although the vaginal mucosa heals and rugae are regained by 3 weeks, the entire postpartum period (6 weeks) is needed for the vagina to complete involution and to gain approximately the same size and contour it had before pregnancy. The vagina does not entirely regain the nulliparous size, however.

● Perineum: After birth, the perineum is the development of edema and generalized tenderness. Portion of the perineum may show ecchymosis from the rupture of surface capillaries. The labia majora and labia minora typically remain atrophic and softened in a woman and never return to their prepregnant state. Many women have episiotomy incisions that are extremely painful.

● Pelvic muscular support: The muscular and fascial support structures of the uterus and vagina may be injured during childbirth. This injury can lead to pelvic relaxation, which is weakening and lengthening of support structures for the uterus, vaginal wall, rectum, urethra, and bladder. Women who practice postpartum pelvic muscle exercises show greater improvement in pelvic muscle strength than those who do not exercise.

Breast

With expulsion of the placenta, the source of all HPL, estrogen and progesterone during pregnancy is suddenly removed. The blood levels of these hormones fall rapidly, but the secretion of prolactin by the anterior pituitary gland continues. Milk is removed from lactiferous sinuses by the newborn's sucking. Sucking is the primary afferent stimulus, but the let-down reflex can be activated by auditory (newborn crying) and visual (seeing the newborn) stimuli. The afferent limb of this pathway is clearly hormonal, because oxytocin that is released from the posterior pituitary causes contraction of the myoepithelial cells of the breasts. Anxiety and tension, severe cold, and pain inhibit the let-down reflex and decrease milk ejection. This underlies the need for a comfortable, relaxed setting in which to breast-feed.

Cardiovascular System

Changes in blood volume after delivery are due to blood loss and post delivery diuresis. There is a transient 15%-25% increase in circulation blood volume after delivery because of the mobilization of extravascular fluid and termination of placenta circulation. It is caused by an increase cardiac output and results in bradycardia during in the 72 h (especial in 24 h) early postpartum period. Gradually, the blood volume decreases and returns to normal level by 2-3 weeks after childbirth.

The white blood cell (WBC) count normally increases after delivery. This leukocytosis is characterized by increased neutrophils and eosinophils and decreased lymphocytes. Clotting factors I, II, VII, IX and X are activated extensively after delivery. These decrease within a few days to pregnant levels, but fibrinogen and thromboplastin return to normal level in 2-4 weeks after birth.

Gastrointestinal System

Digestion and absorption begin to be active again in the gastrointestinal system soon after birth. The new mother usually is hungry because of the energy expended in labor. She usually is thirsty because of the decreased oral intake during labor, the fluid loss from exertion, mouth breathing, and diaphoresis. Besides, constipation is a common problem during the postpartum period.

Urinary System

After birth, an extensive diuresis begins to take place almost immediately following birth to rid the body of the fluid; this increases the daily output of the postpartum women greatly. Urinary-volume may easily rise from a normal level of 1,500 mL to as 3,000 mL during the 2-5 d after birth.

Endocrine System

After expulsion of the placenta, a fairly rapid decline occurs in placental hormones such as estrogen, progesterone, human placental lactogen, and human chorionic gonadotropin. Adrenal hormones such as aldosterone return to pregrenancy levels. If the mother is not breast-feeding, the pituitary hormone prolactin, which stimulates milk secretion, disappears in about 2 weeks. The average time for non-breastfeeding mothers to resume menstruation is 6-10 weeks after childbirth. Breast-feeding delays return of both ovulation and menstruation. The length of the delay depends on the frequency of breast-feeding and the duration of lactation. The longer the period of lactation, the longer the average time to the first menstrual period.

Integumentary System

Following birth, the stretch marks on the abdomen still appear reddened and may be even more prominent. It can be assured that these will fade to a pale white over the next 3-6 months. Excessive pigment on the face and neck and on the abdomen will be barely detectable in 6 weeks.

二 产褥期妇女的心理调适

产褥期妇女的心理调适是指产后产妇从妊娠期和分娩期的不适、疼痛、焦虑中恢复，接纳家庭新成员及新家庭的过程。因为产褥期妇女心理处于脆弱和不稳定状态，面临着潜意识的内在冲突及初为人母的情绪调整，家庭关系改变，经济需求，家庭、社会支持系统的寻求等，故产褥期心理调适指导和支持十分重要。

产褥期妇女的心理调适主要表现在两方面：确立家长与孩子的关系和承担母亲角色的责任。根据鲁宾研究结果，产褥期妇女的心理调适过程一般经历3个时期。

1. 依赖期　产后前3 d。表现为产妇的很多需要是通过别人来满足，如对孩子的关心、喂奶、沐浴等，同时产妇喜欢用语言表达对孩子的关心，较多地谈论自己妊娠和分娩的感受。较好的妊娠和分娩经历、满意的产后休息、丰富的营养摄入和较早较多的与孩子间的对视及身体接触将有助于产妇较快地进入第二期。在依赖期，家人的关心帮助、医务人员的悉心指导极为重要。

2. 依赖-独立期　产后3~14 d。产妇表现出较为独立的行为，开始注意周围的人际关系，主动参与活动，学习和练习护理孩子。但这一时期容易产生压抑，可能由分娩后产妇感情脆弱、太多的母亲责任、新生儿诞生而产生的爱的被剥夺感、痛苦的妊娠和分娩过程、糖皮质激素和甲状腺素处于低水平等因素造成。严重者表现为哭泣，对周围漠不关心，拒绝哺乳和护理新生儿等。此时，应及时提供护理、指导和帮助，促使产妇纠正这种消极情绪。加倍地关心产妇，并督促其家人参与；提供婴儿喂养和护理知识，耐心指导并帮助产妇哺乳和护理新生儿；鼓励产妇表达自己的心情并与其他产妇交流，促进产妇接纳孩子、接纳自己，缓解抑郁状态，平稳地度过这一时期。

3. 独立期　产后2周至1个月。此时，新家庭形成，产妇、家人和婴儿已成为一个完整的系统，形成新的生活形态。夫妇两人共同分享欢乐和责任，开始逐渐恢复分娩前的家庭生活。但是，产妇及丈夫会承受更多的压力，出现兴趣与需要、事业与家庭间的矛盾，哺育孩子、承担家务及维持夫妻关系等各种角色的矛盾。

The birth of a baby event requires such rapid change in family structure and function. Mother progressed through restorative phases to replenish the energy lost during labor and childbirth and gain confidence in her role as mother. Both the mother and the father begin the process of attachment with the newborn. The families must adapt to a new standing in the family structure. Numerous factors influence family adaptation such as previous experience and the availability of a strong support system. So, the role of maternity nurses has gradually expanded from the care of the mother−infant dyad to include the well−being of the entire family. Nurses are concerned with the family's adjustment to childbearing, not only during the hospital stay but also during the early weeks at home as the family makes the transition to parenthood.

任务实施

比较妊娠期及产褥期母体的生理变化,并完成表5-1。

表5-1 妊娠期及产褥期母体的生理变化

生理变化	时期	
	妊娠期	产褥期
生殖系统		
乳房		
血液循环系统		
消化系统		
泌尿系统		
内分泌系统		
腹壁的变化		

任务二　产褥期妇女的护理(Nursing of Postpartum Women)

工作情景

王女士,26岁,发热1d。产妇于4d前自然分娩一3800g女婴,会阴Ⅱ度裂伤,常规修补缝合。查体:体温37.9℃,脉搏85次/min,呼吸18次/min,血压115/70 mmHg。双乳腺触诊轻度肿胀,无发红。子宫在脐下两横指,硬、无压痛,会阴伤口无红肿,恶露量少于月经量,色暗红。

①请明确该产妇的护理诊断。②请陈述对该产妇应实施的护理和健康教育。

任务内容

产褥期护理应考虑到产妇及家庭成员的生理、心理需要,护理人员必须在准确评估产妇生理功能与心理状态的基础上,提供及时、准确的护理。

任务目标

◆ 能叙述产褥期、子宫复旧、恶露的概念。

◆ 能叙述产褥期妇女的临床表现及处理原则。

◆ 能运用所学知识对产褥期妇女进行护理及健康教育。

【概要】

1. 产褥期临床表现

(1)生命体征 产妇体温多数在正常范围内。产妇体温在产后24 h内稍升高，一般不超过38 ℃，可能与产程延长导致过度疲劳有关。产后3～4 d出现乳房血管、淋巴管极度充盈，乳房胀大，伴有37.8～39.0 ℃发热，称为泌乳热，一般持续4～16 h后降至正常，不属于病态，但需要排除其他原因，尤其是感染引起的发热。产后脉率在正常范围内，一般略慢，每分钟在60～70 次，产后呼吸深慢，一般每分钟14～16 次。原因是产后腹压降低，膈肌下降，由妊娠时的胸式呼吸变为腹式呼吸所致。产褥期血压平稳，在正常水平。

(2)子宫复旧 胎盘娩出后子宫圆而硬，宫底在脐下一指，产后第1天略上升至平脐，以后每日下降1～2 cm，至产后第10天降入骨盆腔内。剖宫产产妇子宫复旧所需时间略长。子宫复旧可伴有因宫缩而引起的下腹部阵发性剧烈疼痛，称为产后宫缩痛。经产妇宫缩痛较初产妇明显，哺乳者较不哺乳者明显。宫缩痛常在产后1～2 d出现，持续2～3 d自然消失，不需特殊用药。

(3)恶露 产后随着子宫蜕膜的脱落，血液、坏死的蜕膜等组织经阴道排出称为恶露。恶露有血腥味，但无臭味，持续4～6周，总量为250～500 mL。正常恶露根据颜色、内容物及出现持续时间不同分为血性恶露、浆液性恶露及白色恶露(表5-2)。

表5-2　正常恶露的特点

恶露的类型	持续时间	颜色	大体与镜下成分
血性恶露	产后3 d内	红色	大量血液、坏死蜕膜及少量胎膜
浆液性恶露	产后4～14 d	淡红色	较多坏死蜕膜组织、宫腔渗出液、子宫颈黏液，少量红细胞、白细胞和细菌
白色恶露	产后14 d后	白色	大量白细胞、坏死蜕膜组织、表皮细胞及细菌

(4)褥汗 产后1周内，产妇体内潴留的液体通过皮肤排泄，在睡眠时明显，醒来满头大汗，习称"褥汗"，不属于病态。

2. 处理原则 科学护理产妇，为产妇提供支持和帮助，使其感到舒适，促进产后生理功能恢复，预防产后出血、感染、中暑、抑郁等并发症发生，促进母乳喂养成功。

Signs and Symptoms During Puerperium

• Vital signs: Temperature of 38 ℃ is common during the first 24 h after childbirth and may be caused by dehydration or normal postpartum leukocytosis. If the elevated temperature persists for longer than 24 h or if it exceeds 38 ℃, infection is possible and the fever is reported to the physician. As for pulse, bradycardia, defined as a pulse rate of 60-70 beats per minute, may occur. Respiratory rate may be slow and deep, and 14-16 beats per minute be maintained. Blood pressure generally remains within normal level during pregnancy.

● Fundus (uterus): For the 1st hour after birth, the height of the fundus is at the umbilicus or even slightly above it. It then decreases by about 1 cm or 1 finger breadth per day. By 10 d postpartum, the fundus can no longer be palpated abdominally. The consistency of the fundus should be firm, with a round, smooth shape. A soft fundus indicates atony or sub-involution.

● Lochia: The amount of lochia may increase on early ambulation because of vaginal pooling and increased uterine contractions. Lochia is dark red (lochia rubra) in the first days after delivery and is usually moderate in amount. About the fourth day, it becomes more serous and pink (lochia serosa) with a decrease in flow. After 7-10 d, lochia becomes yellowish-white (lochia alba) with scant flow. Lochia alba persists until 3 weeks postpartum and indicates normal progression of healing.

Principle of Management

Takecare of women scientifically, provide support and help for women, make women feel comfort, promote the recovery of postpartum physiological function. Prevent postpartum bleeding, infection, heat stroke, depression and other complications, and promote the success of breastfeeding.

【护理评估】

1. 健康史　包括对产妇妊娠前、妊娠过程和分娩过程的全面评估。

2. 身心状况

（1）一般情况　评估产妇生命体征、产后出血量及子宫收缩情况。若阴道流血量不多，但子宫收缩不良、宫底上升者，提示宫腔内有积血；若产妇自觉肛门坠胀感，应注意是否有阴道后壁血肿；若子宫收缩好，但仍有阴道流血，色鲜红，应警惕软产道损伤。

（2）生殖系统　应每日在同一时间评估产妇的子宫底高度，子宫不能如期复原常提示异常；阴道分娩后出现的会阴水肿一般在产后2~3 d自行消退，注意观察会阴伤口愈合情况；每日应观察恶露的量、颜色及气味。

（3）排泄　评估产妇产后4 h是否排尿及尿量，对剖宫产术后产妇还应评估尿管是否通畅，尿量及性状是否正常；产妇在产后1~2 d多不排大便，但要注意产后便秘。

（4）乳房　评估有无乳头平坦、内陷及乳头皲裂；有无乳房胀痛及原因；乳汁质量。

（5）心理状态　产妇在产后2~3 d容易发生产后压抑，应注意评估产妇的心理状态。

（6）其他　注意评估产妇的社会支持情况，以及影响母乳喂养的因素等。

3. 辅助检查　必要时进行血常规、尿常规等检查。

【护理诊断】

1. 尿潴留　与产时损伤、活动减少及不习惯床上排尿有关。

2. 母乳喂养无效　与母乳供给不足或喂养技能不熟有关。

【护理措施】

1. 一般护理　为产妇提供空气清新、通风良好、舒适安静的病室环境，保持床单位的清洁、整齐、干净。保证产妇有足够的营养和睡眠，护理活动应不打扰产妇休息。

（1）生命体征　每日测体温、脉搏、呼吸及血压，若体温超过38 ℃，应加强观察，查找原因，并向医生汇报。

（2）饮食　产后1 h鼓励产妇进流质饮食或清淡半流质饮食，以后可进普通饮食。食物应富含营养、足够热量和水分。哺乳产妇应多进蛋白质和汤汁食物，同时适当补充维生素和铁剂，推荐补充铁剂3个月。

（3）排尿与排便　鼓励产妇尽早自行排尿，防止尿潴留及影响子宫收缩引起产后出血。若出现排尿困难，首先要解除产妇担心排尿引起疼痛的顾虑，鼓励产妇坐起排尿，必要时可采用热水熏洗外阴，针刺关元、气海、三阴交等穴位，肌内注射甲硫酸新斯的明等协助其排尿。应鼓励产妇多吃蔬菜，以及早下床活动预防便秘，一旦发生便秘可口服缓泻剂。

（4）活动　产后产妇应尽早开始适宜活动。经阴道自然分娩者产后 6～12 h 可下床轻微活动，产后第 2 天可在室内随意走动，按时做产后健身操。行会阴后－侧切开术或剖宫产术的产妇适当推迟活动时间，鼓励产妇床上适当活动，预防下肢静脉血栓形成。待拆线后伤口不感疼痛时做产后健身操。由于产妇产后盆底肌肉松弛，应避免负重劳动或蹲位活动，以防止子宫脱垂。

2. 症状护理

（1）产后 2 h 的护理　产后 2 h 内极易发生严重并发症，如产后出血、产后心力衰竭、产后子痫等，故产后应严密观察产妇生命体征、子宫收缩情况及阴道出血量，注意宫底高度及膀胱是否充盈。在此期间应该协助产妇首次哺乳。如果产后 2 h 一切正常，将产妇和新生儿送回病室。

（2）观察子宫复旧及恶露　每日在同一时间手测子宫底高度，了解子宫复旧情况。测量前嘱产妇排尿。每日观察恶露的量、颜色和气味。红色恶露增多且持续时间延长应考虑子宫复旧不全，应及时给予子宫收缩剂；若合并感染，恶露有臭味且子宫有压痛，应遵医嘱给予广谱抗生素控制感染。

（3）会阴及会阴伤口护理　每日 2～3 次行会阴及会阴伤口的冲洗，会阴部有缝线者应每日观察伤口周围有无渗血、血肿、红肿、硬结及分泌物，并嘱产妇健侧卧位。

会阴伤口异常的护理：①会阴或会阴伤口水肿者用 50% 硫酸镁湿热敷，产后 24 h 红外线照射外阴；②会阴部小血肿者，24 h 后可湿热敷或远红外线灯照射，大的血肿应配合医师切开处理；③会阴伤口有硬结者可用大黄、芒硝外敷或用 95% 乙醇湿热敷；④会阴切口疼痛剧烈或产妇有肛门坠胀感应及时报告医生，以排除阴道壁及会阴部血肿；⑤会阴部伤口缝线于产后 3～5 d 拆除，伤口感染者，应提前拆线引流，并定时换药。

（4）乳房护理　推荐母乳喂养，按需哺乳。母婴同室，做到早接触、早吸吮。重视心理护理的同时，指导正确的哺乳方法。于产后半小时内开始哺乳，刺激泌乳。乳房应经常擦洗，保持清洁、干燥。每次哺乳前柔和地按摩乳房，刺激泌乳反射。哺乳时应让新生儿吸空乳房，若乳汁充足尚有剩余时，应用吸乳器将剩余的乳汁吸出，以免乳汁淤积影响乳汁分泌，并预防乳腺管阻塞及两侧乳房大小不一等情况。

1）一般护理：哺乳期建议产妇使用大小适中的棉质乳罩。每次哺乳前，产妇应用清水将乳头洗净，乳头处如有痂垢，应先用油脂浸软后再用温水洗净。

2）乳头平坦及凹陷护理：有些产妇的乳头凹陷，一旦受到刺激乳头呈扁平状或向内回缩，婴儿很难吸吮到乳头，可指导产妇做乳头伸展（图 5-1）和乳头牵拉，采取多种喂奶的姿势和使用乳头套以利婴儿含住乳头，也可利用吸乳器进行吸引。在婴儿饥饿时可先吸吮平坦一侧，因此时婴儿吸吮力强，容易吸住乳头和大部分乳晕。

3）乳房胀痛护理：可通过尽早哺乳、外敷乳房、按摩乳房、佩戴乳罩、服用药物等方法进行缓解。

4）乳腺炎护理：轻度乳腺炎者在哺乳前湿热敷乳房 3～5 min，并按摩乳房，哺乳时先喂患侧乳房且应充分吸空乳汁，同时增加哺乳的次数。病情严重者需药物及手术治疗。

5）乳头皲裂护理：轻者可继续哺乳。哺乳前湿热敷乳房 3～5 min，挤出少许乳汁使乳晕变软，让乳头和大部分乳晕含吮在婴儿口中。哺乳后，挤出少许乳汁涂在乳头和乳晕上。疼痛严重者，可用吸乳器吸出乳汁喂给新生儿或用乳头罩间接哺乳，在皲裂处涂抗生素软膏。

6）催乳护理：对于乳汁分泌不足的产妇，应指导其正确的哺乳方法，按需哺乳、夜间哺乳、调节饮食，同时鼓励产妇树立信心。此外，可选用一些催乳方法：①中药涌泉散或通乳丹加减，用猪蹄

2 只炖烂服用;②针刺合谷、外关、少泽、膻中等穴位。

7)退乳护理:产妇因疾病或其他原因不能哺乳时,应尽早退乳。最简单的方法是停止哺乳,不排空乳房,少进汤汁,但有半数产妇会感到乳房胀痛,可口服镇痛药物。此外,可用水煎服生麦芽、芒硝外敷乳房、口服维生素 B$_6$ 等。

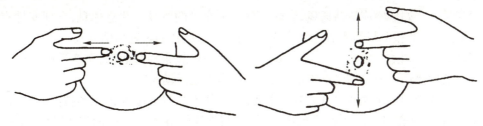

图 5-1　乳头伸展练习

Observing the Uterus Involution

Nurse should assess the height of fundus and characteristics of lochia many times in the first day. After 24 h, the fundus and lochia can be less assessed. Otherwise, the mother will need basic information about involution, including how to assess lochia and how to locate and palpate the fundus. This information allows her to recognize abnormal signs such as prolonged lochia and uterine tenderness, which should be reported to the health care provider.

Perineal Care

The most common method is to fill a squeeze bottle with warm water and spray the perineal area from the front toward the back. Water alone or with a small amount of cleansing solution added is used. During this procedure, water should be avoided to enter the vagina.

Breast Hygiene and Comfort

Instruct the breastfeeding mother to wash her nipples with clear water and to avoid soaps that remove the natural lubrication secreted by Montgomery's glands. Keeping the nipples dry between feedings helps prevent tissue damage, and wearing a good bra provides necessary support as breast size increases. Nurses help women prevent engorgement by assisting them to begin breast-feeding early and feed frequently.

Nipple Trauma

Nipple pain is common during early breast-feeding. Nipple trauma causes more sustained pain. Traumatized nipples appear red, cracked, blistered, or bleeding. Helping the mother with proper positioning may be the most important solution. Increasing air flow to the nipples, feeding with the less inflamed side first, and varying positions for feeding to rotate strain on the nipples also may be helpful. Expressing a small amount of milk to begin the let-down reflex may decrease vigorous suckling on sore nipples.

Flat and Inverted Nipples

Nipple abnormalities should be treated during pregnancy if possible, but interventions can begin after birth if necessary. Use of breast shells can be taught at this time. Nipple rolling just before feeding helps flat nipples become more erect so that the infant can grasp them more readily. A breast pump may help draw out inverted nipples.

Nutrition

Shortly after the delivery, the women may express a desire for something to eat or drink. The postpartum diet should provide for balanced nutrition with enough calories to supply the additional requirements for lactation, if the women will be breastfeeding.

Rest and Sleep

During the puerperium, the mother needs adequate rest and should be encouraged to relax and sleep whenever possible. A quiet, softly lit environment also promotes sleep.

【健康教育】

1. 一般指导　产妇居室应清洁通风,合理饮食保证充足的营养。注意休息,合理安排家务及婴儿护理,注意个人卫生和会阴部清洁。保持良好的心境,适应新的家庭生活方式。

2. 适当活动　经阴道分娩的产妇,产后 6~12 h 内即可起床轻微活动,于产后第 2 天可在室内随意走动。行会阴侧切术或行剖宫产术的产妇,可适当推迟活动时间。

3. 出院后喂养指导　①强调母乳喂养的重要性,评估产妇母乳喂养知识和技能,对知识缺乏的产妇及时进行宣教;②保证合理的睡眠和休息,保持精神愉快并注意乳房的卫生;③上班的母亲可于上班前挤出乳汁存放于冰箱内,婴儿需要时由他人哺喂,下班后及节假日坚持自己喂养;④告知产妇及家属如遇到喂养问题时可选用的咨询方法。

4. 产后健身操　产后健身操(图 5-2)可促进腹壁、盆底肌肉张力的恢复,避免腹壁皮肤过度松弛,预防尿禁失、膀胱直肠膨出及子宫脱垂。根据产妇的情况,运动量由小到大、由弱到强循序渐进。一般在产后第 2 天开始,每 1~2 d 增加 1 节,每节做 8~16 次。出院后继续做产后健身操直至产后 6 周。

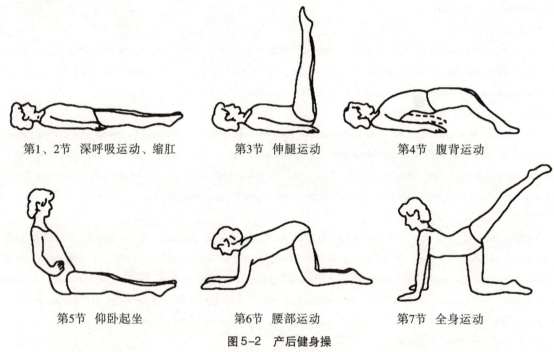

第1、2节　深呼吸运动、缩肛　　　第3节　伸腿运动　　　第4节　腹背运动

第5节　仰卧起坐　　　第6节　腰部运动　　　第7节　全身运动

图 5-2　产后健身操

5. 计划生育　指导产后 42 d 之内禁止性交。根据产后检查情况,恢复正常性生活,并指导产妇选择适当的避孕措施,一般哺乳者宜选用工具避孕,不哺乳者可选用药物避孕。

6. 产后检查

(1)产后访视　由社区医疗保健人员在产妇出院后 3 d 内、产后 14 d、产后 28 d 分别做 3 次产后访视,通过访视可了解产妇及新生儿健康状况。

(2)产后健康检查　告知产妇于产后 42 d 带孩子一起来医院进行一次全面检查,以了解产妇全身情况,特别是生殖器官的恢复情况及新生儿发育情况。

任务实施

产褥期会阴擦洗操作流程见表5–3。

表5–3　产褥期会阴擦洗操作流程

项目	内容
操作前准备	1. 护士准备:衣帽整洁、修剪指甲
	2. 用物准备:治疗车及治疗盘、弯盘2个、镊子2把、无菌镊子缸和镊子、消毒棉球缸、无菌干棉球缸、橡胶单和治疗巾或一次性臀垫、医嘱卡、洗手液
	3. 评估产妇:①产妇情况;②会阴部卫生、皮肤情况,有无留置尿管;③产妇配合程度
	4. 环境:温度、光线适宜,利于保护产妇隐私
操作步骤	1 准备并检查物品,携带用物至床旁
	2. 核对产妇,告知目的,评估并指导产妇,嘱咐产妇排尿
	3. 遮挡产妇
	4. 洗手、戴口罩
	5. 铺一次性臀垫于臀下
	6. 协助产妇取屈膝仰卧位,双膝屈曲向外分开
	7. 脱去对侧裤腿,盖在近侧腿部,并盖上浴巾,对侧腿用盖被遮盖,暴露会阴部
	8. 夹消毒棉球于弯盘内
	9. 将另一弯盘置于两腿间
	10. 两只手各持一把镊子,其中一把用于夹取无菌的消毒棉球,另一把接过棉球进行擦洗
	11. 擦洗顺序:会阴伤口—尿道口和阴道口—小阴唇—大阴唇—阴阜—大腿内侧1/3—会阴体至肛门,由内向外、自上而下。擦2~3遍,直至擦净
	12. 每个棉球限用1次,将用过的棉球放于弯盘内
	13. 干棉球擦干,顺序同前
	14. 撤去用物,协助产妇穿好裤子,整理床单位及用物,交代注意事项并记录
	15. 洗手
注意事项	1. 注意保护产妇隐私
	2. 注意擦洗顺序
	3. 注意观察产妇的反应

微课

课件

练习题及参考答案

（张艳亭）

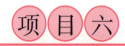

妊娠期并发症妇女的护理（Nursing of Women with Pregnancy Complications）

项目描述

正常妊娠时，胚胎着床在宫腔的适当部位，并继续生长发育，至足月时临产分娩。若胚胎种植在宫腔以外，胚胎或胎儿在宫内生长发育的时间过短或过长，母体出现各种妊娠特有的脏器损害，即为妊娠期并发症。

Childbearing is usually considered a normal process. However, problems can occur during the pregnancy that alter its normal course. Concurrent disorders related solely to pregnancy are called gestational related complications.

任务一 自然流产（Abortion）

工作情景

某女士，30岁，孕11周，出现阵发性下腹痛，阴道排出一大块肉样组织，继而阴道大量出血。目前贫血貌，体温37.2 ℃。妇科检查：宫口已开，有组织堵塞宫口，子宫较孕周略小。

①请列举该患者最可能的临床诊断。②请明确该患者主要的护理问题。③根据目前的情况对患者进行正确的护理。

任务内容

凡妊娠不足28周、胎儿体重不足1 000 g而终止者，称为流产。流产发生于妊娠12周以前者称为早期流产，发生在妊娠12周至不足28周者称为晚期流产。流产又分为自然流产和人工流产，本节内容仅阐述自然流产。自然流产的发生率占全部妊娠的10%～15%，其中80%以上为早期流产。

◆能叙述自然流产的定义及主要病因。

◆能描述自然流产的临床表现并能为患者提供对症护理措施。

【概要】

1. 病因　导致流产的主要原因包括胚胎因素、母体因素、胎盘因素、环境因素。

2. 病理　流产是妊娠物逐渐从子宫壁剥离,然后排出子宫。在妊娠早期,胎盘绒毛发育尚不成熟,与子宫蜕膜联系尚不牢固,因此在妊娠8周以内发生的流产,妊娠产物多数可以完整地从子宫壁分离而排出,出血不多。妊娠8~12周时,胎盘绒毛发育茂盛,与底蜕膜联系较牢固,此时若发生流产,妊娠产物往往不易完整分离排出,常有部分组织残留宫腔内影响子宫收缩,致使出血较多,且经久不止。妊娠12周后,胎盘已完全形成,流产时往往先有腹痛,然后排出胎儿、胎盘。

3. 临床表现　停经、腹痛及阴道出血是流产的主要临床症状。在流产发展的各个阶段,其症状发生的时间、程度也不同。一般流产的发展过程如下。

(1) 先兆流产　先兆流产表现为停经后先出现少量阴道流血,量比月经量少,有时伴有轻微下腹痛或腰背痛。妇科检查:子宫大小与停经周数相符,子宫颈口未开,胎膜未破,妊娠产物未排出。经休息及治疗后,若流血停止或腹痛消失,妊娠可继续进行;若流血增多或腹痛加剧,则可能发展为难免流产。

(2) 难免流产　难免流产由先兆流产发展而来,流产已不可避免。表现为阴道流血量增多,阵发性腹痛加重。妇科检查:子宫大小与停经周数相符或略小,子宫颈口已扩张,但组织尚未排出;晚期难免流产还可有羊水流出或见胚胎组织或胎囊堵于子宫口。

(3) 不全流产　不全流产由难免流产发展而来,妊娠产物已部分排出体外,尚有部分残留于宫内,从而影响子宫收缩,致使阴道出血持续不止,严重时可引起出血性休克。妇科检查:子宫小于停经周数,子宫颈口已扩张,不断有血液自子宫颈口内流出,有时尚可见胎盘组织堵塞于子宫颈口或部分妊娠产物已排出于阴道内,而部分仍留在宫腔内,有时子宫颈口已关闭。

(4) 完全流产　妊娠产物已完全排出,阴道出血逐渐停止,腹痛随之消失。妇科检查:子宫接近正常大小或略大,子宫颈口已关闭。

(5) 稽留流产　又称过期流产,是指胚胎或胎儿已死亡滞留在宫腔内尚未自然排出者。胚胎或胎儿死亡后,子宫不再增大反而缩小,早孕反应消失,若已至妊娠中期,孕妇不感腹部增大,胎动消失。妇科检查:子宫小于妊娠周数,子宫颈口关闭。听诊不能闻及胎心。

(6) 复发性流产　复发性流产指同一性伴侣连续发生3次及3次以上的自然流产。复发性流产大多数为早期流产,少数为晚期流产。早期复发性流产常见原因为胚胎染色体异常、免疫功能异常、黄体功能不全、甲状腺功能减退等;晚期复发性流产常见原因为子宫解剖异常、自身免疫异常等。

(7) 流产合并感染　流产过程中,若阴道流血时间过长、有组织残留于宫腔内或是非法堕胎等,有可能引起宫腔内感染,严重时感染可扩展到盆腔、腹腔乃至全身,并发盆腔炎、腹膜炎、败血症及感染性休克等。

4. 处理原则　不同类型的流产其相应的处理原则亦不同。先兆流产的处理原则是卧床休息,禁止性生活,减少刺激,必要时给予对胎儿危害小的镇静剂。对于黄体功能不足的孕妇,按医嘱每日肌内注射黄体酮(即孕酮)20 mg,以利于保胎,并注意及时进行超声检查,了解胚胎发育情况,避免盲目保胎。难免流产一旦确诊,应尽早使胚胎及胎盘组织完全排出,以防止出血和感染。

不全流产一经确诊,应行吸宫术或钳刮术以清除宫腔内残留组织。完全流产若无感染征象,一般不需特殊处理。稽留流产时应及时促使胎儿和胎盘排出,以防死亡胎儿及胎盘组织在宫腔内稽留日久发生严重的凝血功能障碍。对于复发性流产,在明确病因学诊断后有针对性地给予个性化治疗。流产合并感染的治疗原则为控制感染的同时尽快清除宫内残留物。

Etiology

The main causes of abortion include embryonic factors, maternal factors, placental factors and environmental factors.

Pathology

Hemorrhage into the deciduas basalis and necrotic changes in the tissues adjacent to the bleeding usually accompany abortion. The ovum becomes detached, and this stimulates uterine contractions that result in expulsion. When the sac is opened, fluid is commonly found surrounding a small macerated fetus, or alternatively there may be no visible fetus in the sac, the so-called blighted ovum.

Clinical Classification and Manifestation

Almost invariably the first symptom is bleeding, and the accompanying clinical symptoms are pelvic cramping and low back pain. Spontaneous abortions can be further subdivided based on the signs and symptoms presented.

- Threatened abortion: Vaginal bleeding or spotting occurring in early pregnancy that mayor may not be associated with mild cramps; closed cervix; the process may abate or result in an abortion.

- Inevitable abortion: The above process has progressed such that termination of the pregnancy can not be prevented; bleeding is moderate to copious; uterine cramping is moderate to severe; the membranes may or may not have ruptured; the cervical canal is dilating.

- Incomplete abortion: Part of the products of conception has been passed, but part (usually the placenta) is retained in the uterus; heavy bleeding usually persists until the retained products of conception have been passed; uterine cramping is severe; the cervix is open, with tissue present.

- Complete abortion: All of the products of conception have been expelled; bleeding is slight; uterine cramping is mild.

- Missed abortion: Missed abortion occurs when the fetus dies but is retained in the uterus. When the fetus dies, the early symptoms of pregnancy disappear. The condition may be discovered because fundal height fails to increase, or fetal heart tones are absent.

- Recurrent spontaneous: Abortion recurrent spontaneous abortion usually is defined as three or more spontaneous abortions.

- Septic abortion: A septic abortion is an abortion that is complicated by infection. Infection can happen after a spontaneous abortion, particularly if products of conception are still present. The woman has symptoms of fever and cramp abdominal pain, and her uterus feels tender to palpation. Left untreated, such an infection can lead to toxic shock syndrome, septicemia, kidney failure, and death.

Principle of Management

The pregnant woman should contact her physician or midwife whenever bleeding occurs during pregnancy. The client may be kept at home, and bed rest and sexual abstinence may be prescribed. Occasionally, sedatives are ordered to promote relaxation. If bleeding becomes copious and is accompanied by cramps or uterine contractions, hospitalization may be recommended. IV therapy for fluid replacement or blood transfusions is prescribed as necessary.

【护理评估】

1. 健康史　护士应详细询问孕妇的停经史、早孕反应情况,尤其是阴道流血及腹痛情况。此外,还应全面了解既往病史,以识别发生流产的诱因。

2. 身心状况

(1)一般状况　护士应全面评估孕妇的各项生命体征,判断流产类型,尤其注意与贫血及感染相关的征象。

(2)妇科检查　在消毒条件下进行妇科检查,进一步了解子宫颈口是否扩张、羊膜是否破裂、有无妊娠产物堵塞于子宫颈口内;子宫大小与停经周数是否相符、有无压痛等,并应检查双侧附件有无肿块、增厚及压痛等。

(3)心理状况　流产孕妇的心理状况常以焦虑和恐惧为特征,护士应注意评估。

3. 辅助检查

(1)实验室检查　连续测定血 hCG、人胎盘催乳素、孕激素等动态变化,有助于妊娠诊断和预后判断。

(2)B 型超声显像　超声显像可显示有无胎囊、胎动、胎心等,从而可诊断并鉴别流产及其类型,指导正确处理。

【护理诊断】

1. 有感染的危险　与阴道流血时间过长、宫腔内有残留组织等因素有关。

2. 焦虑　与担心胎儿健康等因素有关。

【护理措施】

1. 先兆流产孕妇的护理　先兆流产孕妇需卧床休息,减少各种刺激,遵医嘱给孕妇适量镇静剂、孕激素等。随时评估孕妇病情变化,如是否腹痛加重、阴道流血量增多等。此外,护士还应注意观察孕妇的情绪反应,加强心理护理。

2. 妊娠不能再继续者的护理　护士应积极采取措施,以及时做好终止妊娠的准备,协助医生完成手术过程,使妊娠产物完全排出,同时建立静脉通路,做好输液、输血准备。并严密监测孕妇的生命体征,观察其腹痛、阴道流血及与休克有关征象。

3. 预防感染　护士应监测患者的体温、血常规及阴道流血、分泌物特征,并严格执行无菌操作规程,加强会阴部护理,指导孕妇维持良好的卫生习惯。当发现感染征象应及时报告医生,并按医嘱进行抗感染处理。

4. 心理护理　由于失去胎儿,孕妇往往会出现伤心、悲哀等情绪反应。护士应给予同情和理解,帮助患者及家属接受现实,顺利度过悲伤期。

Interventions are based on the type of abortion, prognosis, and identified nursing diagnoses. If the client is at home, she is generally placed on restricted activity, and should be instructed to stay in bed, eat a well-balanced diet, save for inspection all perineal pads and all tissue and clots passed, and avoid coitus for 2 weeks following the last incidence of bleeding.

If the client requires hospitalization, nursing care focuses on stabilizing the client. The nurse plays a primary role in reinforcing explanations given by the physician or midwife; monitoring the client's status, including vital signs, amount of bleeding, and comfort level; facilitating diagnostic tests, and preparing the patient for ultrasound or procedures as necessary.

【健康教育】

护士应与孕妇及家属共同讨论此次流产的原因,并向他们讲解流产的相关知识,帮助他们为再次妊娠做好准备。有复发性流产史的孕妇,指导其在下次妊娠确诊后应卧床休息,加强营养,禁止性生活,补充维生素 C、维生素 B、维生素 E 等,治疗期必须超过以往发生流产的妊娠月份。病因明确者,应鼓励患者积极接受对因治疗。

任务实施

列表比较不同类型流产异同点(表 6-1)。

表 6-1　不同类型流产的异同点

流产类型	出血量	下腹痛	组织排出	子官颈口	子官大小	处理原则
先兆流产						
难免流产						
不全流产						
完全流产						
稽留流产						

任务二　异位妊娠(Ectopic Pregnancy)

工作情景

某妇女,28 岁,停经 44 d,在抬重物时突感右下腹剧烈疼痛,伴阴道流血半日。查体:BP 100/50 mmHg,WBC $9.0×10^9$/L,妇科检查见阴道内有少许暗红色血,子官颈举痛明显,后穹隆饱满。

①请列举该患者可能的临床诊断。②请明确该患者主要的护理问题。③根据目前的情况对患者进行正确的护理。

任务内容

受精卵在子官体腔外着床发育时,称为异位妊娠,习称官外孕。异位妊娠以输卵管妊娠最常见(约占 95%),此外还包括卵巢妊娠、腹腔妊娠、子官颈妊娠及阔韧带妊娠等。本节主要阐述输卵管妊娠。

任务目标

◆ 能叙述异位妊娠的定义、病因、临床表现及处理原则。
◆ 能提出异位妊娠患者存在的护理问题并提供相应护理措施。

【概要】

输卵管妊娠是妇产科常见急腹症之一,发病率为 2%～3%,是早期妊娠孕妇死亡的主要原因。

当输卵管妊娠流产或破裂时,可引起腹腔内严重出血,如不及时诊断、处理,可危及生命。输卵管妊娠以壶腹部妊娠最多见,约占78%,其次为峡部、伞部妊娠,间质部妊娠少见(图6-1)。

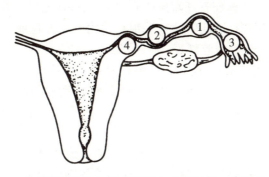

1.壶腹部妊娠;2.峡部妊娠;3.伞部妊娠;4.间质部妊娠。

图6-1　输卵管妊娠的发生部位

1.病因　任何妨碍受精卵正常进入宫腔的因素均可造成输卵管妊娠,包括:输卵管炎症、输卵管发育不良或功能异常、受精卵游走、辅助生殖技术,以及其他如内分泌失调、神经精神功能紊乱、输卵管手术等。

2.病理　输卵管妊娠时,由于输卵管管腔狭窄、管壁薄、蜕膜形成差,受精卵植入后,不能适应孕卵的生长发育,因此当输卵管妊娠发展到一定程度,可出现以下结果。

(1)输卵管妊娠流产　输卵管妊娠流产多见于输卵管壶腹部妊娠,发病多在妊娠8～12周。由于输卵管妊娠时管壁形成的蜕膜不完整,发育中的囊胚常向管腔内突出生长,最终突破包膜而出血,导致囊胚与管壁分离(图6-2),若整个囊胚剥离落入管腔并经输卵管逆蠕动排入腹腔,即形成输卵管完全流产,出血一般不多。若囊胚剥离不完整,有一部分组织仍残留于管腔,则为输卵管不完全流产。此时,管壁肌层收缩力差,血管开放,持续反复出血,量较多,血液凝聚在直肠子宫陷凹,造成盆腔积血和血肿,量多时甚至流入腹腔。

(2)输卵管妊娠破裂　输卵管妊娠破裂多见于输卵管峡部妊娠,发病多在妊娠6周左右。当囊胚生长时绒毛侵蚀管壁的肌层及浆膜,以致穿破浆膜,形成输卵管妊娠破裂(图6-3)。由于输卵管肌层血管丰富,输卵管妊娠破裂所致的出血远较输卵管妊娠流产严重,短期内即可发生大量腹腔内出血使孕妇发生休克,亦可反复出血,形成盆腔及腹腔血肿。

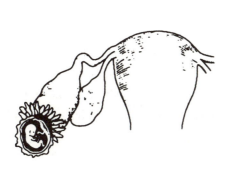

图6-2　输卵管妊娠流产

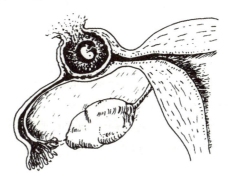

图6-3　输卵管妊娠破裂

(3)陈旧性异位妊娠　有时发生输卵管妊娠流产或破裂后未及时治疗,或内出血已逐渐停止,病情稳定,时间过久,胚胎死亡或被吸收。但长期反复内出血形成的盆腔血肿可机化变硬,并与周围组织粘连,临床上称为"陈旧性宫外孕"。

(4)继发性腹腔妊娠 发生输卵管妊娠流产或破裂后,胚胎被排入腹腔,大部分死亡,不会再生长发育。但偶尔也有存活者,若存活胚胎的绒毛组织仍附着于原位或排至腹腔后重新种植而获得营养,可继续生长发育形成继发性腹腔妊娠。

(5)持续性异位妊娠 近年来,对输卵管妊娠行保守性手术机会增多,若术中未完全清除妊娠物,或残留有存活滋养细胞而继续生长,致术后 β-hCG 不下降或反而上升,称为持续性异位妊娠。

3.临床表现 输卵管妊娠的临床表现与受精卵着床部位、有无流产或破裂、出血量多少及时间长短等有关。

(1)停经 多数患者停经6~8周以后出现不规则阴道流血,但有20%～30%的患者因月经仅过期几天而不认为是停经,或误将异位妊娠时出现的不规则阴道流血误认为月经,可能无停经史主诉。

(2)腹痛 腹痛是输卵管妊娠患者就诊的主要症状,占95%。输卵管妊娠未发生流产或破裂前,常表现为一侧下腹隐痛或酸胀感。输卵管妊娠流产或破裂时,患者突感一侧下腹部撕裂样疼痛,常伴有恶心、呕吐。若血液局限于病变区,主要表现为下腹部疼痛,当血液积聚于直肠子宫陷凹,可出现肛门坠胀感。随着血液由下腹部流向全腹,疼痛亦遍及全腹,血液刺激膈肌,可引起肩胛部放射性疼痛及胸部疼痛。

(3)阴道流血 60%～80%患者会出现阴道流血。胚胎死亡后导致血 hCG 下降,卵巢黄体分泌的激素不能维持蜕膜生长而发生剥离出血,常有不规则阴道流血,色暗红或深褐,量少呈点滴状,一般不超过月经量。少数患者阴道流血量较多,类似月经。阴道流血可伴有蜕膜管型或蜕膜碎片排出,系子宫蜕膜剥离所致。阴道流血常在病灶除去后方能停止。

(4)晕厥与休克 由于腹腔内急性出血及剧烈腹痛,轻者出现晕厥,严重者出现失血性休克。出血量越多越快,症状出现越迅速越严重,但与阴道流血量不成正比。

(5)腹部包块 当输卵管妊娠流产或破裂后所形成的血肿时间过久,可因血液凝固,逐渐机化变硬并与周围器官(子宫、输卵管、卵巢、肠管等)发生粘连而形成包块。

4.处理原则 以手术治疗为主,其次是药物治疗。

(1)手术治疗 应在积极纠正休克的同时,进行手术抢救。根据情况行患侧输卵管切除术或保留患侧输卵管及其功能的保守性手术。

(2)药物治疗 根据中医辨证论治方法,合理运用中药,或用中西医结合的方法,如用化疗药物甲氨蝶呤来抑制滋养细胞增生、破坏绒毛,使胚胎组织坏死、脱落、吸收。

Etiology

A tubal pregnancy may be caused by any condition that narrows the tube or brings about some constriction within it. The following conditions may produce such a narrowing of the fallopian tube: previous pelvic inflammatory disease, previous inflammatory processes of the external peritoneal surfaces of the tube, endometriosis of the tubal wall and lumen, developmental abnormalities resulting in a segmental narrowing of the tubes or excessive length or kinking, previous abdominal or tubal surgery with resultant scarring and adhesions, and previous tubal sterilization.

Pathology

The frequency of tubal abortion depends in part upon the implantation site. Tubal abortion is common in ampullary tubal pregnancy, whereas rupture is the usual outcome with isthmic pregnancy.

● Tubal abortion: The immediate consequence of tubal hemorrhage is further disruption of the connection between the placenta and membranes and the tubal wall. If placental separation is complete, all of the products of conception may be extruded through the fimbriated end into the peritoneal cavity. At this point, hemorrhage may cease and symptoms eventually disappear. Some bleeding usually persists as long as products remain in the oviduct. Blood slowly trickles from the tubal fimbria into the peritoneal cavity and typically pools in the rectouterine cul – de – sac. After incomplete tubal abortion, pieces of the placenta or membranes may remain attached to the tubal wall and, after becoming surrounded by fibrin, give rise to a placental polyp. The process is similar to that in the uterus after an incomplete abortion.

• Tubal rupture: When the fertilized ovum is implanted well within the interstitial portion, rupture usually occurs later. Rupture is usually spontaneous, but it may be caused by trauma associated with coitus or a bimanual examination. With intraperitoneal rupture, the entire conceptus may be extruded from the tube, or if the rent is small, profuse hemorrhage may occur without extrusion. In either event, the woman commonly shows signs of hypovolemia.

• Abdominal pregnancy: If only the fetus is extruded at the time of rupture, the effect upon the pregnancy will vary depending on the extent of injury sustained by the placenta. The fetus dies if the placenta is damaged appreciably, but if the greater portion the placenta retains its tubal attachment, further development is possible. The fetus may then survive for some time, giving rise to an abdominal pregnancy.

Clinical Signs and Symptoms

• Amenorrhea: The woman may at first exhibit the usual early signs of pregnancy and consider herself to be normally pregnant. About a fourth of women do not report amenorrhea; they mistake uterine bleeding that frequently occurs with tubal pregnancy for true menstruation.

• Abdominal pain: Within 3 – 5 weeks after a missed menstrual period, abdominal pain often develops. Pain is the predominant symptom of tubal rupture and may be localized on one side or felt over the entire abdomen. The woman may complain of cramping or sharp, sudden, knifelike pain, often of extreme severity.

• Vaginal bleeding: Vaginal bleeding, which occurs when the embryo dies and the deciduas begins to slough, often appears scant and dark brown, and may be intermittent or continuous.

• Shock and syncope: Hypovolemic shock is a major concern because systemic signs of shock may be rapid and extensive without external bleeding. Women with a ruptured ectopic pregnancy may often present with hypovolemia and shock.

• Pelvic mass: In some cases, there is gradual disintegration of tubal wall followed by slow leakage of blood into the lumen, peritoneal cavity, or both. Gradually, however, trickling blood collects in the pelvis, more or less walled off by adhesions, and a pelvic hematocele results.

Principle of Management

The therapeutic goal of medical management is early diagnosis of ectopic pregnancy based on a detained health history, physical examination, and selected diagnostic tests. Once the diagnosis is made, surgery is usually necessary. If the woman has no history of infertility and no gross evidence of previous salpingitis, a salpingotomy, salpingostomy, or segmental resection and anastomosis may be performed.

【护理评估】

1. 健康史　应仔细询问患者月经史, 以准确推断停经时间。注意不要将不规则阴道流血误认为末次月经。此外, 对不孕、放置宫内节育器、行绝育术、行输卵管复通术、盆腔炎等与发病相关的高危因素予以高度重视。

2. 身心状况　注意评估阴道流血、腹痛及有无休克征象,同时应注意密切观察患者的表现和倾听其诉求。

(1)腹部检查　输卵管妊娠流产或破裂者,下腹部有明显压痛和反跳痛,尤以患侧为甚,轻度腹肌紧张;出血多时,叩诊有移动性浊音;若出血时间较长,形成血凝块,在下腹可触及软性肿块。

(2)盆腔检查　输卵管妊娠未发生流产或破裂者,除子宫略大较软外,仔细检查可能触及胀大的输卵管并有轻度压痛。输卵管妊娠流产或破裂者,阴道后穹隆饱满,有触痛。将子宫颈轻轻上抬或左右摇动时引起剧烈疼痛,称为子宫颈举痛或摇摆痛,是输卵管妊娠的主要体征之一。子宫稍大而软,腹腔内出血多时检查子宫呈漂浮感。

3. 辅助检查

(1)阴道后穹隆穿刺　是一种简单可靠的诊断方法,适用于疑有腹腔内出血的患者。用长针头自阴道后穹隆刺入直肠子宫陷凹,抽出暗红色不凝血为阳性。

(2)妊娠试验　放射免疫法测血中 hCG,尤其是动态观察血 β-hCG 的变化对诊断异位妊娠极为重要,测出异位妊娠的阳性率一般可达 80% ~ 90% 。

(3)超声检查　阴道 B 型超声检查较腹部 B 型超声检查准确性高。异位妊娠的声像特点:宫腔内无妊娠囊,附件区可见轮廓不清的液性或实性包块,内见胚囊或胎心搏动。若结合临床表现及 hCG 测定,对诊断的帮助更大。

(4)腹腔镜检查　适用于输卵管妊娠尚未流产或破裂的早期患者和诊断有困难的患者。

【护理诊断】

1. 疼痛　与输卵管妊娠破裂所致的腹膜炎和腹腔内出血有关。

2. 预感性悲哀　与妊娠失败有关。

【护理措施】

1. 接受手术治疗患者的护理

(1)积极做好术前准备　腹腔镜是近年治疗异位妊娠的主要方法,多数输卵管妊娠可在腹腔镜直视下穿刺输卵管的妊娠囊吸出部分囊液或切开输卵管吸出胚胎,并注入药物;也可以行输卵管切除术。护士在严密监测患者生命体征的同时,配合医生积极纠正患者休克症状,做好术前准备。对于严重内出血并发现休克的患者,护士应立即建立静脉通路,交叉配血,做好输血、输液的准备,以便配合医生积极纠正休克、补充血容量,并按急诊手术要求迅速做好术前准备。

(2)提供心理支持　护士术前向患者及家属解释并解答疑虑,减少和消除患者的紧张、恐惧心理,协助患者接受手术治疗方案。术后,护士应帮助患者以正常的心态接受此次妊娠失败的现实,并向她们讲述异位妊娠的有关知识。

2. 接受非手术治疗患者的护理

(1)严密观察病情　护士需密切观察患者的一般情况、生命体征,并重视患者的主诉,尤应注意阴道流血量与腹腔内出血量不成比例。护士应告诉患者病情发展的一些指征,如出血增多、腹痛加剧、肛门坠胀感明显等,以便当患者病情发展时,医患均能及时发现,给予相应处理。

(2)加强化学药物治疗的护理　化疗一般采用全身用药,也可采用局部用药。在用药期间,应用 B 型超声检查和监测 β-hCG 水平进行严密监护,并注意患者的病情变化及药物毒副反应。

(3)指导患者休息与饮食　患者应卧床休息,避免腹部压力增大,从而减少异位妊娠破裂的机会。此外,护士还应指导患者摄取足够的营养物质,尤其是富含铁蛋白的食物。

(4)监测治疗效果　护士应协助正确留取血标本,以监测治疗效果。

For the patient with a suspected ectopic pregnancy, the nurse should explain the various diagnostic tests and provide support. When acute rupture of a fallopian tube occurs, the situation presents a surgical emergency requiring nursing care aimed at combating shock. An IV infusion is maintained so that blood can be administered as needed to replace losses from the hemorrhage and surgery.

Postoperatively, vital signs should be carefully monitored, fluid replacement administered, and intake and output recorded. Oral intake of foods and fluids should be avoided until bowel function has returned to normal. Early ambulation is encouraged. The nurse must accurately record and assess vaginal bleeding and perineal pad count, continuously-monitoring the client for signs and symptoms of hemorrhage. The surgical site may require special care and dressings. Patients are often given broad-spectrum antibiotics prophylactically.

Emotional care is directed toward facilitating effective coping by encouraging the patient and her family to verbalize their feelings. Information about the causes of ectopic pregnancy may assist them in resolving feelings of guilt and self-blame.

【健康教育】

输卵管妊娠的预后在于防止输卵管的损伤和感染,因此护士应做好患者的健康指导工作,防止发生盆腔感染。教育患者保持良好的卫生习惯,勤洗浴、勤换衣,性伴侣稳定。发生盆腔炎后须立即彻底治疗,以免延误病情。另外,由于输卵管妊娠者中约10%再发和50%~60%不孕,因此,护士需告诫患者,下次妊娠时要及时就医,并且不宜轻易终止妊娠。

任务实施

列表比较流产与异位妊娠临床表现异同点(表6-2)。

表6-2　流产与异位妊娠临床表现异同点

	流产	异位妊娠
停经		
腹痛		
阴道流血		
休克		
盆腔检查		
超声检查		
阴道后穹隆穿刺		

任务三 妊娠期高血压疾病（Hypertensive Disorders of Pregnancy）

工作情景

某初产妇,29 岁,G_1P_0,孕 37 周,头痛、视物不清 2 d,因今日症状加重收入院。查体:血压 140/95 mmHg,脉搏 90 次/min,呼吸 20 次/min,尿蛋白(+)。胎心率 130 次/min,有不规律宫缩。

①请明确该患者主要的护理问题。②根据目前的情况对患者进行正确的护理。

任务内容

妊娠期高血压疾病是妊娠与血压升高并存的一组疾病,发生率为 5%～12%。该组疾病包括妊娠高血压、子痫前期、子痫,以及高血压并发子痫前期和妊娠合并高血压,严重影响母婴健康,是孕产妇及围产儿病死率升高的主要原因之一。

任务目标

◆ 能叙述妊娠期高血压疾病的定义、病因、临床表现及处理原则。
◆ 能提出妊娠期高血压疾病患者存在的护理问题并提供相应护理措施。

【概要】

1.病因　妊娠期高血压疾病的发病原因至今尚未阐明。目前有关病因和发病机制的主要学说有以下几种。

(1)免疫学说　妊娠被认为是成功的自然同种异体移植。从免疫学观点出发,妊娠期高血压疾病病因是胎盘某些抗原物质免疫反应的变态反应,与移植免疫的观点很相似。但与免疫的复杂关系有待进一步证实。

(2)子宫-胎盘缺血缺氧学说　临床发现妊娠期高血压疾病易发生于初产妇、多胎妊娠者、羊水过多者。本学说认为是由于子宫张力增高,影响子宫血液供应,造成子宫-胎盘缺血缺氧。此外,全身血液循环不能适应子宫-胎盘需要的情况,如孕妇有严重贫血、慢性高血压、糖尿病等亦易伴发本病。

(3)血管内皮功能障碍　研究发现,妊娠期高血压疾病者细胞毒性物质和炎症介质含量增高,而前列环素、维生素 E、血管内皮素等减少,诱发血小板凝聚,并对血管紧张因子敏感,血管收缩致使血压升高,并且导致一系列病理变化。此外,气候寒冷、精神紧张也是本病的主要诱因。

(4)营养缺乏及其他因素　据流行病学调查,妊娠期高血压疾病的发生可能与钙缺乏有关。妊娠易引起母体缺钙,导致妊娠期高血压疾病发生,而孕期补钙可使妊娠期高血压疾病的发生率下降,但其发生机制尚不完全清楚。另外,以白蛋白缺乏为主的低蛋白血症及锌、硒等的缺乏与子痫前期的发生发展有关。此外,其他因素(如胰岛素抵抗、遗传等)与妊娠期高血压疾病发生的关系亦有所报道。

2.病理生理　本病的基本病理生理变化是全身小动脉痉挛。小动脉痉挛造成管腔狭窄,周围阻力增大,内皮细胞损伤,通透性增加,体液和蛋白质渗漏,表现为血压上升、蛋白尿、水肿和血液浓缩等。全身各组织器官因缺血、缺氧而受到不同程度损害,严重时脑、心、肝、肾及胎盘等的病理生理变化可导致患者抽搐、昏迷、脑水肿、脑出血、心肾衰竭、肺水肿、肝细胞坏死及被膜下出血,以及胎盘绒毛退行性变、出血和梗死,胎盘早期剥离及凝血功能障碍而导致弥散性血管内凝血(DIC)等。主要病理生理变化简示如下(图6-4)。

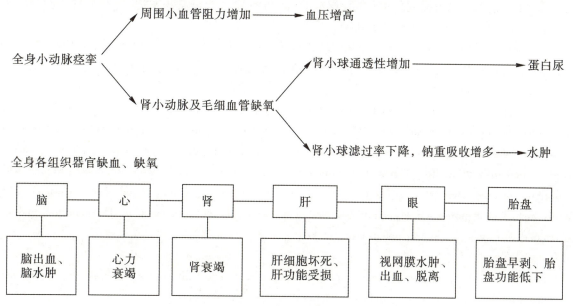

图6-4　妊娠期高血压疾病的病理生理变化

3. 临床表现及分类　妊娠期高血压疾病有以下分类。

(1)妊娠高血压　妊娠期首次出现血压≥140/90 mmHg,并于产后12周内恢复正常;尿蛋白(-);患者可伴有上腹部不适或血小板减少,产后方可确诊。

(2)子痫前期　妊娠20周后出现血压≥140/90 mmHg;尿蛋白≥0.3 g/24 h或随机尿蛋白(+)。

子痫前期出现以下任何一项表现可诊断为重度子痫前期:①血压≥160/110 mmHg和(或)舒张压≥110 mmHg(卧床休息,两次测量间隔时间至少4 h)。②肝功能损害,血清转氨酶水平为正常值2倍以上。③肾功能损害,血肌酐水平大于1.1 mg/dL或为正常值2倍以上。④血小板<10×10⁹/L。⑤肺水肿。⑥新发生的中枢神经系统异常或视觉障碍。妊娠34周以前发病者为早发型子痫前期。

(3)子痫　在子痫前期的基础上出现不能用其他原因解释的抽搐,或伴昏迷,称为子痫。子痫典型发作过程:先表现为眼球固定,瞳孔散大,头扭向一侧,牙关紧闭,继而口角及面部肌肉颤动,数秒后全身及四肢肌肉强直(背侧强于腹侧),双手紧握,双臂伸直,发生强烈的抽动。抽搐时呼吸暂停,面色发绀。持续1 min左右,抽搐强度减弱,全身肌肉松弛,随即深长吸气而恢复呼吸。抽搐期间患者意识丧失。病情转轻时,抽搐次数减少,抽搐后很快苏醒,但有时抽搐频繁且持续时间较长,患者可陷入深昏迷状态。抽搐过程中易发生唇舌咬伤、摔伤甚至骨折等多种创伤,昏迷时呕吐可造成窒息或吸入性肺炎。

(4)高血压并发子痫前期　高血压孕妇于妊娠20周以前无蛋白尿,若孕20周后出现尿蛋白≥0.3 g/24 h,或妊娠20周后突然出现尿蛋白增加、血压进一步升高,或血小板减少(<100×10⁹/L)。

(5)妊娠合并高血压　妊娠前或妊娠20周前血压≥140/90 mmHg,但妊娠期无明显加重;或妊娠20周后首次诊断高血压并持续到产后12周以后。

4. 处理原则　治疗目的是控制病情、延长孕周、尽可能保障母儿安全。处理原则主要为休息、解痉、镇静,有指征地降压、利尿,密切监测母胎情况,适时终止妊娠。根据病情轻重,进行个体化治疗。

(1)妊娠高血压 加强孕期检查,密切观察病情变化,注意休息,调节饮食,采取左侧卧位,以防发展为重症。

(2)子痫前期 患者需要住院治疗,积极处理,防治发生子痫及并发症。治疗原则为解痉、降压、镇静,合理扩容及利尿,适时终止妊娠。

(3)子痫 子痫是本疾病最严重的阶段,直接关系到母儿安危,应积极处理。处理原则:控制抽搐,纠正缺氧和酸中毒,在控制血压、抽搐的基础上终止妊娠。一般抽搐控制后即可考虑终止妊娠。

Risk Factors

Although the cause of hypertensive disorders of pregnancy (HDP) is not understood, several factors are known to increase a woman's risk. HDP tends to occur more frequently in primiparas younger than age 20 years or older than 40 years; women from a low socioeconomic background (perhaps because of poor nutrition); women with multifetal gestation; women with hydramnios; women who are obese; women with underlying disease such as diabetes mellitus, chronic hypertension, chronic renal disease; women with family history of hypertension, especially her mother or sister who had preeclampsia. The condition may be associated with poor calcium or magnesium intake.

Pathology

HDP is systemic peripheral vascular spasm, which affects almost all organs. The vascular spasm may be caused by the action of prostaglandins (notably decreased prostacyclin and increased thromboxane). Increased cardiac output may injure endothelial cells of the arteries, leading to spasm. Normally, blood vessels during pregnancy are resistant to the effects of pressor substances such as angiotensin and norepinephrine so blood pressure remains normal during pregnancy. With hypertension of pregnancy, this reduced responsiveness to blood pressure changes appears to be lost. Vasoconstriction occurs, and blood pressure increases dramatically.

The cardiac system is overwhelmed because the heart is forced to pump against rising peripheral resistance. This reduces the blood supply to organs, most markedly the kidney, liver, brain, and placenta.

Classification and Clinical Manifestation

• Hypertension in pregnancy: Blood pressure first appeared at 140/90 mmHg during pregnancy and returned to normal within 12 weeks postpartum; urinary protein (−); patients with upper abdominal discomfort or thrombocytopenia.

• Preeclampsia: Blood pressure ≥ 140/90 mmHg after 20 weeks of gestation; urinary protein ≥ 0.3 g/24 h or random urinary protein (+).

Severe preeclampsia can be diagnosed with any of the following manifestations. ①Blood pressure ≥ 160/110 mmHg and/or diastolic blood pressure ≥110 mmHg. ②Liver function damage: the level of serum transaminase was more than 2 times of normal value. ③ Impairment of renal function: the level of serum creatinine was more than 1.1 mg/dL or more than 2 times of the normal value. ④Platelets < 10×10^9/L. ⑤Pulmonary edema. ⑥New central nervous system abnormality or visual impairment. Early onset preeclampsia was diagnosed before 34 weeks of gestation.

• Eclampsia: The presence of convulsions on preeclampsia that cannot be explained by other causes, or accompanied by coma. It is divided into prenatal eclampsia, intrapartum eclampsia, and postpartum eclampsia.

The typical attack process of eclampsia: First, the eyes are fixed, the pupils dilated, the head twisted to one side, the teeth are closed, then the mouth and facial muscles tremble, and after a few seconds, whole-body muscle rigidity appears (dorsal stronger than ventral), the hands are clasped, the arms are straight, and strong convulsions occur with apnea. The convulsions last for about 1 min, and then the intensity of convulsions is weakened, the muscles of the whole body are relaxed, and then the patient have the deep inspiration and recovery of breathing. The patient lost consciousness during convulsions. In mild cases, the number of convulsions decreases and recovery occurs soon after convulsions, but sometimes the convulsions are frequent and long lasting, and the patient may fall into a deep coma. In the process of convulsion, many kinds of trauma such as lip and tongue bite, fall and even fracture are easy to occur. Vomiting in coma can cause asphyxia or aspiration pneumonia.

- Chronic hypertension complicated with preeclampsia: Hypertensive pregnant women had no proteinuria before 20 weeks of gestation, and the urine protein ≥0.3 g/24 h after 20 weeks of gestation, or a sudden increase in urinary protein after 20 weeks of gestation, or a further increase in blood pressure, or thrombocytopenia < $100×10^9$/L.

- Pregnancy complicated with chronic hypertension: Blood pressure ≥ 140/90 mmHg before pregnancy or 20 weeks of pregnancy, but no obvious aggravation during pregnancy; or hypertension was first diagnosed after 20 weeks of gestation and continued after 12 weeks postpartum.

Principle of Management

- Mild HDP: If mild symptoms of the disease develop, the client may remain at home and be examined at twice a week. The treatment plan includes the following: restriction of activities, administration of prescribed sedative drugs as necessary; ingestion of a well-balanced diet with ample protein.

- Moderate and severe HDP: The patient is usually hospitalized to prevent convulsions with an anti-convulsant, control the blood pressure within a safe range with an antihypertensive agent, keep sedation, make volume replacement reasonably, use diuretic as necessary, and terminate the pregnancy in good time. The goal of management is to prevent eclampsia and other severe complications while allowing the fetus to mature.

【护理评估】

1. 健康史　详细询问患者于孕前及妊娠 20 周前有无高血压、蛋白尿和(或)水肿及抽搐等征象,既往病史中有无原发性高血压、慢性肾炎及糖尿病等,有无家族史。此次妊娠经过,出现异常现象的时间及治疗经过,特别应注意有无头痛、视力改变、上腹不适等症状。

2. 身心状况　典型的患者表现为妊娠 20 周后出现高血压、水肿、蛋白尿。根据病变程度不同,不同临床类型的患者有相应的临床表现。在评估过程中应注意以下几个方面。

(1)初测血压有升高者,需休息 1 h 后再测,方能正确反映血压情况。同时不要忽略测得血压与其基础血压的比较。而且也可经过翻身试验进行判断,即在患者左侧卧位时测血压直至血压稳定后,嘱其翻身仰卧位 5 min 再测血压,若仰卧位舒张压较左侧卧位≥20 mmHg,提示有发生子痫前期的倾向,其阳性预测值为 33%。

(2)留取 24 h 尿进行尿蛋白检查。凡 24 h 尿蛋白定量≥0.3 g 者为异常。

(3)注意评估妊娠后期水肿发生的原因是否由妊娠期高血压疾病所致。

(4)患者出现头痛、眼花、胸闷、恶心、呕吐等自觉症状时提示病情的进一步发展,即进入子痫前期阶段,护士应高度重视。

(5)抽搐与昏迷是最严重的表现,护士应特别注意发作状态、频率、持续时间、间隔时间、神志情况及有无唇舌咬伤、摔伤,甚至骨折、窒息或吸入性肺炎等。

患者的心理状态与病情的轻重、病程的长短、患者对疾病的认识、自身的性格特点及社会支持系统的情况有关,护士应针对患者及家属的心理状态,提供不同程度的心理支持及疏导。

3. 辅助检查

(1)尿常规检查 根据尿蛋白定量结果确定病情严重程度;根据镜检出现管型判断肾功能受损情况。

(2)血液检查 包括测定血红蛋白、血细胞比容、血浆黏度、全血黏度以了解血液浓缩程度。重症患者应测定血小板计数、凝血时间,必要时测定凝血酶原时间、纤维蛋白原和鱼精蛋白副凝试验(3P 试验)等,以了解有无凝血功能异常。

(3)肝、肾功能测定 如进行丙氨酸氨基转移酶、血尿素氮、肌酐、尿酸等测定。

(4)眼底检查 眼底视网膜小动脉变化是反映妊娠期高血压疾病严重程度的一项重要参考指标。眼底检查可见眼底小动脉痉挛,动静脉管径比例可由正常的 2∶3 变为 1∶2,甚至 1∶4,或出现视网膜水肿、渗出、出血,甚至视网膜脱离,暂时性失明。

(5)其他检查 如心电图、超声心动图、胎盘功能、胎儿成熟度检查等,可视病情而定。

【护理诊断】

1. 组织灌注量改变 与妊娠期高血压疾病致血管痉挛有关。

2. 有(胎儿)受伤的危险 与胎盘灌注不足有关。

3. 有(孕母)受伤的危险 与妊娠期高血压疾病及其治疗或并发症的影响有关。

【护理措施】

1. 妊娠期高血压疾病的预防指导

(1)加强孕期教育 护士应重视孕期健康教育工作,使患者及家属了解妊娠期高血压疾病的知识及其对母儿的危害,从而促使患者自觉于妊娠早期开始接受产前检查,并主动坚持定期检查,以便及时发现异常,以及时得到治疗和指导。

(2)进行休息及饮食指导 患者应采取左侧卧位休息以增加胎盘绒毛血供,保持心情愉快。护士应指导孕妇合理饮食,减少过量脂肪和盐的摄入,增加蛋白质、维生素及富含铁、钙、锌的食物摄入。可从妊娠 20 周开始,每天补充钙剂 1～2 g,可降低妊娠期高血压疾病的发生概率。

2. 一般护理

(1)保证休息 轻度妊娠期高血压疾病患者可住院也可在家休息,但建议子痫前期患者住院治疗。保证充分的睡眠,每日休息不少于 10 h。在休息和睡眠时,以左侧卧位为宜。

(2)调整饮食 轻度妊娠期高血压疾病患者需摄入足够的蛋白质(100 g/d 以上)、维生素、铁和钙剂。食盐量不必严格限制,因为长期低盐饮食可引起低钠血症,对母儿均不利。但全身水肿的患者应限制食盐摄入量。

(3)密切监护母儿状态 护士应询问患者是否出现头痛、视力改变、上腹不适等症状。每日测体重及血压,每日或隔日复查尿蛋白。定期监测血压、胎儿发育状况和胎盘功能。

(4)间断吸氧 可增加血氧含量,改善全身主要脏器和胎盘的氧供。

3. 用药护理 硫酸镁为目前治疗子痫前期和子痫的首选解痉药物,护士应明确硫酸镁的用药方法、毒性反应及注意事项。

(1)用药方法 硫酸镁可肌内注射或静脉给药。

1)肌内注射:25% 硫酸镁溶液 20 mL(5 g),臀部深部肌内注射,1～2 次/d。通常于用药 2 h 后血药浓度达高峰,且体内浓度下降缓慢,作用时间长,但局部刺激性强,注射时应使用长针头行深部肌内注射,也可加利多卡因于硫酸镁溶液中,以缓解疼痛刺激。注射后用无菌棉球或创可贴覆盖针孔,防止注射部位感染,必要时可行局部按揉或热敷,促进肌肉组织对药物的吸收。

2)静脉给药:25%硫酸镁溶液20 mL+10%葡萄糖注射液20 mL,静脉注射,5～10 min内推注完;或25%硫酸镁溶液20 mL+5%葡萄糖注射液200 mL,静脉滴注(1～2 g/h),4次/d。静脉用药后可使血中浓度迅速达到有效水平,用药后约1 h血药浓度可达高峰,停药后血浓度下降较快,但可避免肌内注射引起的不适。

基于不同用药途径的特点,临床多采用两种方式互补长短,以维持体内有效浓度。为了保证患者夜间更好的睡眠,可在睡眠前停用静脉给药,改为肌内注射1次。

(2)毒性反应　硫酸镁的治疗浓度和中毒浓度相近,因此在进行硫酸镁治疗时应严密观察其毒性作用,并认真控制硫酸镁的入量。通常主张硫酸镁的滴注速度以1～2 g/h为宜,24 h不超过25 g,用药时限一般不超过5 d。硫酸镁过量会使呼吸及心肌收缩功能受到抑制甚至危及生命。中毒现象首先表现为膝反射减弱或消失,随着血镁浓度的增加可出现全身肌张力减退及呼吸抑制,严重者心搏可突然停止。

(3)注意事项　护士在用药前及用药过程中均应监测患者血压,同时还应检测以下指标:①膝反射必须存在;②呼吸不少于16次/min;③尿量每24 h不少于400 mL,或每小时不少于17 mL。尿少提示排泄功能受抑制,镁离子易积蓄而发生中毒。由于钙离子可与镁离子争夺神经元上的同一受体,阻止镁离子的继续结合,因此应随时备好10%的葡萄糖酸钙注射液,以便出现毒性作用时及时予以解毒。10%的葡萄糖酸钙10 mL缓慢(5～10 min内推注完)静脉注射,必要时可每小时重复用药1次,直至呼吸、排尿和神经抑制恢复正常,但24 h内不超过8次。

4.子痫患者的护理

(1)协助医生控制抽搐　患者一旦发生抽搐,应尽快控制。硫酸镁为首选药物,必要时可加用强有力的镇静药物。

(2)专人护理,防止受伤　子痫发生后,首先应保持呼吸道通畅,并立即给氧,用开口器或于上、下磨牙间放置一缠好纱布的压舌板,用舌钳固定舌以防咬伤唇舌或舌后坠的发生。患者取头低侧卧位,以防黏液吸入呼吸道或舌头阻塞呼吸道,也可避免发生低血压综合征。必要时用吸引器吸出喉部黏液或呕吐物,以免窒息。在患者昏迷或未完全清醒时,禁止给予饮食和口服药,以防误入呼吸道而致吸入性肺炎。

(3)减少刺激,以免诱发抽搐　患者应安置于单人暗室,保持绝对安静,以避免声、光刺激。一切治疗活动和护理操作尽量轻柔且相对集中,避免干扰患者。

(4)严密监护　密切注意患者血压、脉搏、呼吸、体温及尿量,记录出入量。及时进行必要的血、尿化验和特殊检查,以及早发现脑出血、肺水肿、急性肾衰竭等并发症。

(5)为终止妊娠做好准备　子痫发作后患者多自然临产,应严密观察及时发现产兆,并做好母儿抢救准备。如经治疗病情得以控制仍未临产者,应在患者清醒后24～48 h内引产,或子痫患者经药物控制后6～12 h,考虑终止妊娠。护士应做好终止妊娠的准备。

5.妊娠期高血压疾病患者的产时及产后护理　妊娠期高血压疾病患者的分娩方式应根据母儿的情形而定。

(1)若决定经阴道分娩,需加强各产程护理　在第一产程中,应密切监测患者的血压、脉搏、尿量、胎心、子宫收缩情况及有无自觉症状;血压升高时应及时与医生联系。在第二产程中,应尽量缩短产程,避免产妇用力,初产妇可行会阴侧切并用产钳或胎吸助产。在第三产程中,必须预防产后出血,在胎儿前肩娩出后立即静脉注射缩宫素,禁用麦角新碱,以及时娩出胎盘并按摩宫底,观察血压变化,重视患者的主诉。

（2）建立静脉通路,测量血压　病情较重者于分娩开始即建立静脉通路。胎儿娩出后测患者血压,病情稳定后方可送回病房。在产褥期仍需继续监测血压,产后48 h内应至少每4 h测1次血压。

（3）继续硫酸镁治疗,加强用药护理　重症患者产后应继续硫酸镁治疗1~2 d,产后24 h至5 d内仍有发生子痫的可能,故不可放松治疗及护理。此外,产前未发生抽搐的患者产后48 h亦有发生的可能,故产后48 h内仍应继续硫酸镁的治疗和护理。使用大量硫酸镁的患者,产后易发生子宫收缩乏力,恶露较常人多,因此应严密观察子宫复旧情况,严防产后出血。

During the prenatal period, the nurse should instruct all women about the importance of maintaining a well–balanced diet high in protein intake. In addition, all pregnant women should know the warning signs of HDP, which they should immediately report to the nurse or physician.

The woman manifesting early symptoms of HDP who is managed at home on modified activity or bed rest should be encouraged to position herself frequently in the left lateral position. BP should be monitored regularly by the community health nurse or trained family member.

If symptoms of HDP remain evident or progress, the client is likely to be admitted to the hospital. In establishing a therapeutic hospital atmosphere, the nurse should see that the environment is as comfortable and pleasant as possible. The nurse should see that the equipment necessary for safe and efficient care of the client is immediately available in the client's room and is in good working order. Equipment for catheterization and administration of appropriate medications should be readily available. Frequent observations are made for progressive symptoms or changes in condition, with special attention to visual disturbances, headaches, and epigastric pain. Urine should be tested for protein, using a clean – catch, midstream specimen.

Other necessary supplies for the care of the HDP woman may include padded side rails, suction apparatus for aspirating mucus, and equipment for administering oxygen, in case cyanosis or depressed respiration indicate the need. An emergency medication tray should be immediately accessible, including items such as $MgSO_4$, calcium gluconate ($MgSO_4$ antagonist), sodium bicarbonate, hydralazine, and epinephrine.

Because serious side effects may occur with $MgSO_4$ administration, it is essential for the nurse to monitor urinary output, deep tendon reflexes, and respiratory rate prior to, during, and after $MgSO_4$ administration. Mg^{2+} serum levels are drawn every 6 h.

【健康教育】

对妊娠期高血压患者,应进行饮食指导并嘱其注意休息,以左侧卧位为主,加强胎儿监护,自数胎动,掌握自觉症状,加强产前检查,定期接受产前保护措施。对子痫前期患者,应使患者学会识别不适症状及用药后的不适反应,还应掌握产后的自我护理方法,加强母乳喂养的指导。同时,注意家属的健康教育,使孕妇得到心理和生理的支持。

任务四　早产(Preterm Labor)

任务内容

早产是指妊娠满28周至不满37足周之间分娩。此时娩出的新生儿称为早产儿,出生体重多在1 000～2 499 g,各器官发育尚不够成熟。据统计,早产儿中约有15%于新生儿期死亡,而且,围产儿死亡中与早产有关者占75%,防止早产是降低围产儿死亡率的重要环节之一。

任务目标

◆能叙述早产的定义、病因、临床表现及护理措施。
◆能分析早产患者的健康需求,针对性提供健康教育。

【概要】

1.病因　①孕妇因素:孕妇如合并感染性疾病(尤其性传播疾病),子宫畸形,子宫肌瘤,急、慢性疾病及妊娠并发症时易诱发早产。②胎儿、胎盘因素:胎膜早破、绒毛膜羊膜炎、子宫过度膨胀以及胎盘因素如前置胎盘、胎盘早期剥离等,均可致早产。

2.临床表现　早产的临床表现主要是子宫收缩,最初为不规则宫缩,常伴有少许阴道血性分泌物或出血。胎膜早破的发生较足月临产多,继之可发展为规律有效宫缩,与足月临产相似,使子宫颈管消失和宫口扩张。

3.处理原则　若胎儿存活,无胎儿窘迫、胎膜未破,通过休息和药物治疗控制宫缩,尽量维持妊娠至足月;若胎膜已破,早产已不可避免时,则应尽可能地预防新生儿合并症以提高早产儿的存活率。

Etiology

There are certain conditions to be associated with the initiation of preterm labor:uterine overdistention by conditions such as polyhydramnios and twins, uterine anomalies, history of uterine surgery, fetal anomalies,maternal infections such as asymptomatic bacteriuria (almost twice the risk of entering preterm labor as women without bacteria in their urine),cocaine, smoking, psychological stress, long employment hours,and fatigue.

Clinical Signs and Symptoms

Preterm labor has three defining characteristics:onset of labor after 28 weeks and before 37 weeks,regular uterine contractions occurring once or more every 10 min for 1 h, and cervical change (dilatation is less than 3 cm).

Principle of Management

Indications for inhibition of labor include factors that prove the necessity for prolonging the in utero time. If the decision is made to attempt to halt the labor,a combination of supportive and pharmacologic interventions will probably be implemented.

【护理评估】

1.健康史　详细评估可致早产的高危因素,如孕妇以往有流产、早产史或本次妊娠期有阴道流血则发生早产的可能性大,应详细询问并记录患者既往出现的症状及接受治疗的情况。

2. 身心状况　妊娠满28周后至37周前出现有明显的规律宫缩(至少1次/10 min)伴有子宫颈管缩短,可诊断为先兆早产。如果妊娠28～37周,出现20 min≥4次且每次持续≥30 s的规律宫缩,并伴随子宫颈管缩短≥75%,子宫颈进行性扩张2 cm以上者,可诊断为早产临产。

早产已不可避免时,患者常会不自觉地把一些相关的事情与早产联系起来而产生自责感;由于妊娠结果的不可预知,恐惧、焦虑、猜疑也是早产孕妇常见的情绪反应。

3. 辅助检查　通过全身检查及产科检查,结合阴道分泌物的生化指标检测,核实孕周,评估胎儿成熟度、胎方位等;观察产程进展,确定早产的进程。

【护理诊断】

1. 有窒息的危险　与早产儿发育不成熟有关。

2. 焦虑　与担心早产儿预后有关。

【护理措施】

1. 药物治疗的护理　先兆早产的主要治疗为抑制宫缩,与此同时,还要积极控制感染、治疗合并症和并发症。护理人员应能明确具体药物的作用和用法,并能识别药物的毒副作用,以避免毒性作用的发生,同时,应对患者做相应的健康教育。常用抑制宫缩的药物有以下几类。

(1) β肾上腺素受体激动剂　其作用为激动子宫平滑肌β受体,从而抑制宫缩。此类药物的副作用为心率加快、血压下降、血糖增高、血钾降低、恶心、出汗、头痛等。常用药物:利托君、沙丁胺醇等。

(2) 硫酸镁　镁离子直接作用于肌细胞,使平滑肌松弛,抑制子宫收缩。首次量为5 g,加入25%葡萄糖注射液20 mL中,在5～10 min内缓慢注入静脉(或稀释后半小时内静脉滴注),以后以每小时2 g静脉滴注,宫缩抑制后继续维持4～6 h后改为每小时1 g,直到宫缩停止后12 h。使用硫酸镁时,应密切观察患者有无中毒迹象。

(3) 钙通道阻滞剂　阻滞钙离子进入肌细胞而抑制宫缩。常用硝苯地平10 mg舌下含服,每6～8 h 1次。用药时必须密切监测患者心率及血压的变化,对已用硫酸镁者应慎用,以防血压急剧下降。

(4) 前列腺素合成酶抑制剂　前列腺素有刺激子宫收缩和软化子宫颈的作用,其抑制剂则有减少前列腺素合成的作用,从而抑制宫缩。常用药物有吲哚美辛、阿司匹林等。但此类药物可通过胎盘抑制胎儿前列腺素的合成与释放,可能导致胎儿动脉导管过早关闭而造成胎儿血液循环障碍,因此,临床已较少用。必要时仅在孕34周前短期(1周内)选用。

2. 预防新生儿合并症的发生　在保胎过程中,应每日进行胎心监护,教会患者自数胎动,有异常时及时采取应对措施。对妊娠35周前的早产者,在分娩前按医嘱给予患者糖皮质激素如地塞米松、倍他米松等,可促胎肺成熟,明显降低新生儿呼吸窘迫综合征的发病率。

3. 为分娩做准备　若早产已不可避免,应尽早决定合理分娩的方式,如臀位、横位,估计胎儿成熟度低,而产程又需较长时间者,可选用剖宫产术结束分娩;经阴道分娩者,应考虑使用产钳和会阴切开术以缩短产程,从而减少分娩过程中对胎头的压迫。同时,充分做好早产儿保暖和复苏的准备,临产后慎用镇静剂,避免发生新生儿呼吸抑制的情况;产程中应给患者吸氧;新生儿出生后,立即结扎脐带,防止过多母血进入胎儿循环造成循环系统负荷过重。

4. 为患者提供心理支持　护士可安排时间与患者进行开放式的讨论,让患者了解早产的发生并非她的过错,有时甚至是无缘由的。但也要避免为减轻患者的负疚感而给予过于乐观的保证。由于早产是出乎意料的,患者多没有精神和物质准备,对产程中的孤独感、无助感尤为敏感,因此,家人和护士在身旁提供支持较足月分娩更显重要,并能帮助患者重建自尊,以良好的心态承担早产儿母亲的角色。

The woman with preterm labor and her family can be expected to have a high level of anxiety. Support from a primary nurse who can be with them through the admission process and provide information about what is and will be happening can be helpful in allaying their anxiety. Bed rest in the side-lying position and adequate hydration, either orally or intravenously, are usually instituted while the decision on further treatment is being made. An intake and output record should be kept. Comfort measures as with any labor should be used, and analgesic medications should be avoided or kept to a minimum.

Care of the Woman Receiving Tocolytic Therapy

The nurse plays an important role in the care of the client receiving a tocolyticagent by IV infusion. The nurse is usually responsible for starting the IV and preparing the infusion. The protocol varies with the institution, the doctor's orders, and the drug to be used. The solution should be administered with the use of an infusion pump so the dosage can be carefully titrated. If uterine contractions are successfully inhibited, the woman may be put on oral maintenance therapy. The initial oral dose should be given 30 minutes before the IV ritodrine is discontinued. Vital signs should be taken every 2 h for the first 24 h, then every 4 h. Uterine activity and side effects also should be monitored.

Home Monitoring and Care

When a client is being monitored at home, nursing responsibilities include daily evaluation and reporting of uterine activity, responses to treatment, and general health. The client is given a schedule for when to attach her monitor and transmit electronically the information, enabling the nursing service to "observe" her uterine activity at various points throughout the day. If they see increased uterine activity, they contact her physician regarding appropriate orders for tocolysis or the need for an office of hospital examination. The nurse also educates the client about monitoring, pregnancy nutrition, and stress management.

【健康教育】

孕妇良好的身心状况可减少早产的发生,突然的精神创伤亦可诱发早产。因此,应做好孕期保健工作,指导孕妇加强营养,保持平静的心情。避免诱发宫缩的活动,如抬举重物、性生活等。高危孕妇必须多卧床休息,以左侧卧位为宜,以增加子宫血液循环,改善胎儿供氧。慎做肛查、阴道检查等,积极治疗合并症,子宫颈内口松弛者应于孕14~16周或更早些时间做子宫内口缝合术,防止早产的发生。

任务五　过期妊娠(Post Term Pregnancy)

任务内容

平时月经周期规律,妊娠≥42周(≥294 d)尚未分娩,称为过期妊娠,其发生率占妊娠总数的3%~15%。近年来由于对妊娠超过41周孕妇的积极处理,过期妊娠的发生率明显下降。

任务目标

◆ 能叙述过期妊娠的定义、病因、临床表现及护理措施。

◆ 能分析过期妊娠患者的健康需求，提供针对性健康教育。

【概要】

1. 病因　确切病因不清楚。过期妊娠的发生可能与胎盘分泌雌激素功能缺陷有关。雌激素缺乏降低了子宫对缩宫素的敏感性，进而发生过期妊娠。

2. 病理

(1)胎盘　过期妊娠的胎盘病理有两种类型，即胎盘功能正常、胎盘功能减退。

(2)羊水　妊娠42周后羊水量迅速减少约30%，减至300 mL以下；羊水粪染率明显增高，是足月妊娠的2~3倍，若同时伴有羊水过少，羊水粪染率达71%。

(3)胎儿　过期妊娠胎儿生长模式与胎盘功能有关，可分以下3种。

1)正常生长及巨大胎儿：胎盘功能正常者，能维持胎儿继续生长，约25%成为巨大胎儿。

2)胎儿过熟综合征：过熟儿表现出过熟综合征的特征性外貌，与胎盘功能减退、胎盘血流灌注不足、胎儿缺氧及营养缺乏等有关。典型表现为皮肤干燥、松弛、起皱、脱皮，身体瘦长，胎脂消失，容貌似"小老人"。因为羊水减少和胎粪排出，胎儿皮肤黄染，羊膜和脐带呈黄绿色。

3)胎儿生长受限：小样儿可与过期妊娠共存，后者更增加胎儿的危险性，约1/3过期妊娠死产儿为生长受限小样儿。

3. 对母儿的影响

(1)对围产儿影响　除上述胎儿过熟综合征外，胎儿窘迫、胎粪吸入综合征、新生儿窒息及巨大胎儿等围产儿疾病发病率及死亡率均明显增高。

(2)对母体影响　产程延长和难产率增高，使手术产率及母体产伤明显增加。

4. 处理原则　妊娠40周以后胎盘功能逐渐下降，42周以后明显下降，因此，在妊娠41周以后，即应考虑终止妊娠，尽量避免过期妊娠。若妊娠41周后无任何并发症(妊娠期高血压疾病、妊娠糖尿病、胎儿生长受限、羊水过少等)，也可密切观察，继续等待。一旦妊娠过期，则应终止妊娠。终止妊娠的方式应根据胎儿安危状况、胎儿大小、子宫颈成熟度综合分析，恰当选择。

Etiology

The actual physiologic cause of post term pregnancy is still obscure. There is some evidence that a placental estrogen deficiency may be a possible cause.

Pathology

• Placental dysfunction：When the placenta ages, depositing fibrin and calcium, intervillous hemorrhagic infarcts occur and basal membrane of the placental blood vessels thickens and degenerates, affecting diffusion of oxygen. These changes have been noted in the post term placenta.

• Amniotic fluid：Decreased amniotic fluid, or oligohydramnios, is the factor most frequently associated with post term pregnancy. Decreased amniotic fluid below 400 mL can reduce the cushioning effect of the fluid. As a result it becomes far more likely that the fetus will entrap or compress its own cord, shutting off blood flow to and from itself for intermittent intervals.

Meconium contamination：When the fetus is post term, the expulsion of meconium into the already diminished volume of amniotic fluid causes the meconium to thicken, inhibits the normal antibacterial properties of the amniotic fluid and promotes stiffening of the cord.

Maternal, Fetal and Neonatal Effects

- Fetal and neonatal effects: The increase risk for macrosomia, fetal hypoxia, meconium aspiration syndrome, hypoglycemia, polycythemia, birth injury.
- Maternal effects: It includes physical exhaustion and the increase cesarean delivery risk.

Principle of Management

Women should be informed of the benefits and risks of induction of labor and expectant management. The woman's preferences should be considered in the plan of management. Individualize the plan of care with the goal of not pushing nature too soon, but do not allow variables to develop that will decrease tolerance to labor, such as decreased, meconium-stained amniotic fluid, a hard fetal head, and macrosomia.

【护理评估】

1. 健康史　应仔细询问患者停经史、早孕反应及胎动出现时间,准确核实妊娠周数。

2. 身心状况　注意观察患者胎动及羊水量的变化,评估是否有胎儿窘迫、胎动减少等情况。发生过期妊娠时,患者和家属常常表现出惊慌、焦虑,应注意观察患者的表现和倾听其诉求。

3. 辅助检查　根据超声检查核实妊娠周数;根据胎动情况、电子胎心监护及超声检查判断胎儿宫内安危状况。

【护理诊断】

1. 有母体与胎儿双方受干扰的危险　与羊水过少、异常分娩等有关。

2. 焦虑　与担心胎儿安危及预后有关。

【护理措施】

1. 减少恐惧感　鼓励患者及其家属表达愤怒、挫折、极度疲惫的感觉及对胎儿情况的担心。与患者和家属讨论预产期的意义,预产期只是一个月的中位数,在这个月中90%的产妇会分娩。在做胎心监护时,提供机会让产妇听胎心、看胎心率的反应。

2. 促进胎儿气体交换

(1)产前　告知患者数胎动的方法及其重要意义,告知患者及家属医疗计划的内容(包括每周1次子宫颈评分、评价子宫颈成熟度)及其原因。通过做胎儿监护,评估胎儿窘迫的征兆。让患者做好配合各种医疗干预(如引产、产钳分娩或剖宫产)的准备。

(2)产时　谨慎使用镇痛剂和镇静剂,使用连续胎心监护,以及早发现胎儿窘迫的征兆。为分娩做准备,随时做好剖宫产和产钳终止分娩的准备,同时做好新生儿窒息抢救配合的准备。胎膜破裂时,评估胎心率,注意羊水的量和颜色变化。出现胎儿窘迫时,应及时通知医生。

3. 减少胎儿损伤　使用超声诊断方法排除巨大儿,使用产程图及早发现因大于胎龄儿或因胎儿颅骨过熟而造成的难产。如果出现羊水粪染,通知新生儿科工作人员到场,做好新生儿窒息抢救配合的准备工作。人工破膜时发现羊水粪染,胎心监护发现胎心基线异常或出现变异减速、晚期减速,或胎心变异消失,应及时通知医生。

Alleviating Fear

Encourage the patient and her family to openly express their anger, frustrations, feelings regarding the extreme fatigue, and fears related to fetal well-being. Provide opportunities for the patient to listen to the fetal heart rate (FHR) and see evidence of FHR reactivity during fetal surveillance studies.

Maintaining Fetal Gas Exchange

During antepartum, instruct the patient about the importance of weekly cervical examinations and how to assess for daily-fetal activity. Assess for signs of fetal compromise by carrying out the ordered fetal surveillance studies. Prepare the patient for potential medical interventions. During intrapartum, use pain medications and sedatives very cautiously. Use continuous fetal monitoring to recognize early evidence of a nonreassuring FHR change.

Alleviating Fetal Injury

Assist with ultrasound to rule out macrosomia. Graph the labor against the normal labor curve to detect early signs of labor dystocia related to large-for-gestational-age fetus or advanced bone maturation of the fetal skull. Notify pediatric personnel for presence during delivery if meconium is noted in the amniotic fluid. Confirm findings with the attending physician if meconium is noted on amniotomy. Also notify the physician if there is a nonreassuring change in the FHR baseline, nonreassuring decelerations are noted, or loss of variability develops. In the presence of a nonreassuring FHR pattern, meconium in the amniotic fluid is a critically important sign.

【健康教育】

①教会患者自测胎动。②加强宣教,使患者及家属认识过期妊娠的危害。③行母乳喂养相关知识指导。

微课　　　　　　　课件　　　　　练习题及参考答案

（张艳亭）

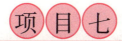

项目七

胎儿及附属物异常妇女的护理
（Nursing of Fetal and appendage abnormalities）

项目描述

妊娠是一个复杂的生理过程,妊娠期受各种内、外因素的影响,可能会出现一些影响母体和胎儿健康的异常状况,如多胎妊娠、巨大胎儿、胎儿窘迫及新生儿窒息、前置胎盘、胎盘早剥、羊水量异常、胎膜早破等胎儿及附属物的异常。

Pregnancy is a complex physiological process, and it is affected by a variety of internal and external factors. Some abnormal conditions will affect the health of the mother and fetus, such as multiple pregnancy, giant fetus, fetal distress and neonatal asphyxia, placenta previa, placenta abruption, amniotic fluid, premature rupture of membranes and other fetal and accessory abnormalities.

任务一　多胎妊娠（Multiple Pregnancy）

工作情景

患者,26 岁,G_2P_0,双胎,妊娠 24 周,因近 2 d 肚皮时常发紧来院就诊。体格检查:各项生命体征正常,心肺听诊无异常。产科检查:宫高脐上三横指(27 cm),腹围 90 cm,胎心正常。

①请明确该患者主要的护理问题。②根据目前的情况对患者进行正确的护理。

任务内容

一次妊娠宫腔内同时有两个或两个以上胎儿为多胎妊娠。临床上以双胎妊娠多见。

任务目标

◆能叙述双胎妊娠的分类及特点、临床表现及处理原则。
◆能对双胎妊娠者进行正确评估。

【概要】

1. 分类

（1）双卵双胎　由两个卵子分别受精而形成的双胎妊娠，约占双胎妊娠的 2/3。两个胎儿的遗传基因不同，其性别、血型、容貌可相同或不同。胚胎各自形成胎盘和胎囊，两者血液互不相通，胎盘可紧贴在一起似融合，但两个胎囊之间隔有两层羊膜和两层绒毛膜，有时两层绒毛膜可融为一层。

（2）单卵双胎　由一个受精卵分裂而形成的双胎妊娠，约占双胎妊娠的 1/3。两个胎儿的遗传基因相同，其性别、血型相同，容貌相似。多数为共同的胎盘，两个胎儿血液循环相通。根据受精卵发生分裂的时间不同，形成双羊膜囊双绒毛膜、双羊膜囊单绒毛膜、单羊膜囊单绒毛膜、连体双胎 4 种类型。

2. 临床表现　妊娠期早孕反应较重。体重增加迅速，子宫增大明显。妊娠晚期常有呼吸困难、活动不便、胃部胀满、食欲减退等不适，孕妇感到极度疲劳和腰背部疼痛，常出现下肢水肿、静脉曲张等。

3. 处理原则　双胎妊娠易引起妊娠期高血压疾病、妊娠期肝内胆汁淤积症、贫血、胎膜早破及早产、产后出血、胎儿发育异常、双胎输血综合征、选择性生长受限等并发症，应按照高危妊娠进行管理。预产期前提前住院待产，根据孕妇的健康情况、胎儿大小、胎方位、产道情况等选择合适的分娩方式，并积极预防产后出血。

Clinical Signs and Symptoms

Women with multiple pregnancy have severe morning sickness, significantly enlarged uterus, and gain weight rapidly. In the third trimester of pregnancy, women with multiple pregnancy usually experience breathing difficulties, stomach fullness, loss of appetite, extreme fatigue, back pain, lower limb edema, varicose veins and other discomforts.

Principle of Management

Because of the prenatal and perinatal risk, early diagnosis is very important. The mother needs to be monitored carefully during the prenatal period, and should be hospitalized ahead of date of delivery. A decision about the route of delivery must be made, it should be taken into account the maternal health status, fetal size, fetal position, and birth canal conditions. Postpartum hemorrhage should be actively prevented.

【护理评估】

1. 健康史　孕妇的年龄、胎次、家族中有无双胎妊娠史，是否因不孕症使用了促排卵药物。本次妊娠经过，孕妇是否出现并发症有关的症状及诊治情况，产前检查情况等。

2. 身心状况　双胎妊娠属于高危妊娠，孕妇常常既喜悦，又担心母儿的安危，表现出紧张、焦虑的状态。询问其早孕反应程度，有无呼吸不畅、食欲减退、焦虑等。评估有无下肢水肿、静脉曲张及表现程度。子宫底高度大于正常孕周，妊娠中晚期腹部可触及两个胎头及多个肢体，在腹部不同部位可听到两个不同速率的胎心音，每分钟相差 10 次以上，或其间隔有无音区。

3. 辅助检查　B 型超声检查于妊娠 6 周后可见宫腔内有两个原始心管搏动。妊娠中晚期可筛查胎儿结构畸形如连体双胎、开放性神经管畸形。B 型超声检查还可确定两个胎儿的胎方位。

【护理诊断】

1. 营养失调：低于机体需要量　与营养摄入不足，满足不了双胎发育需要有关。

2. 潜在并发症　如早产、妊娠期高血压疾病、前置胎盘、胎盘早剥、产后出血等。

【护理措施】

1.一般护理　嘱孕妇加强产前检查,多休息,尤以左侧卧位为宜。妊娠晚期多卧床,减少活动,禁止性生活,尽量避免胎膜早破与早产。加强营养,少量多餐,补充富含蛋白质、维生素、必需脂肪酸、铁、钙、叶酸的饮食等,预防并发症发生。

2.病情观察　监测孕妇的宫高、腹围、体重,观察胎儿生长发育情况及胎心、胎方位。观察并及时发现双胎妊娠常见的并发症,如早产、妊娠期高血压疾病、前置胎盘、胎盘早剥、羊水过多等。

3.治疗护理　分娩期应督促产妇进食进水、保证睡眠,以保持良好体力。密切观察产程进展、宫缩情况,勤听胎心,做好抢救新生儿的准备。第一个胎儿娩出后,立即断脐,助手协助在腹部固定第二个胎儿为纵产式,注意观察有无脐带脱垂、胎盘早剥等并发症。第一胎娩出后20 min左右,第二个胎儿自然娩出。第二个胎儿娩出后,在产妇腹部放置沙袋加压,防止腹压骤降引起休克,并给予缩宫素肌内注射或静脉滴注预防产后出血。若第一胎娩出后等待15 min仍无宫缩,可行人工破膜并给予低剂量缩宫素静脉滴注,促进子宫收缩。产程中须注意预防胎头交锁或胎头嵌顿。

The mother needs to be monitored more frequently during the prenatal period, and needs frequent rest periods using the side-lying position. Diet is regulated to allow for adequate weight gain, protein, iron and folic acid intake. The latter weeks of a multiple pregnancy are likely to be associated with heaviness of the lower abdomen, back pains and swelling of the feet and ankles. The nurse can be helpful in giving the woman anticipatory guidance regarding these matters during the prenatal period. As with any client, she needs to be taught signs and symptoms of preterm labor.

During labor, steps are taken to ensure a successful outcome for the woman and fetuses. Two staff members with at least one skilled in resuscitation are needed for each fetus at the time of delivery. Fetal heart rates, the uterine contraction and maternal vital signs must be monitored continuously. To accomplish the vaginal delivery of twins, the first twin is delivered either by vertex or assisted breech delivery. The position of the second twin is ascertained, and it is brought into position by a combination of vaginal and abdominal manipulation, 15 min after the first baby is born, if there is a second sac, it is carefully ruptured to allow a slow loss of fluid and to guard against cord prolapse and abruption. A spontaneous or a prophylactic forceps vertex delivery is preferred.

【健康教育】

①指导孕妇加强营养,注意休息及休息体位。②注意观察子宫复旧及恶露的情况,有异常及时就诊。③指导产妇母乳喂养,以及时采取恰当的避孕措施。

任务实施

双胎妊娠管理流程见表7-1。

表7-1　双胎妊娠管理流程

项目	内容
双绒毛膜双胎产检安排	孕22~24周大畸形筛查后,每4周产检1次。B型超声检查直至32周后,每2周检查1次。至36周后,每周检查1次,至38周分娩

续表 7-1

项目	内容
单绒毛膜双胎产检安排	孕 20~22 周大畸形筛查后，每 2 周产检 1 次直至 30 周后。孕 28 周常规促胎肺成熟。30 周后每周产检 1 次至 34 周，情况良好可至 36~37 周分娩。有相关胎儿母体风险因素，适时终止妊娠
超声检测指标	生长监测、最大羊水池深度；两胎儿体重相差大于 10% 或较小胎儿体重小于第 10 百分位，或羊水量>8 cm，<2 cm 则须加测两胎儿的脐动脉、静脉血流，静脉导管血流及大脑中动脉血流
分娩方式选择	可以经阴道分娩，需注意第二胎儿手术产可能 剖宫产指征：①第一胎儿为肩先露、臀先露；②宫缩乏力致产程延长，经保守治疗效果不佳，胎儿窘迫，短时间内不能经阴道结束分娩；③联体双胎孕周>26 周；④严重妊娠并发症需尽快终止妊娠

任务二　胎儿窘迫（Fetal Distress）

工作情景

患者，女，29 岁，G_2P_1，因停经 40^{+2} 周未临产，自觉胎动减少 1 d 入院。平素月经规律，既往体健，无急、慢性病史。孕期如期行产前检查，无异常发现。产科检查：腹围 90 cm，宫高 34 cm，胎方位 ROA，胎心率 145 次/min，先露 S-2，子宫颈口未开，骨盆测量无异常。B 型超声提示胎盘Ⅲ级。家属要求阴道分娩终止妊娠，即采取缩宫素引产。产程进展顺利，子宫颈口开全 1 h 后，胎心率减慢，经吸氧后未改善，胎心率 106 次/min，检查见先露位置 S+3。

①请明确该患者主要的护理问题。②根据目前的情况对患者进行正确的护理。

任务内容

胎儿窘迫是指胎儿在子宫内因缺氧危及其健康与生命的综合症状，发病率为 2.70%~38.5%。临床上分为急性与慢性胎儿窘迫，急性胎儿窘迫主要发生在临产过程中，慢性胎儿窘迫多发生在妊娠晚期。

任务目标

◆ 能叙述胎儿窘迫的分类、临床表现及处理原则。
◆ 能对胎儿窘迫进行正确评估。

【概要】

1. 病因　①母体因素：缺氧性疾病、妊娠并发症、缩宫素使用不当、子宫不协调性收缩、急产、产程延长等。②胎儿因素：宫内肺炎、先天性心血管疾病、母儿血型不合、胎儿畸形、产程延长使胎头受压过久等。③脐带、胎盘因素：脐带脱垂、脐带缠绕是急性胎儿窘迫最常见原因。

2.临床表现

（1）急性胎儿窘迫　常发生在分娩期。

1）胎心率异常：缺氧初期可表现为胎心率加快，胎心率>160 次/min，甚至>180 次/min；缺氧严重时胎心率减慢而不规则，甚至<100 次/min，可出现频繁晚期减速，严重者胎死宫内。

2）胎动异常：缺氧早期胎动频繁，随缺氧程度加重胎动逐渐由强变弱，次数减少甚至消失。胎动消失常常出现在胎心消失之前。

3）羊水胎粪污染：缺氧加重时胎儿迷走神经兴奋，肠蠕动亢进，肛门括约肌松弛，胎粪排出污染羊水。羊水污染分为 3 度：Ⅰ度羊水呈浅绿色、质地稀薄；Ⅱ度羊水呈黄绿色、质地较稠厚；Ⅲ度羊水呈棕黄色、质厚呈糊状。10%～20%的产妇分娩中会出现胎粪污染，因此单纯羊水胎粪污染不是胎儿窘迫的表现。出现羊水胎粪污染时，若伴有胎心异常，提示胎儿窘迫；若继续待产，容易发生胎粪吸入，造成不良胎儿结局。

（2）慢性胎儿窘迫　发生在妊娠晚期，临床常见于妊娠期高血压疾病、胎儿生长受限、羊水过少、过期妊娠等。早期表现为胎动减慢，<10 次/2 h 或减少 50%者提示胎儿缺氧可能。电子胎心监护显示无应激试验（NST）异常。

3.处理原则　急性胎儿窘迫者，在吸氧、改变体位的同时，积极对因治疗，纠正或改善胎儿缺氧状态，并及时终止妊娠。慢性胎儿窘迫者，结合病因、妊娠周数、胎儿成熟度、胎儿缺氧程度等综合考虑，或期待治疗或终止妊娠。

Etiology

- Maternal oxygenation：An inadequate oxygen content of the maternal blood may result from poor gas exchange in the lungs，cardiac failure，or anemia.

- Uterus：The most important factor is abnormal uterine action of the hypertonic type.

- Fetus：There may be distress due to infection，cardiac disorders，anemia.

- Placenta：The most important conditions are pre-eclampsia/eclampsia，chronic，hypertension/renal disease，and diabetes，which may result in some compromise in blood flow.

- Umbilical cord：This is the final supply link to the fetus，and blood flow may be entanglements about the body of the fetus，knotting，presentation，or prolapse.

Clinical Signs and Symptoms

- Changes in fetal heart rate：It is the indicator of acute fetal distress. Tachycardia is the first change observed，but is not constant；a rate over 160 beats/min is indicative of early hypoxia. For bradycardia，the fetal heart rate is less than 100 beats/min，which indicates severe hypoxia.

- Changes in acid base status：The degree of acidosis can be measured quite accurately with the technique of fetal blood sampling（usually scalp）. A value below 7.20 is the indicator of fetal suffering from hypoxia.

- Meconium in the amniotic fluid：The pathological explanation proposes that fetuses pass meconium is response to hypoxia. Meconium passage is due to relaxation of the sphincter anus muscle induced by faulty aeration of the fetal blood. Severe meconium passage is a potential warning of fetal asphyxia.

Principle of Management

Look for possible cause and remove the cause if possible. Repositioning of patient and administration of oxygen to the mother，and timely termination of pregnancy should be ordered.

【护理评估】

1.健康史　了解孕妇年龄、孕产史，是否有吸烟、酗酒、吸毒等不良嗜好，有无内科疾病史，本次妊娠经过是否顺利,是否有妊娠并发症,子宫是否过度膨胀,胎儿有无畸形或生长发育迟缓等。了解分娩过程是否顺利,产程中缩宫素或镇静剂、麻醉剂等是否使用不当。

2.身心状况　评估情绪状态,患者及家属常因担忧胎儿及新生儿的安危而紧张、焦虑不安。了解胎心率、胎动、羊水的量与性状,以判断胎儿窘迫程度。

3.辅助检查

(1)B型超声检查　监测胎心、胎动、羊水、胎儿呼吸运动、胎儿肌张力等。

(2)胎儿电子监护　无应激试验为无反应型,缩宫素激惹试验阳性或分娩过程中出现晚期减速、变异减速,提示胎儿有宫内窘迫。

(3)胎儿头皮血气分析　胎儿头皮血 pH<7.20(正常值为 7.25～7.35),PO_2<10 mmHg(正常值为 15～30 mmHg),PCO_2>60 mmHg(正常值为 35～55 mmHg),可诊断为代谢性酸中毒,提示胎儿危险。

(4)羊膜镜检查　如见羊水浑浊,呈浅绿色、黄绿色或棕黄色,提示有胎儿缺氧的可能。

(5)胎盘功能检查　对慢性胎儿窘迫者,于妊娠晚期测定尿雌三醇(E_3),如 24 h 尿 E_3 值急骤减少 30%～40%,或连续多次<10 mg/24 h,提示胎盘功能减退。

【护理诊断】

1.有胎儿受伤的危险　与子宫胎盘的功能不良致胎儿缺氧有关。

2.焦虑　与担心胎儿宫内安危有关。

3.预感性悲哀　与胎儿可能死亡有关。

【护理措施】

1.一般护理　指导孕妇改变体位,以左侧卧位为宜。急性胎儿窘迫时可用面罩或鼻导管吸氧,氧流量为 10 L/min,每次 30 min,间隔 5 min。

2.病情观察　密切监测胎心,每 15 min 听 1 次,胎膜破裂时注意立即听胎心并观察流出羊水的性状。对于慢性胎儿窘迫者,教会孕妇自我计数胎动,及时进行胎盘功能检查。必要时行胎儿电子监护。

3.心理护理　向孕妇及家属提供相关信息,以减轻他们的焦虑。对于胎儿不幸死亡的,为其安排一个远离其他新生儿和产妇的房间,可让他们为死产婴儿做一些事情,也可以提供孩子的足印卡、床头卡等作纪念。应鼓励他们诉说悲伤,并提供支持性关怀。

4.治疗护理　遵医嘱正确用药,临床常用50%葡萄糖注射液 80～100 mL,维生素 C 0.5～1.0 g 静脉滴注,以提高胎儿对缺氧的耐受力。出现酸中毒时静脉滴注 5% 碳酸氢钠 100～200 mL。因胎儿出生后易发生新生儿窒息,还需做好新生儿窒息复苏术的准备工作。若胎儿缺氧加重或治疗无效,应及时做好阴道助产或剖宫产终止妊娠的护理配合。

Repositioning of patient and administration of oxygen to the mother. Discontinuation of uterine stimulants and correction of uterine hyperstimulation.

Vaginal examination to rule out prolapsed cord. Notification of anesthesia the need for emergency delivery. Monitoring of fetal heart rate by electronic fetal monitoring in the operating room prior to abdominal preparation. If the scalp pH is less than 7.20, fetal monitoring show variable deceleration or late deceleration, fetal heart rate is less than 100 beats/min, or more than 180 beats/min, with meconium in amniotic fluid, immediate delivery is indicated. Request that qualified personnel be in attendance for newborn resuscitation and care.

【健康教育】

①加强产前检查,有高危因素者应酌情增加产前检查次数,提前住院待产。②加强营养,合理饮食,减少孕期糖尿病和贫血的发生。③休息时采取左侧卧位,教会孕妇自我计数监护胎动,发现问题及时到医院诊治。

任务实施

电子胎心监护操作方法见表7-2。

表7-2　电子胎心监护操作方法

项目	内容
操作目的	1. 监测胎儿宫内储备能力
	2. 检测胎心率
评估要点	评估产妇孕周、胎方位,腹部皮肤状况、腹形,有无宫缩、胎动情况
操作准备	1. 产妇准备:协助产妇排空膀胱,取舒适体位
	2. 护士准备:着装整洁规范,仪表端庄大方
	3. 操作用物:胎心监护仪、纸巾、耦合剂,必要时备屏风
操作步骤	1. 核对医嘱
	2. 核对产妇信息(床号、姓名、住院号、床头卡、手腕带),做好解释,取得配合
	3. 洗手,戴口罩,携用物至产妇床旁,再次核对产妇
	4. 根据情况帮助产妇取舒适体位,保护隐私
	5. 暴露腹部,用四步触诊法确定胎儿背的位置
	6. 涂耦合剂在胎心探头上,打开监护仪开关,将胎心探头置于适当部位;宫缩间歇置宫缩探头于子宫底部,腹带固定,松紧适宜,告知产妇胎动探头使用方法及注意事项
	7. 监护20 min,观察监护情况,发现异常告知医生,根据情况酌情延长监护时间
	8. 监护完毕,撤去监护探头,擦净产妇皮肤,帮助产妇取舒适卧位
	9. 关闭监护仪,询问产妇需要,整理床单位,清理用物
	10. 洗手,取口罩,将监护结果报告医生,并粘贴于报告单上。操作时间25 min
指导要点	1. 指导产妇如何正确自测胎动
	2. 指导产妇监测注意事项及配合要点
注意事项	1. 尽量避免仰卧,避免空腹监护,注意保护隐私
	2. 固定带松紧适宜,注意探头是否有滑脱现象,以及时调整部位。每次检测20 min,发现异常可适当延长监护时间,并报告医生
	3. 宫缩探头严禁涂耦合剂

任务三　新生儿窒息（Neonatal Asphyxia）

工作情景

患者,女,26岁,G_1P_0,足月妊娠,腹痛2 h入院。平时月经规律,孕期无异常,平素体健。查体:一般情况可,发育正常,营养中等。心肺(−),肝脾未触及,下肢水肿(+)。产科检查:腹围100 cm,宫高35 cm,LOA,先露S−1,骨盆外测量正常。入院后14 h子宫颈口开全,宫口开全40 min,发现胎心减慢,102次/min,吸氧后无明显改善,即行产钳助产,娩出一女婴,新生儿Apgar评分4分。经紧急复苏抢救后,出生后5 min第二次Apgar评分8分。

①请明确该患者主要的护理问题。②根据目前的情况对患者进行正确的护理。

任务内容

新生儿窒息是指分娩前及分娩过程中的各种因素导致新生儿出生后不能建立正常呼吸,引起缺氧、酸中毒并导致多器官损害的一种病理生理状况。新生儿窒息是胎儿出生后的紧急情况,须立即实施新生儿窒息复苏急救,以降低新生儿死亡率和伤残率。

任务目标

◆ 能叙述新生儿窒息的分类、临床表现及处理原则。
◆ 能对新生儿窒息进行正确评估及护理。

【概要】

1.病因　①胎儿窘迫延续。②呼吸中枢受到抑制或损害:分娩过程中使用镇静剂、麻醉剂不当,使呼吸中枢受抑制;产程延长、阴道助产术操作不当、剖宫产器械损伤等使胎儿脑部长时间缺氧或损伤,发生颅内出血,使呼吸中枢受到损害。③呼吸道阻塞:分娩过程中胎儿吸入黏液、羊水、胎粪等阻塞呼吸道,出生后气体交换受阻。④其他:早产、宫内肺炎、肺发育不良、呼吸道畸形等使新生儿呼吸循环功能受影响。

2.临床表现　根据胎儿娩出后1 min Apgar评分,将新生儿窒息分为轻度窒息和重度窒息两类。重度窒息者在出生后5 min进行第二次Apgar评分,根据评分结果可判断预后,如5 min Apgar评分仍<3分,则新生儿死亡率及以后发生脑部后遗症的概率明显增加。

(1)轻度窒息　又称青紫窒息,Apgar评分为4~7分。患儿表现:新生儿面部及四肢皮肤呈青紫色,呼吸表浅或不规则,心跳规则、强而有力,心率通常减慢(80~100次/min),肌张力好,对刺激有反应。

(2)重度窒息　又称苍白窒息,Apgar评分为0~3分。患儿表现:新生儿全身皮肤苍白,无呼吸或仅有喘息样微弱呼吸,心跳不规则、慢而弱,心率<80次/min,肌张力松弛,对刺激无反应。

3.处理原则　以预防为主,估计胎儿娩出后有窒息的危险时应做好复苏准备。一旦发生新生儿窒息,应立即实施新生儿复苏计划(neonatal resuscitation program,NRP),以降低新生儿死亡率,预防远期后遗症。

Etiology

● Continuation of fetal distress：Various causes lead to fetal intrauterine hypoxia, which is not corrected before birth, and fetal hypoxia persists after birth. The respiratory center is suppressed or damaged.

● Respiratory center depression：The use of sedatives and anesthetics in the process of childbirth is improper, so that the respiratory center is inhibited. Prolonged labor, improper operation of vaginal midwifery, caesarean section instrument injury and so on make fetal brain long time hypoxia or injury, intracranial hemorrhage, so that the respiratory center is damaged.

● Obstructed respiratory tract：During labor, the fetus inhales mucus, amniotic fluid, meconium and other obstructed respiratory tract, so that the postnatal gas exchange is blocked.

● Other：Premature births, intrauterine pneumonia, lung dysplasia, and respiratory tract malformations affect the respiratory and circulatory function of newborns.

Clinical Signs and Symptoms

Apgar score remains a useful clinical tool to classify newborn health immediately after birth and to assess the effectiveness of resuscitative measures. Each of five easily identifiable characteristics—heart rate, respiratory effort, muscle tone, reflex irritability and color, is assessed and assigned a value of 0, 1, or 2. In the currently recommended expanded form, concurrent resuscitation interventions are also recorded over time. The total score, based on the sum of the five components, is determined in all neonates at 1 min and 5 min after delivery. In those with a score <7, the score may be calculated at further 5-minute intervals until a 20-minute Apgar score is assigned or resuscitation efforts are halted.

With oxygen deprivation and carbon dioxide (CO_2) elevation, there is a transient period of rapid breathing, and if it persists, breathing stops, which is termed primary apnea. This stage is accompanied by a fall in heart rate and loss of neuromuscular tone. Simple stimulation will usually reverse primary apnea. If oxygen deprivation and asphyxia persist, however, the newborn will develop deep gasping respirations, followed by secondary apnea. This latter stage is associated with a further decline in heart rate, fall in blood pressure, and loss of neuromuscular tone. Neonates in secondary apnea will not respond to stimulation and will not spontaneously resume respiratory efforts. Unless ventilation is assisted, death follows.

Principle of Management

Prevention first, the fetus should be prepared for recovery at the risk of asphyxia after delivery. Once the neonatal asphyxia occurs, the neonatal resuscitation program should be performed immediately to reduce neonatal mortality rates and to prevent long-term sequelae.

【护理评估】

1. 健康史　了解是否存在胎儿窘迫的危险因素,了解分娩过程是否顺利及有无不恰当处理,胎儿娩出后是否及时清理呼吸道,娩出孕周,胎儿发育有无异常,有无发生宫内感染。

2. 身心状况　产妇因担心新生儿出现意外,常表现出紧张、焦虑或悲伤等。对新生儿应在其娩出后立即进行第一次评估,以决策新生儿是否需要复苏,然后根据新生儿出生后 1 min 内呼吸、心率、皮肤颜色、肌张力、对刺激的反射状况进行 Apgar 评分,根据评分结果判断有无窒息及窒息程度。

3. 辅助检查

(1)血气分析　检测血液 pH(正常值 7.35～7.45)、PaO_2(正常值 60～90 mmHg)、$PaCO_2$(正常值 35～45 mmHg),可评估患儿低氧血症程度、呼吸功能和体液酸碱平衡状况,指导氧疗和机械通气。

（2）影像检查　头颅 B 型超声、CT 或磁共振可帮助评估缺血缺氧性脑病及颅内出血。

【护理诊断】

1.清理呼吸道无效　与呼吸道被羊水、黏液、胎粪阻塞有关。

2.气体交换受损　与各种因素导致不能建立自主呼吸有关。

3.有受伤的危险　与新生儿脑部长时间缺氧、复苏抢救操作有关。

4.有感染的危险　与抢救操作、免疫功能低下有关。

5.焦虑/预感性悲哀　与担心新生儿生命安全及预后有关。

【护理措施】

1.心理护理　安慰、鼓励产妇及家属，选择适宜的时间告知新生儿情况，争取其理解、支持和配合，减轻其担忧和焦虑情绪。提供情感支持，避免抢救时大声喧哗，以免加重其恐惧心理。

2.复苏前准备　估计胎儿娩出后可能发生窒息的，提前做好新生儿复苏准备，包括人员（须有儿科医生在场）、复苏器械、药品及其他用物等。产房设置温度在 25～28 ℃，调节新生儿远红外辐射台温度为 32～34 ℃（足月儿）。

3.复苏的步骤及护理配合　复苏的基本程序是评估—决策—措施，在整个复苏中不断重复。评估主要基于以下 3 个体征：呼吸、心率、脉搏氧饱和度。通过评估 3 个体征中的每一项来确定每一步是否有效，其中心率是最重要的。在 ABCDE 复苏原则下，采取以下步骤进行复苏。

（1）快速评估　出生后立即快速评估 4 项指标：①足月吗？②羊水清吗？③有呼吸或哭声吗？④肌张力好吗？如 4 项指标答案均为"是"，应快速擦干，进行常规护理。若 4 项中有 1 项为"否"，则需进行初步复苏。

（2）初步复苏

1）保暖：用预热的毛巾包裹新生儿放在辐射保暖台上，避免高温引发的呼吸抑制。

2）摆好体位：将新生儿肩部垫高 1～2 cm，使新生儿头呈轻微伸仰位。

3）清理呼吸道：必要时（分泌物多或有气道梗阻时）用吸球或吸管（12F 或 14F）先口咽后鼻腔清除分泌物及羊水，时间<10 s，吸引器负压<100 mmHg。当羊水胎粪污染时，首先评估新生儿有无活力，若肌张力低、无呼吸或喘息样呼吸、心率<100 次/min，为无活力。新生儿无活力时，应协助医生采用气管插管（图 7-1）吸取胎粪，要求在 20 s 内完成。插管时动作要轻柔，避免因负压过大损伤气道黏膜。若不具备气管插管条件，应清理口鼻后立即开始正压通气。

4）擦干和刺激：快速彻底擦干头部、躯干和四肢，拿掉湿毛巾。彻底擦干也是对新生儿的刺激，可以诱发自主呼吸。若仍无呼吸时，可轻拍新生儿足底 1～2 次或摩擦背部 2 次，以刺激呼吸。

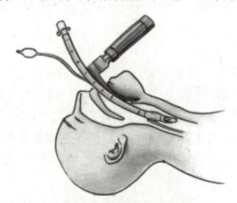

图 7-1　咽喉镜气管插管

（3）气囊面罩正压通气　新生儿复苏的关键是建立充分的正压通气。其指征为：①呼吸暂停或喘息样呼吸；②心率<100 次/min。要求在 1 min 内实施有效的正压通气。通气压力通常为 20～25 cmH$_2$O，少数病情严重的新生儿可采取 2～3 次 30～40 cmH$_2$O 压力进行通气，频率 40～60 次/min。国内新生儿自动充气式气囊容量 250 mL，用前要检查减压阀，有条件的最好配备压力表。持续气囊面罩正压通气>2 min，可产生胃充盈，应常规经口插入 8F 胃管，用注射器抽气并保持胃管远端处于开放状态。

无论足月儿或早产儿，正压通气均要在脉搏氧饱和度仪的检测指导下进行。足月儿开始用空气进行复苏，早产儿开始用 30%～40% 浓度的氧，根据血氧饱和度调整给氧浓度，使氧饱和度达到目标值。若无气囊面罩，可立即采取口对口人工呼吸。口对口人工呼吸方法：将一块纱布叠成4 层，置于新生儿口鼻上，一只手托起新生儿颈部，另一只手轻压上腹部防止气体进入胃内，对准患儿口鼻处轻轻吹气，见到其胸部微微隆起时停止吹气，将口移开，放于腹部的手轻轻向下按压协助排气，一吹一压为 1 次，每分钟 30 次，直至面色红润、停止吹气能见到胸部自主起伏、恢复呼吸为止。

（4）评估及决策

1）评估心率：可触摸新生儿脐带搏动或用听诊器听心跳，计数 6 s，乘以 10 即得每分钟心率。有条件者的可用 3 导联心电图测量心率。

2）判断有效通气：有效的正压通气表现为胸廓起伏良好，心率迅速增快。

3）评估后决策：①矫正通气步骤。若达不到有效通气，需要矫正通气步骤。包括检查面罩和面部接触是否紧密，再次通畅气道（如调整头的位置为鼻吸气位，清除分泌物，使新生儿口张开）及增加气道压力。若心率仍<100 次/min，可采取气管插管或使用喉罩气道。②决定下一步措施。经30 s 有效正压通气后，若出现自主呼吸且心率≥100 次/min，可逐渐减少并停止正压通气，根据脉搏氧饱和度值确定是否常压给氧，若需常压给氧，鼻内插管法流量<2 L/min，5～10 个气泡/s；若心率<60 次/min，采取气管插管正压通气的同时，开始胸外心脏按压。

（5）胸外心脏按压　有效正压通气 30 s 后心率<60 次/min，在气管插管正压通气同时应协助医生进行胸外心脏按压，此时氧浓度增加至 100%。胸外心脏按压方法：新生儿仰卧，用两手拇指法（图7-2）或单手示、中指法（图7-3），放于胸骨下 1/3（两乳头连线中点下方）按压，避开剑突。按压深度约为胸廓前后径的 1/3（使胸骨下降 1～2 cm），按压后即放松，按压时间稍短于放松时间。胸外心脏按压和正压通气的比例为 3∶1，即 90 次/min 按压和 30 次/min 人工呼吸，达到每分钟 120 个动作，每个动作 0.5 s。45～60 s 重新评估心率，心率仍<60 次/min，除继续胸外心脏按压外，考虑使用肾上腺素。

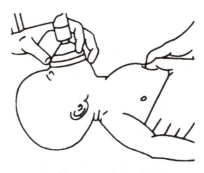

图 7-2　两手拇指法按压

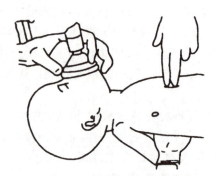

图 7-3　单手示、中指法按压

(6)药物治疗　新生儿窒息复苏时,很少需要用药。新生儿心动过缓通常是肺通气不足或严重缺氧所致,纠正心动过缓的最重要步骤是充分的正压通气。

1)肾上腺素:若经正压通气和胸外心脏按压 45 ~ 60 s,心率持续<60 次/min,遵医嘱予 1：10 000 肾上腺素脐静脉或气管内注入,脐静脉用量为 0.1 ~ 0.3 mL/kg,气管内用量为 0.5 ~ 1.0 mL/kg,必要时 3 ~ 5 min 重复 1 次。

2)扩容剂:有低血容量,怀疑失血或休克的新生儿,用其他复苏措施无效时,采用 0.9% 氯化钠注射液进行扩容,首次剂量 10 mL/kg,经脐静脉或外周静脉缓慢(5 ~ 10 min)注射。必要时重复扩容 1 次。

3)其他药物:在分娩现场新生儿复苏时,一般不使用碳酸氢钠。因碳酸氢钠的高渗透性和产生的 CO_2 可对心肌和大脑功能造成损害。若正压人工呼吸使新生儿心率和肤色恢复正常后,仍有严重的呼吸抑制,且母亲在分娩前 4 h 有用麻醉药史,给予麻醉药拮抗剂纳洛酮肌内或静脉注射,剂量为 0.1 mg/kg。

4.复苏后护理

(1)继续保暖,密切监护新生儿体温、呼吸、心率、脉搏、皮肤颜色、排尿等,发现异常及时反馈、及时处理。

(2)保持呼吸道畅通,随时吸出呼吸道内液体,新生儿取交替侧卧位以避免再次窒息。

(3)适当延迟哺乳,其间静脉补液维持营养;保持新生儿安静,各种护理和治疗操作须轻柔,应用维生素 K、维生素 C 等预防颅内出血;遵医嘱应用抗生素预防感染。

(4)一旦完成复苏,应定期检测血糖,低血糖者静脉给予葡萄糖。

(5)合并中、重度缺氧缺血性脑病者,有条件的单位给予亚低温治疗并做好相应的护理。

Initialsteps of warming the newborn can be done on the mother's chest or abdomen. Direct skin-to-skin contact with the mother and drying and covering the newborn with a warm blanket will help maintain newborn's temperature (36.5–37.5 ℃). Additional routine care steps include drying, gentle stimulation by rubbing the newborn's back, and continued observation during the transition period. If not vigorous or if preterm, the neonate is carried to aprewarmed radiant warmer for the initial newborn care steps. At the radiant warmer, newborns must be positioned to maximally open the airway, with mild extension of the neck. If the newborn is apneic or has copious secretions that it cannot clear, a bulb syringe or suction catheter may be used to clear the mouth and then the nose. Intubation and suction are reserved for suspected airway obstruction.

After completion of the initial stabilization steps, apnea, gasping respirations, or heart rate ≤100 beats per minute (bpm) should prompt immediate administration of positive-pressure ventilation with room air. Assisted ventilation by facemask at a rate of 40-60 breaths per minute is recommended. Oxygen saturation is monitored by pulse oximetry. If the heart rate remains ≤100 bpm after 5-10 positive pressure breaths, the attempted ventilation is inadequate and corrective steps must be taken. The two most common problems are mask leak due to an ineffective seal and malposition of the airway. If corrective steps do not improve the heart rate, either intubation with an endotracheal tube or placement of a laryngeal mask airway is required.

Alternative airway: If mask ventilation is ineffective or prolonged, an alternative airway is placed. For tracheal intubation, a laryngoscope with a straight blade-size 0 for a preterm newborn and size 1 for a term neonate is used. Gentle cricoid pressure may be useful. An increasing heart rate and $ETCO_2$ detection after several breaths are the primary methods of confirming intubation of the trachea and not the esophagus. Once in place, the tube is used for tracheal suctioning only for a suspected obstructed airway. Otherwise, an positive-pressure device is attached to the endotracheal tube. Air puffs are delivered at a rate of 40-60 per minute with a force adequate to stabilize the heart rate.

Chest compressions: Most commonly, effective ventilation is all that is required to stabilize the newborn in the delivery room. If the heart rate remains <60 bpm despite ventilation corrective steps, including placement of tracheal tube, chest compressions are initiated. Once the tracheal tube has been secured, compressions are done from the head of the bed rather than the side so that space is opened for a provider to have umbilical venous access. When compressions are initiated, the oxygen concentration is increased to 100 percent. With the two-thumb compression method, hands encircle the chest, while the thumbs depress the sternum. Compressions are delivered on the lower third of the sternum at a depth sufficient to generate a palpable pulse. This is typically one third of the anterior-posterior diameter of the chest. A 3 : 1 compressions-to-ventilation ratio is recommended, and 90 compressions and 30 breaths achieve approximately 120 events each minute. Coordinated chest compressions and ventilations should continue until the spontaneous heart rate is ≥60 bpm.

Epinephrine: Intravenously administered epinephrine is indicated if the heart rate remains ≤60 bpm after adequate ventilation and chest compressions. The recommended intravenous dose is 0.01-0.03 mg/kg. Epinephrine may be given through the endotracheal tube if venous access has not been established, but its action is less reliable. If given through the endotracheal tube, higher doses are employed 0.05-0.1 mg/kg.

Discontinuation of resuscitation: ILCOR (the International Liaision Committee on Resuscitation) concludes that it is reasonable to discontinue resuscitative efforts for a neonate who remains without a heartbeat despite at least 10 min of continuous and adequate resuscitative efforts. Notably, the decision to continue or discontinue resuscitative efforts must be individualized.

【健康教育】

①产褥期注意休息,加强营养,注意情绪调节,避免过度受刺激影响机体康复。②指导母乳喂养的方法、注意事项及护理婴儿的一般知识。③指导产妇及家属注意观察新生儿的身体状况,发现异常现象及时报告医护人员。

任务实施

新生儿窒息复苏流程见图7-4。

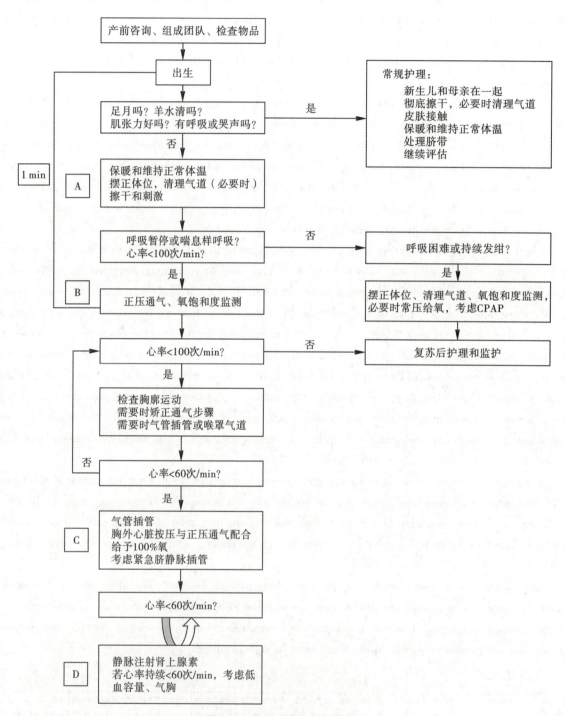

图7-4 新生儿窒息复苏流程

任务四　前置胎盘(Placenta Previa)

工作情景

患者,女,28 岁,G_1P_0,以"宫内孕 39 周,阴道出血 2 d"为主诉入院。2 d 前无任何原因阴道出血,量少呈暗红色,无腹痛。产科检查,子宫大小与妊娠月份相符合,胎心率 140 次/min,胎方位 LOA,先露部为头高浮,并在耻骨联合上听到吹风样杂音,腹部无压痛。B 型超声检查:宫内胎儿,胎位 LOA,胎心音好,有胎动;羊水厚度为 7 cm,胎盘位于子宫前壁,下缘距子宫颈内口 3.5 cm,厚度为 2.6 cm。

①请明确该患者主要的护理问题。②根据目前的情况对患者进行正确的护理。

任务内容

妊娠 28 周后,胎盘附着于子宫下段,位置低于胎儿先露部,其下缘达到或覆盖子宫颈内口,称为前置胎盘,是妊娠晚期常见的阴道流血原因。

任务目标

◆ 能叙述前置胎盘的病因、分类、临床表现及处理原则。

◆ 能对前置胎盘进行正确评估及护理。

【概要】

1.病因　可能与下列因素有关。①子宫内膜病变与损伤:分娩、剖宫产、多次流产、刮宫、产褥感染等可致子宫内膜受损或炎症,子宫蜕膜血管生长不良,受精卵着床后为摄取足够的营养,胎盘伸展到子宫下段。②胎盘面积过大或胎盘异常:见于多胎妊娠、巨大儿,或有副胎盘。③受精卵滋养层发育迟缓。④其他:辅助生殖技术受孕、孕妇不良生活习惯(吸烟、吸毒)等。

2.分类　依据胎盘边缘与子宫颈内口的关系,将前置胎盘分为 3 种类型(图 7-5)。

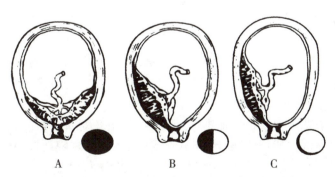

A.完全性前置胎盘;B.部分性前置胎盘;C.边缘性前置胎盘。

图 7-5　前置胎盘的类型

（1）完全性前置胎盘　又称中央性前置胎盘,子宫颈内口完全被胎盘组织覆盖。

（2）部分性前置胎盘　子宫颈内口部分被胎盘组织覆盖。

（3）边缘性前置胎盘　胎盘附着于子宫下段,边缘达到但未超越子宫颈内口。若胎盘附着于子宫下段,边缘距子宫颈内口的距离<20 mm,称为低置胎盘。若妊娠中期超声检查发现胎盘接近或覆盖子宫颈内口时,不诊断为前置胎盘,而称为胎盘前置状态。因胎盘边缘与子宫颈内口的关系随妊娠的不同时期而改变,临床上以处理前最后一次检查结果确定其分类。

3.临床表现　典型症状是妊娠晚期或临产时,孕妇发生无诱因、无痛性反复阴道流血。阴道流血的发生时间、出血量、发生次数与前置胎盘类型有关。

4.治疗原则　止血、纠正贫血、预防感染,适时终止妊娠。根据妊娠周数、胎儿情况、产次、前置胎盘类型、阴道流血量等综合做出判断,降低早产率与围产儿死亡率。

Etiology

There is no known cause of placenta previa. However, certain risk factors have been associated with the increased risk of developing placenta previa. These include multiparity, advancing maternal age, multiple gestation, previous cesarean birth, and uterine incisions. It is thought to occur whenever the placenta is forced to spread to find an adequate exchange surface.

Classification

Placenta previa is classified as complete (total), partial, or marginal implantation by the location of the placenta in the lower uterine segment and the degree to which the internal cervical os is covered.

- Total placenta: Previa occurs when the placenta completely covers the internal cervical os.

- Partial placenta: Previa occurs when the placenta partially covers the internal cervical os.

- Marginal placenta: Previa occurs when the placenta attaches on the region of the lower uterine segment but does not extend beyond the margin of the internal os.

Clinical Signs and Symptoms

The most characteristic event in placenta previa is abrupt, painless, and bright red hemorrhage, which usually does not appear until near the end of the second trimester or after. Usually the bleeding ceases spontaneously, only to recur.

Principle of Management

Medical interventions are determined by the location of the placenta, the amount of bleeding, and the gestational age of the fetus. The goal of medical management is to ensure the birth of a mature neonate without complications to the client or fetus.

【护理评估】

1.健康史　评估孕妇是否有前置胎盘的危险因素,询问其阴道流血的发生经过、诊治情况。

2.身心状况　因突然阴道流血,担心母婴双方的安全,孕妇及家属常感到紧张、恐慌,应注意观察其情绪反应,以及时安慰鼓励。

（1）症状　完全性前置胎盘阴道出血早、出血量多,多在妊娠28周左右发生,甚至1次出血就发生失血性休克。边缘性前置胎盘出血晚、量较少,多发生在妊娠晚期或临产后,一些孕妇产后检查胎盘胎膜才被发现。部分性前置胎盘出血时间、出血量介于两者之间。

（2）体征　大量出血可出现失血性休克征象。腹部检查:子宫大小与妊娠周数相符,质软,无压痛,胎先露高浮或伴胎位异常。

3.辅助检查

（1）B型超声检查　可显示子宫壁、胎盘、胎先露及子宫颈的位置,明确前置胎盘及类型的诊断。

（2）产后检查胎盘胎膜　若前置部位的胎盘有黑紫色陈旧血块附着,胎膜破口距胎盘边缘距离<7 cm,可诊断为前置胎盘。

【护理诊断】

1.舒适度减弱　与病情需要绝对卧床有关。

2.组织灌注量改变　与周围血容量减少有关

3.有感染的危险　与出血多致抵抗力下降及病原体经前置胎盘剥离面侵入有关。

【护理措施】

1.一般护理　嘱孕妇多休息,以左侧卧位为宜,血止后可轻微活动。指导孕妇加强营养,多摄入高蛋白、高热量、高维生素、富含铁的食物,纠正贫血。加强会阴护理,保持会阴清洁、干燥,预防发生感染。

2.病情观察　密切观察孕妇的生命体征,观察阴道流血量、色及出血时间,监测胎儿宫内情况。注意识别病情危重的指征如休克表现、胎心或胎动异常等。

3.心理护理　耐心向孕妇及家属解释病情,消除其紧张焦虑的心情,使其保持平静心态,并能积极配合治疗。

4.治疗护理

（1）期待疗法的护理　期待疗法适用于妊娠<36周、胎儿存活、阴道流血量少、一般情况良好的孕妇。孕妇应绝对卧床休息,严密观察其出血情况,监护胎儿宫内情况。禁止肛门检查和不必要的阴道检查。遵医嘱备血、用药,如补血剂、宫缩抑制剂、镇静剂,必要时输血。给予广谱抗生素预防感染。对于病情加重、出血量增多或早产者,做好终止妊娠的相关准备、新生儿抢救准备。

（2）终止妊娠的护理　终止妊娠的指征:反复发生多量出血甚至休克者,无论胎儿成熟与否,应终止妊娠;出现胎儿窘迫征象,或胎儿电子监护发现胎心异常者;胎龄超过36周,或胎儿成熟度检查提示胎肺成熟者,或分娩已发动者均应终止妊娠。

根据前置胎盘的类型和孕妇、胎儿的情况选择终止妊娠的方法。剖宫产者,积极做好术前准备、纠正贫血、预防感染等措施,并做好预防产后出血及新生儿窒息的准备工作。阴道分娩者,在做好紧急抢救的准备下,协助人工破膜、腹部包扎腹带,迫使胎头下降,减少出血。

Plans for nursing intervention vary, depending on whether conservative or active medical management is prescribed. However, continuous close monitoring of maternal and fetal status is essential.

The client who is being managed at home or who is being discharged after an initial bleeding episode may require a referral for homemaking services. Assistance in these areas is likely to facilitate client compliance with bed rest or restricted activities.

Ongoing assessments of maternal and perinatal status should be performed by the nurse to detect changes. Any indication of compromise to the client or the fetus should be alert for the possibility of infection and continued bleeding after delivery.

The client experiencing an excessive blood loss prior to or during delivery often requires this loss to be replaced. Packed red blood cells, fresh frozen plasma may be given to replace clotting factor deficiencies. It also may be necessary to administer oxygen to prevent maternal and fetal hypoxia.

【健康教育】

①加强知识宣教,减少影响子宫内膜血运的情况发生。如避免多次刮宫、引产、多产或宫内感

染,摒弃不良习惯,戒烟、戒毒、戒酒。②重视产前检查,以便及时发现异常及时诊治。妊娠期发生出血者,应及时就诊。③产后注意休息、加强营养、保持心情愉悦,促进身体尽快康复。

任务实施

前置胎盘大出血的抢救流程见图7-6。

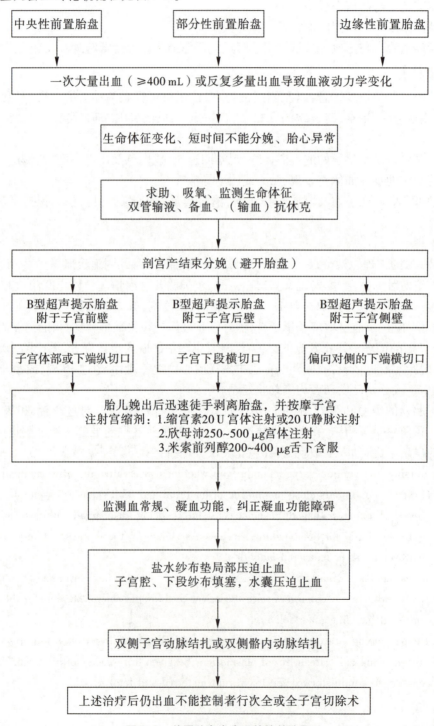

图7-6 前置胎盘大出血的抢救流程

任务五 胎盘早剥（Placental Abruption）

工作情景

患者，女，31 岁，G_2P_1，妊娠 32 周，腹部持续疼痛 2 h 入院。本次妊娠经过：孕 24 周出现下肢水肿，孕 30 周出现头痛、头晕，测血压 150/90 mmHg，服用抗高血压药后好转，未进一步诊治。今日在家不小心滑倒，于 2 h 前突然出现腹部疼痛，阵发性加剧，无阴道出血及其他症状。体格检查：患者表情痛苦，面色苍白，心率 98 次/min，BP 130/75 mmHg，宫高 31 cm，腹围 87 cm，子宫质硬，有明显压痛，胎位触不清，未闻及胎心音。肛诊：子宫颈展平，子宫颈口未开，先露部高浮。

①请明确该患者主要的护理问题。②根据目前的情况对患者进行正确的护理。

任务内容

胎盘早剥是指妊娠 20 周后或分娩期，正常位置的胎盘在胎儿娩出前部分或全部从子宫壁剥离，是妊娠晚期常见的出血原因之一，起病急，进展快，出血严重者危及母儿安全，是妊娠期的严重并发症。

任务目标

◆ 能叙述胎盘早剥的病因、分类、临床表现及处理原则。
◆ 能对胎盘早剥进行正确评估及护理。

【概要】

1. 病因　可能与下列因素有关。

（1）血管病变　各种血管病变致子宫蜕膜螺旋小动脉缺血或硬化，使远端毛细血管缺血、坏死、破裂出血，形成底蜕膜层血肿，导致胎盘剥离，如妊娠期高血压疾病、慢性肾脏病或全身血管病变等。孕晚期长时间仰卧位休息，致子宫静脉压升高，蜕膜静脉破裂，也会引起胎盘剥离。

（2）机械性因素　腹部受到外伤（挤压、撞击或摔伤）、脐带过短的牵拉可造成胎盘早剥。

（3）宫腔内压力突然下降　羊水过多者破膜后羊水流出速度过快、双胎妊娠的第一胎娩出过快，使宫腔压力骤减，发生胎盘早剥。

（4）其他　高龄多产、有血栓形成倾向、胎盘早剥史、辅助生殖技术助孕、吸烟、吸毒等。

2. 病理　主要病理变化是底蜕膜出血，形成血肿，使胎盘自附着处剥离。剥离形式有 3 种类型（图 7-7），分别是显性剥离、隐性剥离、混合性出血。

隐性剥离、混合性出血者，内出血严重时，血液渗入子宫肌层，使肌纤维分离、断裂、变性，血液甚至侵入浆膜层，使子宫表面出现紫蓝色瘀斑，特别是胎盘附着处更明显，称为子宫胎盘卒中。大量内出血者，胎盘剥离处的蜕膜和绒毛产生大量组织凝血活酶，进入母血激活凝血系统，并进一步激活纤维蛋白溶解系统，导致母体发生凝血功能障碍。

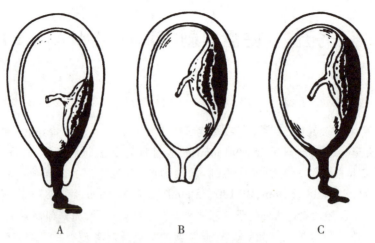

A. 显性剥离；B. 隐性剥离；C. 混合性出血。
图7-7 胎盘早剥的分类

3.临床表现及分级 典型临床表现是阴道流血、腹痛，可伴有子宫张力增高和子宫压痛，尤以胎盘剥离处更明显。阴道出血量往往与疼痛程度、胎盘剥离程度不一定符合，尤其是后壁胎盘的隐性剥离。早期表现通常以胎心率异常为首发征象，宫缩间歇期子宫呈高张状态，胎位触诊不清。严重时子宫呈板状，压痛明显，胎心率改变或消失，甚至出现恶心、呕吐、出汗、面色苍白、脉搏细弱、血压下降等休克征象。

在临床上推荐按照胎盘早剥的 Page 分级标准评估病情的严重程度。

0 级：分娩后回顾性产后诊断。

Ⅰ级：外出血，子宫软，无胎儿窘迫。

Ⅱ级：胎儿窘迫或胎死宫内。

Ⅲ级：孕妇出现休克症状，伴或不伴弥散性血管内凝血（DIC）。

出现胎儿宫内死亡的患者胎盘剥离面积常超过 50%；接近 30% 的胎盘早剥会出现凝血功能障碍。

4.处理原则 早期识别，积极纠正休克，及时终止妊娠，控制 DIC，防治并发症。终止妊娠的时机和方式根据孕周、病情程度、有无并发症、母儿状况等决定。

Etiology

The causative mechanism of abruptio placenta is not known. However, it may be due to an inherent weakness or anomaly in the spiral arterioles, it includes preeclampsia, gestational hypertension, chronic hypertension, and chronic renal disease. Certain conditions are believed to be contributing factors, some factors include multiple gestation, short umbilical cord, hydramnios and abdominal trauma.

Pathology and Classification

Placental abruption is initiated by hemorrhage into the deciduas basalis. The deciduas then splits, leaving a thin layer adherent to the myometrium. The types are divided into overt abruptio placenta, covert abruptio placenta and mixed hemorrhage.

● Overt abruptio placenta: When a separation occurs at the margin, blood passes between the uterine wall and fetal membranes, creating an external hemorrhage. This type is also called revealed abruptio placenta.

● Covert abruptio placenta：It is also called concealed abruptio placenta，is characterized by central separation that entraps lost blood between the uterine wall and the placenta. In this situation，a concealed hemorrhage often masks the seriousness of the problem.

● Mixed hemorrhage：Part of the separation is near the edge，and part is concealed in the center area. Blood also may infiltrate the myometrium，causing a blue discoloration of the uterus，known as a couvelaire uterus（uteroplacental apoplexy）.

Clinical Signs and Symptoms

Abruptio placenta may be classified by degree of placental separation，in terms of heavy or light type：light type is marginal abruption with external bleeding；heavy type includes partial abruption with concealed bleeding or complete abruption with concealed bleeding.

The manisfestations of an abruption are dark vaginal bleeding；abdominal pain，often sudden，severe，and "knifelike"；and a firm，tender uterus. The pain is produced by the accumulation of blood behind the placenta，with subsequent distention of the uterus. Because of the almost woody hardness of the uterine wall，fetal parts may be difficult to palpate. The contraction pattern typical of an abruptio placenta is frequent，low-amplitude contractions with an increase in resting tone. Shock is often out of proportion to visible blood loss，as manifested by a rapid pulse，dyspnea，yawning，restlessness，pallor，syncope，and cold，clammy perspiration.

Principle of Management

Treatment for placental abruption will vary depending upon gestational age and status of the mother and fetus. If the fetus is alive and at or near term，prompt delivery by cesarean birth is used for moderate to severe abruption. If the fetus has already succumbed，usually an indication of an extensive placental separation，vaginal delivery is preferred.

【护理评估】

1.健康史　询问孕妇是否有胎盘早剥的危险因素，询问其阴道流血的发生经过、诊治情况。

2.身心状况　因病情进展快情况危急，担心母儿安全，孕妇及其家属常常感到高度紧张或恐惧。

胎盘早剥的典型症状是腹痛、阴道出血。根据其腹痛的程度、失血征象与阴道流血是否相符、子宫质地及大小、胎方位、胎心音等表现评估其剥离的类型及病情严重程度。观察是否出现 DIC、急性肾衰竭、子宫胎盘卒中、羊水栓塞、产后出血等并发症。

3.辅助检查

（1）B 型超声检查　典型的图像显示在胎盘与子宫壁之间出现液性低回声区。须注意的是，若检查结果阴性也不能完全排除胎盘早剥。

（2）实验室检查　了解孕妇贫血程度及有无凝血功能异常，包括血常规、凝血功能、肝肾功能、电解质、DIC 筛选试验等。

（3）电子胎儿监护　了解胎儿在宫内的安危状况，检查可出现胎心基线变异消失、变异减速、晚期减速、胎心缓慢等。

【护理诊断】

1.疼痛　与胎盘后血肿刺激子宫有关。

2.组织灌注量改变　与出血、DIC 有关。

3.潜在并发症　子宫胎盘卒中、DIC、羊水栓塞、产后出血等。

4.胎儿有受伤的危险　与胎盘灌注量减少有关。

【护理措施】

1. 一般护理　绝对卧床,以左侧卧位为宜。定时间断吸氧,改善胎儿血氧供应。加强会阴部护理,减少感染概率。

2. 病情观察　监测生命体征,观察腹痛情况、子宫质地及大小、阴道流血及贫血程度。监测胎儿宫内情况。注意观察是否出现子宫胎盘卒中、DIC、急性肾衰竭、产后出血等并发症。

3. 心理护理　向孕妇及家属解释病情及所采取措施的目的,取得积极的配合。加强心理疏导,对胎儿不幸死亡的,予以安慰、支持,帮助孕妇及家属走出悲伤的情绪状态。

4. 治疗护理

(1)迅速开放静脉通道,以及时补充血容量,改善血液循环,并注意给氧、保暖等。

(2)确诊Ⅱ、Ⅲ级胎盘早剥应及时终止妊娠。根据病情程度、母儿状况、产程进展等决定终止妊娠的方式。

1)阴道分娩:适应于0~Ⅰ级胎盘早剥,以外出血为主,孕妇一般情况良好,估计短时间内可结束分娩者。人工破膜使羊水缓慢流出,缩小子宫容积,用腹带包裹腹部压迫胎盘,使其不再继续剥离,必要时滴注缩宫素。密切观察,一旦发现异常及时改行剖宫产术结束分娩。

2)剖宫产术:适应于Ⅰ级胎盘早剥,发生胎儿窘迫者;Ⅱ、Ⅲ级胎盘早剥,短时间内不能结束分娩者或产妇病情恶化;破膜后产程无进展者。护理人员配合做好阴道分娩或剖宫产术的相关准备、预防感染措施,并做好抢救新生儿的准备。

Nursing interventions should be based on the presenting symptomatology and appropriate nursing diagnoses, in conjunction with any additional workups or therapies ordered by the physician. If the abruption is mild and the fetus is immature, careful and continuous nursing observation is necessary to detect evidence of progressive maternal blood loss or changes in fetal status. In more acute situations, hourly intake and output should be recorded. Oxygen may be administered by face mask at 8−10 L/min to prevent or minimize fetal hypoxia.

Observations should be made for signs and symptoms of maternal hypovolemia and hypoxemia, such as tachycardia and shortness of breath. It also is essential for the nurse to assess the client for adverse reactions to blood transfusions.

In cases of moderate to severe abruption and a live fetus, the nurse should provide preoperative teaching about the possibility of a cesarean delivery and birth of a preterm infant.

Following delivery, the nurse should continue assessing fluid−volume balance and vital signs. The uterus should be palpated frequently for atony. The client should be evaluated for signs of excessive blood loss.

【健康教育】

①有妊娠期高血压疾病、肾脏病等危险因素者,应积极治疗控制病情,加强妊娠期监护。②注意自我保护,避免腹部外伤。妊娠晚期避免长时间仰卧位休息。③出院后注意休息,加强营养。

任务实施

胎盘早剥和前置胎盘的鉴别见表7-3。

表7-3　胎盘早剥和前置胎盘的鉴别

疾病	发病时期	病史	发病	腹痛	典型症状	子宫检查	胎儿检查
胎盘早剥	多见于分娩期	妊娠期高血压疾病、外伤史	起病急	突发性剧烈腹痛	剧烈腹痛,胎心变化,阴道出血量无或不多	子宫板状硬,宫缩间歇期不能松弛	胎位不清、胎心音可消失
前置胎盘	妊娠晚期或临产	多次刮宫、分娩史	无明显诱因	无腹痛	无痛性反复阴道流血,有外出血表现	子宫软、无压痛,子宫大小与妊娠周数相符	胎先露高浮,易发生胎位异常

任务六　羊水量异常(Abnormal Amniotic Fluid)

工作情景

患者,女,25岁,以"宫内孕28周,自觉腹部增大迅速"来就诊。近半月感觉腹部增大明显,出现心悸、气短,不能平卧休息。下肢出现水肿,休息后水肿消失。检查:腹壁紧张,皮肤透亮,腹部有液体震颤感,胎位扪不清,胎心音遥远不清晰,腹围98 cm。

①请明确该患者主要的护理问题。②根据目前的情况对患者进行正确的护理。

任务内容

正常妊娠时,羊水处于边产生边吸收的动态平衡中。如果这种动态平衡失衡,则会出现羊水量过多或过少。羊水量过多是指妊娠期间羊水量超过2 000 mL。

任务目标

◆ 能叙述羊水过多的病因、临床表现及处理原则。

◆ 能对羊水过多进行正确评估。

【概要】

1.病因

(1)胎儿疾病　明显的羊水过多常伴有胎儿畸形,以神经系统和消化道畸形最常见。其中,神经管缺陷性疾病最常见,约占50%,如无脑儿、脑膨出、脊柱裂;消化道畸形约占25%,主要为食管或小肠闭锁。

(2)多胎妊娠　发生率约为单胎妊娠的10倍。

（3）胎盘脐带病变　胎盘绒毛血管瘤、巨大胎盘、脐带帆状附着等也可导致羊水过多。

（4）妊娠期疾病　妊娠糖尿病、母儿 Rh 血型不合、胎儿免疫性水肿、胎盘绒毛水肿等。

（5）其他　约 30% 为特发性羊水过多。

2.临床表现

（1）急性羊水过多　多发生在妊娠 20～24 周，较少见。羊水量在数日内迅速增多，子宫急剧增大，因腹压增加而出现明显的压迫症状。孕妇感腹胀、食欲减退，出现呼吸困难，不能平卧，甚至发绀。查体可见腹壁皮肤绷紧发亮，子宫明显大于妊娠周数，胎位扪不清，胎心音遥远或听不清。下肢及外阴部水肿或静脉曲张。

（2）慢性羊水过多　多发生于妊娠晚期，较多见。羊水在数周内逐渐增多，孕妇多能适应，症状较缓和。产检时发现腹部过度膨隆，腹壁皮肤发亮、变薄，有液体震颤感，子宫大于妊娠周数，胎位不清，胎心音遥远或听不到。

3.处理原则　根据是否合并胎儿畸形、妊娠周数、孕妇自觉症状程度等综合考虑。合并胎儿畸形者，尽早终止妊娠；胎儿正常者，寻找病因并积极治疗，适时终止妊娠。

Etiology

Underlying causes of hydramnios include fetal anomalies—either structural abnormalities or genetic syndromes—in approximately 15% , and diabetes in 15%–20%. Congenital infection, red blood cell alloimmunization, and placental chorioangioma are less frequent etiologies. Infections that may present with hydramnios include cytomegalovirus, toxoplasmosis, syphilis, and parvovirus. Hydramnios is often a component of bydrops fetalis, and several of the above causes—selected anomalies, infections, and alloimmunization may result in a hydropic fetus and placenta.

Clinical Signs and Symptoms

Unless hydramnios is severe or develops rapidly, maternal symptoms are infrequent. With chronic hydramnios, amniotic fluid accumulates gradually, and a woman may tolerate excessive abdominal distention with relatively little discomfort. Acute hydramnios, however, tends to develop earlier in pregnancy. It may result in preterm labor before 28 weeks or in symptoms that become so debilitating as to necessitate intervention.

Symptoms may arise from pressure exerted within the over–distended uterus and upon adjacent organs. When distention is excessive, the mother may suffer dyspnea and orthopnea to such a degree that she may be able to breathe comfortably only when upright. Edema may develop as a consequence of major venous system compression by the enlarged uterus, and it tends to be most pronounced in the lower extremities, vulva, and abdominal wall. Rarely, oliguria may result from ureteral obstruction by the enlarged uterus.

Principle of Management

Treatment is directed to the underlying cause. Occasionally, severe hydramnios may result in early preterm labor or the development of maternal respiratory compromise. In such cases, large–volume amniocentesis–termed amnio reduction may be needed. 1,000–2,000 mL of fluid is slowly withdrawn over 20 min, depending on the severity of hydramniosand gestational age.

【护理评估】

1.健康史　询问孕妇是否有导致羊水过多的母儿疾病存在，如妊娠糖尿病、多胎妊娠、严重贫血、母儿血型不合等。

2.身心状况　询问有哪些不适症状、出现的时间及程度。了解腹围、宫高及胎儿情况。孕妇及家属常因担心胎儿可能会有某种畸形而感到紧张、焦虑,甚至恐惧。

3.辅助检查

(1)B型超声检查　可测量羊水池深度,检查有无多胎妊娠、胎儿畸形等情况。诊断标准:①羊水最大暗区垂直深度(AFV)>8 cm可确诊。其中AFV在8~11 cm为轻度羊水过多,12~15 cm为中度羊水过多,>15 cm为重度羊水过多。②羊水指数(AFI)>25 cm可确诊。其中AFI 25~35 cm为轻度羊水过多,36~45 cm为中度羊水过多,>45 cm为重度羊水过多。

(2)甲胎蛋白测定　合并胎儿开放性神经管缺损时,母血、羊水中甲胎蛋白水平明显增高。

【护理诊断】

1.舒适度的改变　与子宫过度增大、腹压升高有关。

2.潜在并发症　胎膜早破、脐带脱垂、胎盘早剥、产后出血等。

3.预感性悲哀　与胎儿畸形有关。

【护理措施】

1.一般护理　注意休息,指导孕妇采取左侧卧位,有呼吸困难、腹胀等压迫症状者取半卧位,协助孕妇做好日常生活护理。低钠饮食,减少饮水量,多食蔬菜和水果,防止便秘。减少增加腹压的活动。

2.病情观察　定期测量孕妇的体重、宫高、腹围,了解病情进展。注意观察是否出现胎膜早破、胎盘早剥和脐带脱垂的征象,以及时发现异常。

3.心理护理　耐心解释病情,对孕妇及家属提供心理支持,使其理解、配合治疗。

4.治疗护理　羊水过多合并胎儿畸形者,须及时终止妊娠。可行羊膜腔穿刺放羊水后,注入乳酸依沙吖啶引产,或人工破膜放羊水终止妊娠。胎儿正常、妊娠不足37周而压迫症状严重者,可行羊膜腔穿刺放羊水缓解不适症状,必要时可3~4周后再次放羊水以减轻宫腔内压力。

配合、协助医生完成放羊水的工作。羊膜腔穿刺放羊水应在B型超声引导下进行,防止损伤胎盘及胎儿。注意无菌操作,预防感染。人工破膜应采用高位破膜器,控制羊水以每小时500 mL的速度缓慢流出,避免宫腔压力骤减导致胎盘早剥。放羊水后,为避免腹压骤降引起休克,应于腹部放置沙袋或腹带包扎。

羊水过少

【健康教育】

①注意休息,营养均衡,低钠饮食。②预防便秘,减少增加腹压的活动,如用力咳嗽、屏气、情绪激动等。③再次妊娠应加强产前检查。如有遗传性疾病,妊娠前及时进行相关检查。

任务实施

羊水过多的诊断及处理流程见图7-8。

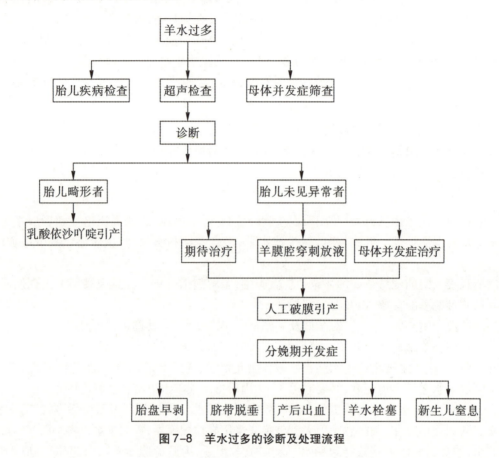

图7-8　羊水过多的诊断及处理流程

任务七　胎膜早破(Premature Rupture of Membrane)

工作情景

患者,女,28岁,G_1P_0,宫内孕34周,感冒后咳嗽3 d,于3 h前咳嗽时突然阴道流液,量少但持续不断,不能控制,无腹痛及阴道流血。入院检查:一般情况好。宫底位于剑突下三指,LOA,无宫缩,胎心率148次/min,先露部高浮,骨盆外测量正常,阴道口有少量清亮液体流出。阴道检查:子宫颈口未开。

①请明确该患者主要的护理问题。②根据目前的情况对患者进行正确的护理。

任务内容

胎膜早破是指临产前胎膜自然破裂。发生在妊娠37周及以后的为足月胎膜早破;妊娠未达37周发生的为未足月胎膜早破,后者常引起早产,使围产儿死亡率增加。

任务目标

◆ 能叙述胎膜早破的病因、临床表现及处理原则。

◆ 能对胎膜早破者进行正确评估。

【概要】

1.病因　胎膜早破的发生常常是多因素影响的结果。

(1)胎膜炎症　病原微生物上行感染引起胎膜炎症,是胎膜早破的主要原因。

(2)胎先露与骨盆入口衔接不良　如骨盆狭窄、头盆不称、胎位异常等,胎先露与骨盆入口不能紧密衔接,胎膜受力不均,当宫腔压力进一步增高时引起胎膜破裂。

(3)羊膜腔压力增高　常见于多胎妊娠、羊水过多等。

(4)子宫颈内口松弛　子宫颈发育异常或产伤或手术损伤致子宫颈内口松弛,使胎膜失去应有的支持力而易发生胎膜早破。

(5)机械性刺激　羊膜腔穿刺不当、腹部受到撞击、性生活刺激等可导致胎膜早破。

(6)营养因素　缺乏维生素、铜、锌等,胎膜发育不良、抗张能力下降。

2.临床表现　孕妇突感有液体自阴道流出,腹压增加时,阴道流液量增加。肛诊或阴道检查触不到前羊膜囊,上推胎先露时阴道流液增多。有时可在阴道流液中见到白色块状物。

3.处理原则　及时住院治疗,根据孕周、破膜时间、有无感染、母儿情况等采取保胎或终止妊娠的处理措施。

Etiology

The cause of premature rupture of membrane (PROM) is unknown in most cases. Increased intrauterine pressure with multiple gestation and polyhydramnios, inflammatory processes such as cervicitis and amnionitis, placenta previa, abruptio placentae, abnormalities of the internal cervical os, multiple amniocenteses, and therapeutic abortions are factors that are at times associated with PROM. It was once believed that an inherently weak fetal membrane might be a cause of PROM. Current information reveals that a bacterial invasion can often precede and may possibly be the cause of PROM in 30% –40% of the cases.

Clinical Signs and Symptoms

The patient feels gushing of fluid from vagina, and fluid leakage increases with movement change. Differential diagnosis will be urinary incontinence and vaginal discharge.

Principle of Management

Timely hospitalization is important, and measures should be taken to prevent the pregnancy or terminate the pregnancy according to the gestational age, rupture time, infection, maternal and child conditions.

【护理评估】

1.健康史　询问发生胎膜早破的诱因,既往有无生殖系统炎症病史及诊治经过,了解胎膜破裂的时间、孕周。

2.身心状况　孕妇常因担心早产和早产儿的安全而紧张、焦虑。

询问其阴道流出液体的情况,是否在咳嗽、打喷嚏时流液量增多,或取某一种体位时液体流出增多。检查触不到前羊膜囊,上推胎儿先露部可见到流液量增多。

3.辅助检查

（1）阴道流液酸碱度检测　正常阴道 pH 为 4.5～5.5,羊水 pH 为 7.0～7.5。如果测得阴道流液 pH≥7 可诊断,但是子宫颈黏液、精液、血液、尿液污染可能会出现假阳性。

（2）阴道流液干燥涂片检查　阴道流液干燥涂片检查可见羊齿植物叶状结晶。

（3）羊水培养　诊断是否发生绒毛膜羊膜炎。在超声引导下行羊膜腔穿刺抽取羊水,进行羊水涂片革兰氏染色检查、细菌培养、白细胞计数、葡萄糖测定。

【护理诊断】

1.有感染的危险　与胎膜破裂后病原体沿生殖道黏膜上行感染有关。

2.胎儿有受伤的危险　与脐带脱垂、宫内肺炎、胎儿窘迫有关。

3.焦虑/恐惧　与胎膜早破引起早产、担心胎儿安危有关。

【护理措施】

1.一般护理　保持会阴部清洁。先露部未衔接者应绝对卧床,抬高臀部,预防脐带脱垂。避免不必要的肛查和阴道检查。

2.病情观察　观察孕妇生命体征、子宫有无宫缩,监护胎心、胎动,观察流出羊水的性状,有无条索状物经阴道脱出,以及时发现感染、早产和胎儿窘迫等征象。

3.心理护理　了解孕妇及家属的想法及感受,提供心理支持,减轻紧张、焦虑。

4.治疗护理　破膜超过 12 h 者应预防性应用抗生素。足月胎膜早破者,如破膜后未临产,常于破膜 12 h 后引产或剖宫产终止妊娠。未足月胎膜早破者,如妊娠<24 周,以引产为宜;妊娠 24～27^{+6}周,综合考虑新生儿成活概率、孕妇及家属意愿等决定是否终止妊娠;妊娠 28～33^{+6}周,符合保胎条件的可行期待治疗;妊娠 34～36^{+6}周者或出现绒毛膜羊膜炎、胎儿窘迫等并发症者应终止妊娠。

期待治疗即保胎治疗,孕妇应绝对卧床,勤换消毒会阴垫,出现宫缩时应用宫缩抑制剂。早产不可避免时用地塞米松或倍他米松肌内注射,促进胎肺成熟。妊娠 24～27^{+6}周保胎者,因保胎过程长、风险大,应充分告知治疗过程中的风险。

Preventing Infection

Teach the importance of perineal care after each voiding and stool. Perform no vaginal examinations until the patient is in active labor. Notify the physician if temperature is greater than 38 ℃ ,fetal or maternal tachycardia develops,foul-smelling amniotic fluid develops, or amniotic fluid changes from straw color. If signs of an intra-amniotic infection are manifested,be prepared to begin broad-spectrum antibiotic therapy.

Maintaining fetal gas exchange

● Prenatal:Reposition mother,and administer oxygen by mask if variable decelerations occur. Instruct patient to report any decrease in fetal activity. Prepare the patient for ordered fetal well-being and maturity studies.

● Intrapartum:Use continuous fetal monitoring for early detection of nonreassuring FHR changes. Assess amniotic fluid for meconium. Notify the physician at the first signs of a nonreassuring FHR change. Once delivery is imminent,notify the intensive care nursery of a possible high risk infant.

● Alleviating fear:Encourage expectant parents to communicate openly about their feelings and concerns.

【健康教育】

①注意妊娠期卫生保健,保持会阴部清洁。②妊娠晚期禁止性交,避免腹部受撞击、重压。③重视产前检查,子宫颈内口松弛者应于妊娠 12～14 周行子宫颈内口环扎术。

任务实施

胎膜早破急救流程见图7-9。

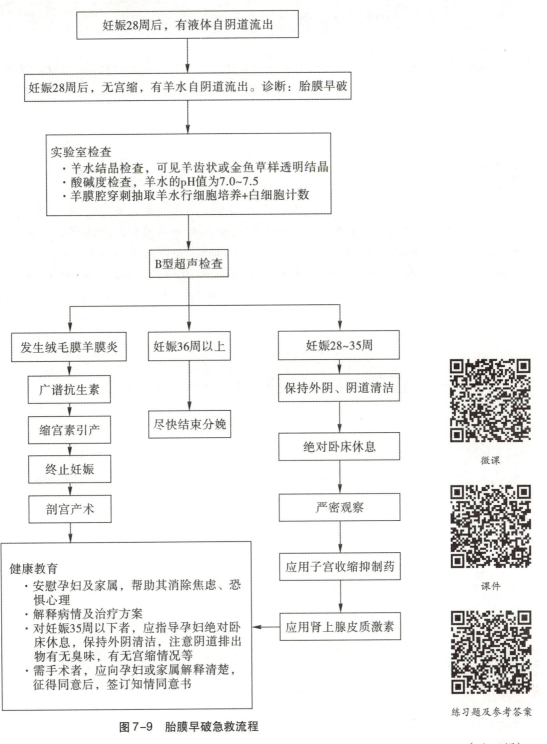

图7-9 胎膜早破急救流程

微课

课件

练习题及参考答案

（王珏辉）

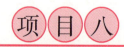

项目八

妊娠合并症妇女的护理
（Nursing of Women in Pregnance Complications）

项目描述

妊娠合并症是产科临床较常见的病理现象，合并症与妊娠之间相互影响，若处理不当，可使母婴安全受到威胁。临床常见有妊娠合并心脏病、糖尿病、病毒性肝炎、贫血等。

Pregnance comorbidities are the common pathology phenomenon in obstetrics. The comorbidities and pregnancy affect each other. If they are handled improperly, the safety of mother and infant can be threatened. Common clinical pregnance comorbidities include pregnance with heart disease, diabetes, viral hepatitis, anemia, etc.

任务一　心脏病（Cardiac Disease）

工作情景

患者，女，29岁，G_1P_0，妊娠10周，从事家务劳动后感胸闷、气短、心悸，近1周来半夜常因胸闷而起床。查体：P 116次/min，R 23次/min，心界向左扩大，心尖区有收缩期Ⅲ级杂音，性质粗糙，肺底有细湿啰音，下肢水肿阳性。

①请明确该患者主要的护理问题。②根据目前的情况对患者进行正确的护理。

任务内容

妊娠合并心脏病是严重的妊娠合并症，以合并先天性心脏病最多见，在我国孕妇死亡原因中居第二位，占非直接产科死因的第一位。欧美国家发病率为1%～4%，我国发病率约为1%，死亡率约为0.73%。妊娠、分娩及产褥期机体变化均可加重心脏负担而诱发心力衰竭（简称心衰）。

任务目标

◆能叙述妊娠与心脏病的相互影响、早期心力衰竭的表现及处理原则。

◆能对心脏病患者能否妊娠进行正确评估。

◆能对患者提供正确护理。

【概要】

1.妊娠、分娩与心脏病的相互影响

（1）妊娠、分娩对心脏病的影响

1）妊娠期：由于血容量和血流动力学等方面的变化，心脏负担加重，易发生心力衰竭。①血容量增加：血容量自妊娠第 6 周开始逐渐增加，至妊娠 32～34 周达高峰，总血容量比非妊娠期增加 30%～45%，此后维持较高水平。②心排出量增加和心率加快：血容量增加使心排出量较孕前平均增加 30%～50%，休息时心率平均每分钟增加 10～15 次。③心脏位置改变：妊娠晚期子宫增大，膈肌升高，心脏向左前、向上发生移位，心脏大血管扭曲，使心脏负荷进一步加重。

2）分娩期：是孕妇血流动力学变化最显著的阶段。①第一产程：每次子宫收缩有 250～500 mL 的血液被挤入体循环，使血容量增加、回心血量增加，心排出量增加 20% 左右，同时血压升高、脉压增大及中心静脉压升高。②第二产程：除子宫收缩外，腹肌和骨骼肌的收缩，使外周循环阻力增加；分娩时产如屏气用力，使肺循环压力增加；屏气时腹压升高，使血液从内脏向心脏回流增加。第二产程心脏负担最重。③第三产程：胎儿娩出后，子宫突然缩小，腹腔内压骤降，大量血液流向内脏器官，回心血量减少；同时，胎盘循环停止，子宫血窦内约有 500 mL 血液进入体循环，回心血量骤增。这两种血流动力学的急剧变化，使产妇心脏难以耐受，极易诱发心力衰竭。

3）产褥期：产后 3 d 内，仍是心脏负担较重的时期。子宫收缩使一部分血液进入体循环，孕期组织间潴留的液体也开始回到体循环，加重心脏负担，心脏病产妇仍易发生心力衰竭。

综上所述，妊娠 32～34 周、分娩期及产褥期的最初 3 d 内，心脏病孕产妇因心脏负担加重，是最易发生心力衰竭的危险时期。

（2）心脏病对妊娠、分娩的影响　　心脏病不影响受孕。心功能良好者，在严密监护下可以妊娠；心功能低下不宜妊娠者，因缺血、缺氧使胎儿发育受影响，易导致胎儿窘迫、流产、早产甚至死胎发生。围产儿死亡率明显升高。

2.心脏病心功能分级

（1）主观感受分级　　常用纽约心脏病协会（NYHA）分级标准，将心脏功能分为 4 级。

Ⅰ级：一般体力活动不受限制。

Ⅱ级：一般体力活动稍受限制，活动后心悸、轻度气短，休息时无症状。

Ⅲ级：一般体力活动显著受限制，休息时无不适，轻微活动即感不适、心悸、呼吸困难，或既往有心力衰竭史。

Ⅳ级：不能进行任何体力活动，休息时仍有心悸和呼吸困难等症状，活动时加重。

（2）客观评价　　根据 1994 年美国心脏病协会（AHA）标准委员会修订标准，用心电图、运动负荷试验、X 射线、超声心动图等检查结果来评价心脏病的严重程度。

A 级：无心血管病的客观依据。

B 级：客观检查显示有轻度心血管疾病。

C 级：有中度心血管疾病的客观依据。

D 级：有重度心血管疾病的表现。

轻、中、重度心血管疾病标准未做出明确规定，由医生根据检查结果进行判断，将患者的两种分级并列，如心功能Ⅱ级 C 等。

3.早期心力衰竭的临床表现　　出现下列症状与体征，应考虑为早期心力衰竭：①轻微活动后即有胸闷、心悸、气短。②休息时心率超过 110 次/min，呼吸超过 20 次/min。③夜间常因胸闷而坐起，或需到窗口呼吸新鲜空气。④肺底部出现少量持续性湿啰音，咳嗽后不消失。

4.处理原则　首先确定患者是否可以妊娠,不宜妊娠者应指导患者采取有效措施严格避孕,如已妊娠,根据孕周采取适当措施终止妊娠。可以妊娠者,严密监护母儿情况,预防心力衰竭与感染,适时选择合适方式终止妊娠。

(1)能否妊娠的指征　①可以妊娠:心脏病变较轻,心功能Ⅰ～Ⅱ级,既往无心力衰竭史,且无其他并发症者,在严密监护下可以妊娠。②有下列情况者一般不宜妊娠:心脏病变较重、心功能Ⅲ～Ⅳ级、既往有心力衰竭病史、有肺动脉高压、右向左分流型先天性心脏病、严重心律失常、围生期心肌病遗留有心脏扩大、风湿热活动期、并发细菌性心内膜炎。

(2)妊娠期处理　①不宜妊娠者:应在妊娠12周前行人工流产术。如妊娠12周以上,应在密切监护下继续妊娠。发生心力衰竭者应先控制心力衰竭之后再终止妊娠。②可以妊娠者:加强孕期保健,预防心力衰竭,动态观察心功能,适时终止妊娠。

(3)分娩期处理　妊娠晚期应提前选择适宜的分娩方式。①阴道分娩:心功能Ⅰ、Ⅱ级,胎儿不大,胎位正常,子宫颈条件良好者,可考虑在严密监护下经阴道分娩。②剖宫产:胎儿偏大,产道条件不佳及心功能Ⅲ～Ⅳ级者,均应择期剖宫产,或阴道分娩产程进展不顺利、心功能不全进一步恶化者,也应及时采取剖宫产终止妊娠;不宜再妊娠者,同时行输卵管结扎术。

(4)产褥期处理　注意休息,预防产后出血、感染、心力衰竭等并发症。

Classification

The American Heart Association has developed a classification system for heart disease based on the woman's functional capacity.

- Ⅰ: Cardiac disease with no limitation of physical activity. Absence of symptoms of cardiac insufficiency and anginal pain.

- Ⅱ: Cardiac disease with slight limitation of physical activity. Comfortable at rest. Fatigue, palpitation, dyspnea, or anginal pain with ordinary physical activity.

- Ⅲ: Cardiac disease with moderate to marked limitation of physical activity. Comfortable at rest. Excessive fatigue, palpitation, dyspnea, or anginal pain with less than ordinary-physical activity.

- Ⅳ: Cardiac disease with inability to perform any physical activity without discomfort. Symptoms of cardiac insufficiency or of the anginal syndrome may occur at rest and with any physical activity.

Clinical Signs and Symptoms

Signs and symptoms include dyspnea, syncope (fainting) with exertion, hemoptysis, paroxysmal nocturnal dyspnea, and chest pain with exertion. Additional signs that confirm the diagnosis: cyanosis; clubbing; diastolic, presystolic, or continuous heart murmur; cardiac enlargement; a loud, harsh systolic murmur associated with a thrill; serious arrhythmias.

Principle of Management

With appropriate management, women in class Ⅰ and Ⅱ generally are able to experience anormal pregnancy with no or few problems, whereas women in class Ⅲ and Ⅳ are at higher risk of significant hemodynamic morbidity and mortality. Whenever possible, class Ⅲ and Ⅳ women with correctable lesions should be counseled to undergo cardiac surgery before conception. For women with class Ⅲ or Ⅳ heart disease, the primary goal of management is to prevent cardiac decompensation and development of congestive heart failure. Also, every effort is made to protect the fetus from hypoxia and intrauterine growth retardation (IUGR), which can occur if placental perfusion is inadequate.

【护理评估】

1.健康史　有无心脏病史及诱发心力衰竭的因素。了解既往病史,有无先天性心脏病、风湿性心脏病、风湿热病史等,既往诊疗经过,有无心力衰竭史、心脏手术史等。了解妊娠经过,有无重度贫血、上呼吸道感染、妊娠期高血压疾病、过度疲劳、睡眠不好等诱发心力衰竭的因素存在。

2.身心状况　由于担心病情危及母儿的生命安全,孕产妇及家属常存在焦虑、恐惧等心理。

了解是否出现胸闷、气短、心悸、乏力、活动受限等与心脏病有关的症状,有无水肿、发绀、心脏增大、肝大等体征。评估心功能,特别注意评估有无早期心力衰竭的表现。评估胎儿生长发育是否正常,有无宫内缺氧。评估临产后宫缩及产程进展情况,以及产后子宫缩复情况,恶露的量、色及性状,母乳喂养及出入量等。

3.辅助检查

(1)心电图检查　可提示各种心律失常、ST 段改变。

(2)胸部 X 射线检查　显示有心界扩大。

(3)超声心动图　可显示心脏结构、各瓣膜变化。

(4)B 型超声检查　了解胎儿生长发育情况。

(5)胎儿电子监护仪　了解胎儿宫内储备能力。

【护理诊断】

1.活动无耐力　与心功能差有关。

2.自理能力缺陷　与心功能差活动受限及需卧床休息有关。

3.潜在并发症　心力衰竭、洋地黄中毒。

4.母乳喂养中断　与心功能差不能耐受母乳喂养有关。

5.焦虑/恐惧　与担心胎儿与自身安全有关。

【护理措施】

1.非孕期护理　心脏病患者妊娠前应先来医院咨询,根据心脏病种类、病变程度、心功能、孕期监护及医疗条件等考虑能否妊娠。

2.妊娠期护理

(1)加强产前检查　从孕早期开始,定期进行产前检查,酌情增加产前检查次数。妊娠风险低者,产前检查频率同正常妊娠。每次检查应进行妊娠风险评估,妊娠风险分级增高,产前检查次数增加。妊娠 32 周后,发生心力衰竭的概率增加,产前检查应每周 1 次。发现早期心力衰竭征象应及时入院治疗。孕期经过顺利者,也应在妊娠 36~38 周提前住院待产。

(2)预防心力衰竭　避免过度劳累及情绪激动,保证休息,休息时以左侧卧位或半卧位为宜,每日睡眠 10 h,注意增加午休。指导高蛋白、高维生素、低盐、低脂肪饮食,妊娠 16 周以后,每日食盐量不超过 5 g;体重每月增加不超过 0.5 kg,整个孕期不宜超过 12 kg。预防引起心力衰竭的各种诱因,如避免受凉、上呼吸道感染,纠正贫血和心律失常等。定期进行心脏功能检查,出现心力衰竭时积极药物治疗,注意药物剂量与毒性反应。妊娠晚期心力衰竭的患者,待心力衰竭控制后再行产科处理;严重心力衰竭经内科积极治疗效果不佳者,可边控制心力衰竭边紧急行剖宫产,以抢救患者生命。

3.分娩期护理

(1)第一产程　安慰及鼓励产妇,消除其紧张情绪,可适当应用地西泮、哌替啶等镇静剂。每 15 min 测血压、脉搏、呼吸、心率 1 次。一旦发现心力衰竭征象,应给予产妇高浓度面罩吸氧,取半卧位,遵医嘱用西地兰 0.4 mg 加 25% 葡萄糖注射液 20 mL 缓慢静脉注射,必要时间隔 4~6 h 重复给药 1 次。产程开始后即应预防性使用抗生素。密切监护胎儿情况,每 30 min 测胎心率 1 次。

(2)第二产程　指导产妇不屏气用力加腹压,鼓励产妇以呼吸及放松技巧减轻不适感,必要时给予硬膜外麻醉。子宫颈口开全后,应行会阴切开术、胎头吸引或产钳助产术,尽可能缩短第二产程。

(3)第三产程　胎儿娩出后,产妇腹部应立即放置1~2 kg重沙袋持续24 h,防止腹压骤降而诱发心力衰竭。为防止产后出血过多诱发心力衰竭,可用缩宫素10~20 U静脉或肌内注射,禁用麦角新碱,以防静脉压升高。产后出血过多者,应遵医嘱适当输血、输液,注意输液速度不可过快。

4.产褥期护理

(1)预防感染　预防性应用广谱抗生素,至产后1周左右无感染征象时停药。注意外阴部清洁卫生。加强营养,增强抵抗力,避免过劳、受凉。

(2)预防心力衰竭　产后3 d内,产妇需充分休息,尤其产后24 h内应绝对卧床休息。密切监测生命体征及心功能变化,以及早发现早期心力衰竭症状。病情轻者,24 h后根据心功能适当下床活动,以减少血栓的形成。

(3)预防便秘　合理膳食,多吃蔬菜、水果,必要时应用缓泻剂。

(4)指导母乳喂养　心脏病妊娠风险低且心功能Ⅰ级者建议哺乳。对于疾病严重的心脏病产妇,即使心功能Ⅰ级,也建议人工喂养。不宜哺乳者,应及时回乳,指导家属人工喂养的方法。

5.心理护理　解释病情,告知应对措施,减轻产妇及家属的紧张、恐惧心理。鼓励产妇树立信心,积极配合治疗及护理措施。鼓励产妇适度地参加照顾婴儿的活动,促进亲子互动。

6.急性心力衰竭的急救护理

(1)体位　患者取坐位,双腿下垂,必要时应用四肢轮流结扎法,以减少静脉回心血量,减轻心脏负担。

(2)吸氧　高流量面罩或加压给氧,为增加气体交换面积,可用50%的乙醇加入氧气过滤瓶中。严重者采用持续气道正压通气(continuous positive airway pressure,CPAP)。

(3)配合医生药物治疗　按医嘱应用镇静剂、强心剂、利尿剂、血管扩张剂、支气管扩张剂等。注意观察药物疗效与不良反应。

Nursing intervention is directed toward assisting the client to minimize the workload on the cardiovascular system and reduce the risks of complications developing during pregnancy and the postpartum period. Information obtained from preconception cardiac assessment of the woman with congenital heart disease is particularly helpful in managing nursing and medical care. The nurse should review the signs and symptoms of cardiac decompensation and other complications (e. g. , PIH, preterm labor) with all clients. Nursing care for the pregnant client with cardiac disease focuses on activity and rest, nutrition, medications, and prevention of infection. The nurse also must be aware of specific obstetric considerations throughout the pregnancy.

【健康教育】

①介绍疾病的相关知识,使产妇能正确地自我照顾,避免诱发心力衰竭的因素,早期发现心力衰竭的表现及时就诊。②不宜再妊娠的患者,心功能良好者可在产后1周行绝育术,有心力衰竭者待病情控制后行绝育术。未绝育者应严格避孕。

任务实施

妊娠合并心脏病处理流程见图8-1。

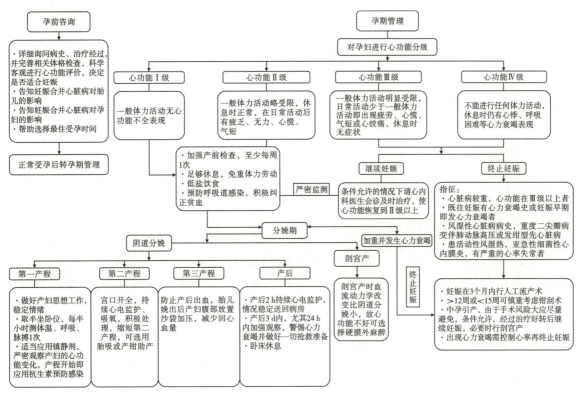

图8-1　妊娠合并心脏病处理流程

任务二　糖尿病(Diabetes Mellitus)

工作情景

患者,女,27岁,G_1P_0,宫内妊娠30^{+5}周。近1周来饭量较前明显增加,并有多饮、多尿现象,前来就诊。行口服葡萄糖耐量试验(OGTT),结果分别为5.3 mmol/L、10.7 mmol/L、8.6 mmol/L。查体:T 36.6 ℃,P 70 次/min,R 20 次/min,BP 120/80 mmHg。宫高在脐与剑突之间,胎心率148 次/min,骨盆外测量无异常。身高160 cm,体重85 kg。既往体健,无糖尿病病史。

①请明确该患者主要的护理问题。②根据目前的情况对患者进行正确的护理。

任务内容

糖尿病是多种因素引起的以慢性血糖水平升高为特征的全身性慢性代谢性疾病。妊娠合并糖尿病有两种类型,一种是妊娠前已有糖尿病,称为糖尿病合并妊娠;另一种是妊娠后才发生或首次发现糖尿病,称为妊娠糖尿病;以后者多见,约占糖尿病孕妇的80%以上。妊娠合并糖尿病是妊娠期常见的内科合并症,母婴的并发症较多,应引起重视。

任务目标

◆ 能叙述妊娠与糖尿病的相互影响、妊娠合并糖尿病的表现及处理原则。
◆ 能对妊娠合并糖尿病进行正确评估及护理。

【概要】

1. 妊娠、分娩与糖尿病的相互影响

(1)妊娠期糖代谢特点 ①妊娠早期,早孕反应使孕妇摄入量减少、胎儿从母体摄取葡萄糖增加,雌激素、孕激素增加母体对葡萄糖的利用等原因导致孕妇空腹血糖降低。②胰岛素需要量增加和糖耐量降低:妊娠后血容量逐渐增加,血液稀释使胰岛素相对不足;胎盘分泌的雌激素、孕酮、人胎盘催乳素、胎盘胰岛素酶等使机体对胰岛素抵抗作用增强,孕妇对胰岛素的敏感性随妊娠周数增加而降低,从而降低糖耐量。③肾糖阈降低:孕期母体肾血流量及肾小球对糖的滤过率增加,肾小管对糖的重吸收率下降,使肾糖阈降低。

(2)妊娠、分娩对糖尿病的影响 妊娠期糖代谢的变化复杂,妊娠可使既往无糖尿病的孕妇发生妊娠期糖尿病(gestational diabetes mellitus,GDM),也可使隐性糖尿病显性化,使原有糖尿病患者的病情加重。由于妊娠期孕妇体内激素水平变化,脂解作用增强,酮体生成增加,而低血糖可使脂解作用进一步加强,若应用胰岛素治疗的孕妇未及时调整用量,可能会出现血糖过低或过高,孕妇极易发生低血糖昏迷或酮症酸中毒。分娩过程中体力消耗大,产妇进食量少;胎盘娩出后,胎盘产生的抗胰岛素物质迅速消失,如果不及时调整胰岛素用量,很易发生低血糖休克。

(3)糖尿病对妊娠、分娩的影响 影响取决于糖尿病病情及血糖控制水平。①对孕妇的影响:受孕率降低,流产率升高,妊娠期高血压疾病发生率高,感染率高尤以尿路感染最常见,羊水过多发生率较非糖尿病孕妇高10倍,难产、手术产、产道损伤增多,易发生产后出血,易发生酮症酸中毒。②对胎儿、新生儿的影响:巨大胎儿发生率较非糖尿病孕妇者高出3~4倍,胎儿畸形发生率为非糖尿病孕妇3~5倍,胎儿生长受限发生率增加,新生儿呼吸窘迫综合征发生率增加,新生儿低血糖发生率增加。新生儿脱离母体高血糖环境后,高胰岛素血症仍存在,若不及时补充糖,易发生低血糖,围产儿死亡率高。

2. 临床表现 多数孕妇无明显的临床表现。如果妊娠期出现"三多"症状(多饮、多食、多尿),或出现外阴阴道假丝酵母菌病反复发作难以治愈,或孕妇体重过度增长,或并发羊水过多或巨大胎儿,应警惕合并糖尿病的可能性。

3. 处理原则 允许妊娠者,加强孕期监护,在内科、产科密切监护下,尽可能将孕妇血糖控制在正常或接近正常范围内,注意监测胎儿宫内情况,适时终止妊娠,防止并发症的发生。

Clinical Signs and Symptoms

• Hyperglycemia:If a woman's insulin amount is insufficient,glucose cannot be used by body cells.

The cells register their glucose want, and the liver quickly converts stored glycogen to glucose to increase the serum glucose level. Because of the insulin insufficiency, however, the body cells still cannot use the glucose, and the serum glucose levels continue to rise.

- Glycosuria: When the level of blood sugar of the woman rises to 8. 3 mmol/L (normal is 4. 4 - 6. 6 mmol/L), the kidneys begin to excrete quantities of glucose in the urine in an attempt to lower the level.
- Polyuria: Because of osmotic action, the increased amount of glucose in the urine reduces fluid absorption in the kidney, and large quantities of fluid are lost in urine.

Principle of Management

Both women with gestational diabetes and those with overt diabetes need more frequent prenatal visits than usual so they can be more frequently monitored than others to regulate glucose values.

【护理评估】

1.健康史　评估有无妊娠合并糖尿病的高危因素,如糖尿病家族史、孕前体重>90 kg、反复自然流产,是否有死胎、畸形儿、呼吸窘迫综合征(RDS)足月儿或巨大儿等病史。了解本次妊娠经过,是否有反复发作的外阴阴道假丝酵母菌病、胎儿是否偏大、有无羊水过多等。了解患者的病情控制及治疗情况、有无糖尿病并发症等。

2.身心状况　了解孕妇及家属对病情的认知程度、情绪反应和心理状态,是否存在担心、焦虑、恐惧等心理,是否掌握相关的自我保健及护理知识。

(1)妊娠期　重点评估孕妇有无糖代谢紊乱症候群、糖尿病并发症及胎儿发育情况。病情轻者,"三多一少"(多饮、多食、多尿、体重下降)症状不明显;重者,除"三多一少"外,常出现皮肤瘙痒、外阴阴道假丝酵母菌病等。注意评估是否有视网膜病变、糖尿病性肾病、妊娠期高血压疾病、羊水过多等。了解胎儿宫内发育情况,有无胎儿生长受限、胎儿窘迫、畸形或巨大儿等。

(2)分娩期　除监测产程和胎儿安危外,注意评估产妇是否出现低血糖及酮症酸中毒症状,表现为头晕、心悸、面色苍白、出汗、恶心、呕吐、烦躁、视力模糊、呼吸快、呼气有烂苹果味等。

(3)产褥期　着重评估产妇有无产后出血及感染征象,有无低血糖或高血糖症状,新生儿有无低血糖、呼吸窘迫综合征。

3.辅助检查

(1)心电图检查　可提示各种心律失常、ST 段改变。

(2)胸部 X 射线检查　显示心界扩大。

(3)超声心动图　显示心脏结构、各瓣膜变化。

(4)B 型超声检查　了解胎儿生长发育情况。

(5)胎儿电子监护仪　了解胎儿宫内储备能力。

【护理诊断】

1.有感染的危险　与糖尿病患者抵抗力下降有关。

2.胎儿有受伤的危险　与糖尿病可能导致胎盘供血不足、畸形儿、胎儿肺泡表面活性物质不足、巨大儿、低血糖等有关。

3.潜在并发症　如低血糖、酮症酸中毒。

4.焦虑　与担心身体状况及胎儿安全有关。

【护理措施】

1.一般护理

(1)饮食控制　轻症患者仅需饮食控制即可维持血糖在正常范围。妊娠早期,糖尿病孕妇需要

妇产科护理学 Obstetric and Gynecological Nursing

热量与孕前相同;孕中期后,每周所需热量增加3%~8%,其中碳水化合物占40%~50%、蛋白质占20%~30%、脂肪占30%~40%。建议多食粗粮、豆类、绿叶蔬菜、低糖水果等,每日热量分配比例是早餐25%、午餐30%、晚餐30%、睡前点心(含蛋白质及碳水化合物)15%。控制餐后1 h血糖值<8 mmol/L。另外,每日补充钙剂1.0~1.2 g、叶酸5 mg、铁15 mg。

(2)合理运动:运动可提高外周组织对胰岛素的敏感性,促进葡萄糖的利用,有利于控制病情。指导选择适宜的运动方式,如散步或中速步行,每日至少1次,每次20~40 min,餐后1 h进行。

2.病情观察　定期行血糖、尿酮体监测,眼底检查,注意观察孕产妇有无低血糖表现、感染征兆和产后出血迹象。密切监测胎儿发育情况和胎盘功能。

妊娠合并糖尿病患者
血糖控制目标

3.心理护理　介绍疾病的相关知识、目前病情、治疗措施及其必要性,以及低血糖的症状和紧急应对措施,使孕妇及家属消除紧张或焦虑,能积极配合治疗。耐心倾听孕妇表达其内心感受,关心、鼓励孕妇以积极的心态面对问题。及时提供新生儿各种信息,创造亲子互动机会,促进母婴亲情发展。

4.用药护理　对于非药物疗法不能有效控制血糖的GDM患者,为避免低血糖和酮症酸中毒的发生,首选胰岛素进行药物治疗,一般从小剂量开始,并根据病情、妊娠时期、血糖值进行调整。

5.产科护理配合

(1)孕前护理　确定糖尿病患者是否能妊娠。根据White分类法,分期达D、F、R级者母儿危险较大,不宜妊娠,如已妊娠应尽早终止。器质性病变较轻、血糖控制良好者,可在积极治疗、密切监护下继续妊娠。

(2)妊娠期护理　密切监测血糖变化,以及时调整胰岛素用量。妊娠早期应每周检查1次至妊娠第10周;妊娠中期应每2周检查1次,一般妊娠20周时胰岛素的需要量开始增加,应及时进行调整。重视产前检查,定期行B型超声检查胎儿发育情况、有无畸形、羊水量。加强对糖尿病并发症的监护,定期行眼底检查、肾功能检查和测定糖化血红蛋白含量。

(3)分娩期护理

1)选择合适的时间终止妊娠:在控制血糖、确保母儿安全的情况下,尽量在接近预产期(39周后)终止妊娠。若血糖控制不良,伴有血管病变、严重感染、胎儿窘迫等,在采取促胎肺成熟措施后及时终止妊娠。

2)指导分娩方式的选择:妊娠合并糖尿病并非剖宫产的指征,如病情轻、无其他产科指征可阴道分娩;如果病情重,并发血管病变,或有骨盆狭窄、胎位异常、胎儿窘迫、巨大儿等应行剖宫产。

3)产程中护理:密切监测血糖、尿糖、尿酮体和胎儿情况。控制血糖不低于5.6 mmol/L,必要时可按每4 g葡萄糖加1U胰岛素的比例进行输液,预防发生低血糖。阴道分娩者,如产程大于16 h易发生酮症酸中毒,故应严密观察,避免产程延长,产程时间不超过12 h为宜,如产程中发现产程进展缓慢或胎儿窘迫,应考虑改行剖宫产。

(4)产后护理

1)及时调整胰岛素用量:分娩后24 h内胰岛素用量应减至原用量的1/2,48 h应减少到原用量的1/3。

2)预防性应用广谱抗生素,保持外阴部或腹部伤口清洁,防止产褥感染。

3)新生儿护理:糖尿病产妇的新生儿,无论体重大小均按早产儿护理。注意保温、吸氧,以及早喂糖水,早开奶。新生儿出生时取脐血检测血糖,出生后30 min开始定时滴服25%葡萄糖注射液,10~15滴/min,防止低血糖,并注意预防低血钙、高胆红素血症及新生儿呼吸窘迫综合征发生。多数新生儿在出生后6 h内血糖值可恢复至正常。

Adequate control of pregnant women with GDM or pregestational diabetes is of primary concern when planning nursing interventions to prevent or lessen the incidence of perinatal mortality and morbidity.

Nutrition

Diabetic women who anticipate pregnancy will follow a prescribed well–balanced dietary regimen before conception and will be in a state of good metabolic control.

Exercise

Research findings suggest that pregnant women in supervised diet and cardiovascular exercise programs have lower levels of glycemia than those managed on a regimen of diet alone. Furthermore, exercise in combination with diet is an effective alternative to insulin for controlling GDM. Low – to – moderate intensity exercise is believed to be safe and beneficial.

Blood Glucose Monitoring

Control of diabetes is now assessed by home blood glucose monitoring. Client education should focus on specific guidelines for using the machine, when to test blood glucose, how to perform the finger stick, and how to record the results. The client should enter all blood glucose levels in the home record keeping system, which also includes insulin doses, weight, and diet.

Insulin Administration

The goal of treatment with insulin is euglycemia, blood glucose levels as near the normal range as possible. Maintaining optimal blood glucose levels requires meticulous regulation of medication, adherence to the prescribed diet, and carefully planned activity.

Obstetric Considerations

Under optimum circumstances, the diabetic woman should deliver near term, usually between 38 and 40 weeks' gestation. Assessment of the phosphatidylglycerol (PG) content in amniotic fluid is often performed to verify fetal lung maturity prior to delivery unless gestational age dating has been well established. When PG is present, delivery is planned. Vaginal delivery is usually possible for diabetic women who have maintained well–controlled plasma glucose levels. Oxytocin induction may be attempted when labor does not begin spontaneously by 40 weeks' gestation, the cervix is considered favorable, and the fetus is not macrosomic. Cesarean section is indicated for cases of fetal compromise, macrosomia, or an unfavorable cervix. Early delivery is necessary only for deteriorating fetal condition or in selected cases of maternal vascular disease, hypertension, and previous stillbirth.

During labor and delivery, an intravenous infusion of regular insulin and glucose using a calibrated pump is used to control maternal glucose in insulin–dependent diabetics. Uterine activity and fetal heart are monitored continuously. Following delivery, insulin is administered as indicated by blood glucose monitoring, and the client is closely observed for insulin reactions.

【健康教育】

①产后及时复查血糖。妊娠期空腹血糖异常明显者,产后应尽早复查空腹血糖,血糖值仍异常者,应诊断为糖尿病合并妊娠;空腹血糖正常的 GDM 患者,应于产后 6～12 周行 OGTT 检查,如果异常,考虑是产前漏诊的糖尿病,正常者仍应每 3 年复查 1 次血糖。②如再妊娠,再次发生 GDM 的概率高达 60%～70%,因此,产后应长期做好避孕措施,可使用安全套或手术结扎,不宜用宫内节育器或避孕药。③用胰岛素治疗的产妇,哺乳对婴儿没有影响,鼓励实施母乳喂养。

任务实施

妊娠糖尿病门诊管理流程见图8-2。

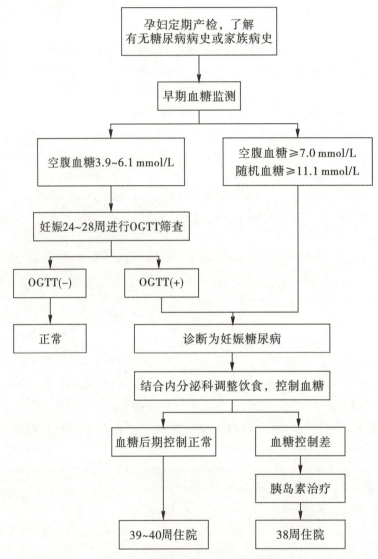

图8-2　妊娠糖尿病门诊管理流程

OGTT 正常范围:空腹血糖<5.1 mmol/L,餐后 1 h 血糖<10.0 mmol/L,餐后
2 h 血糖<8.5 mmol/L。

任务三　病毒性肝炎(Viral Hepatitis)

工作情景

患者,女,25 岁,G_1P_0,孕 34^{+6} 周,自觉乏力、食欲差伴腹胀 1 周,近 3 d 症状加重。查体:BP 130/80 mmHg,T 37.1 ℃,全身皮肤及巩膜黄染,心肺无异常,宫底位于剑突下三指。血液检查:血胆红素 51.3 μmol/L,HBsAg 阳性。

①请明确该患者主要的护理问题。②根据目前的情况对患者进行正确的护理。

任务内容

病毒性肝炎是肝炎病毒引起的以肝脏病变为主的传染性疾病,妊娠的任何时期都有被肝炎病毒感染的可能。已确定的肝炎病毒有 5 种:甲型肝炎病毒(HAV)、乙型肝炎病毒(HBV)、丙型肝炎病毒(HCV)、丁型肝炎病毒(HDV)及戊型肝炎病毒(HEV),其中以 HBV 感染最常见。国内外报告孕妇病毒性肝炎的发病率为 0.8%~17.8%,其发病率约为非孕妇的 6 倍,孕期肝炎发展到重症肝炎的发生率较非孕妇高,重症肝炎仍是我国孕产妇主要的死亡原因之一。

任务目标

◆ 能叙述妊娠与病毒性肝炎的相互影响、妊娠合并病毒性肝炎的表现及处理原则。
◆ 能对妊娠合并病毒性肝炎进行正确评估及护理。

【概要】

1. 妊娠、分娩与病毒性肝炎的相互影响

(1)妊娠、分娩对病毒性肝炎的影响　妊娠期肝脏的生理变化使其负担加重,原有肝损坏进一步加重,容易发展成重症肝炎。①妊娠期增多的雌激素需在肝内灭活,妨碍肝脏对脂肪的代谢,胎儿代谢产物需经母体肝内解毒,增加了肝脏负担。②因妊娠反应,母体摄入减少,体内蛋白质等营养物质相对不足;而妊娠期机体新陈代谢率高,营养物质消耗增多,肝内糖原储备降低,使肝脏抗病能力下降。③分娩时体力消耗、出血、麻醉、缺氧、酸性代谢产物增多等可进一步加重肝脏负担。

(2)病毒性肝炎对妊娠、分娩的影响　①对孕产妇的影响:产科并发症发生率高,早孕反应加重,妊娠期高血压疾病发病率增高,容易发生严重的产后出血;重症肝炎的发生率高,为非孕妇女的 66 倍,易导致产后大出血、消化道出血、感染等,最终诱发肝性脑病和肝肾综合征,威胁母婴生命安全。②对围产儿的影响:胎儿畸形发病率约升高 2 倍;部分在围生期感染的婴儿,可转为慢性病毒携带者,将来容易发展为肝硬化或原发性肝癌;近年研究发现,病毒性肝炎与唐氏综合征(21 三体综合征)的发病密切相关;肝功能异常的孕产妇,流产、早产、死胎、死产和新生儿死亡率明显增加,死亡率高达 46‰。

2. 临床表现　患者可有全身酸痛、乏力、畏寒、发热、尿色深黄、食欲减退、恶心、呕吐、腹部不适、右上腹疼痛、腹胀、腹泻等症状,皮肤和巩膜黄染、肝区叩击痛。

3. 处理原则　原则上肝炎患者不宜妊娠。感染 HBV 的育龄妇女在妊娠前应行肝功能检查、血清 HBV-DNA 检测、肝脏 B 型超声检查。最佳受孕时机是肝功能正常、血清 HBV-DNA 低水平、肝脏 B 型超声无特殊改变时。轻症急性肝炎，经积极治疗后好转者可继续妊娠。慢性活动性肝炎患者妊娠后可加重，对母儿危害较大，治疗后效果不好应考虑终止妊娠。治疗主要采用护肝、对症、支持疗法。

Clinical Manifestation

Patients may have general pain, fatigue, chills, fever, dark yellow urine, poor appetite, nausea, vomiting, abdominal discomfort, right upper abdominal pain, abdominal distension, diarrhea and other symptoms. The patient had yellow skin and sclera and percussion pain in the liver.

Principle of Management

If HBsAg is positive, liver function tests and a complete hepatitis panel should be performed. Pregnant women at high risk for hepatitis B infection should be offered vaccination. Available vaccines are produced by recombinant DNA technology and aretherefore safe for use in pregnancy. The newborn is recommended to give hepatitis immunoglobulin and hepatitis vaccine soon after delivery, which reduces the risk for infection to less than 10%.

【护理评估】

1. 健康史　评估孕妇有无与肝炎患者密切接触史，或输血、注射血制品史，有无肝炎病家族史及当地有无肝炎流行史等。了解其妊娠经过、疾病诊疗经过、用药情况及病情控制情况。

2. 身心状况　由于缺乏疾病的相关知识和对自身病情不了解，患者及家属常表现出担心、焦虑甚至恐惧等心理。

评估孕妇是否出现不能用妊娠反应或其他原因解释的消化系统症状，如食欲减退、恶心、呕吐、腹胀、厌油腻、乏力、肝区痛等。黄疸型肝炎患者可表现出黄疸，小便深黄色。评估孕妇是否有重症肝炎的表现，如出现畏寒，发热，皮肤巩膜、尿色黄染且逐渐加重，极度乏力，腹胀，频繁呕吐，有肝臭气味，甚至嗜睡、烦躁、神志不清、昏迷等。

查体可触及肝大、触痛，肝区叩击痛阳性；妊娠晚期受增大子宫影响，肝脏不易被触及，如能触及应想到异常。重症患者肝脏进行性缩小。

3. 辅助检查

（1）肝功能检查　血清中丙氨酸氨基转移酶（ALT）明显升高，特别是数值大于正常值 10 倍以上而且持续时间较长，排除其他原因外，对病毒性肝炎有诊断价值。血清胆红素明显上升 [>17 μmol/L(1 mg/dL)]、尿胆红素阳性对诊断病毒性肝炎有价值。

（2）血清病原学检测　可确定病毒性肝炎的类型。

（3）其他　凝血功能检查及胎盘功能检查。

【护理诊断】

1. 营养失调:低于机体需要量　与食欲减退、恶心、呕吐、营养摄入减少有关。

血清病原学检测及其意义

2. 潜在并发症　产后出血、肝性脑病。

3. 焦虑/恐惧　与产妇担心自身安危、担心传染给胎儿有关。

【护理措施】

1. 一般护理　注意休息，每日保证 9 h 睡眠和适当的午休，避免劳累。加强营养，保证高蛋白、高维生素、富含碳水化合物和纤维素的低脂饮食。保持大便通畅，避免便秘发生。重症肝炎者应严格限制蛋白质的摄入，每日摄入量应<0.5 g/kg，可增加碳水化合物，使每日热量维持在 1 800 kcal

（1 kcal＝4.186 kJ）以上。

2.病情观察　密切观察孕产妇消化道症状、黄疸情况，监测肝炎病毒血清病原学标志物及肝功能。监测凝血功能，注意观察孕产妇有无口、鼻、皮肤黏膜出血倾向。重症肝炎者应严密监测生命体征，密切观察有无性格改变、行为异常、扑翼样震颤等肝性脑病前驱症状，严格限制液体入量，并记录出入量。

3.心理护理　向孕产妇及家属解释病情和治疗方案，减轻孕产妇及家属的焦虑或恐惧心理，使其能积极配合治疗及护理措施。鼓励孕产妇表达出其内心感受，给予理解和安慰。

4.产科护理配合

（1）妊娠期护理

1）妊娠早期感染者，若为轻型应积极保肝治疗，可继续妊娠；若为重型待孕产妇病情好转后行人工流产术终止妊娠；妊娠中、晚期感染者不宜终止妊娠，若经积极治疗后病情无好转，可考虑终止妊娠。

2）落实消毒隔离制度，防止交叉感染：需开设隔离诊室为肝炎孕妇进行产前检查，用过的医疗用物应用 2 000 mg/L 含氯制剂浸泡消毒，防止交叉感染。

3）预防加重肝炎的诱因：妊娠合并重症肝炎时，应积极保肝治疗，预防及治疗肝性脑病，如用高血糖素－胰岛素－葡萄糖、6 合氨基酸等。避免应用损害肝脏的药物，预防各种感染。限制蛋白质的摄入，增加碳水化合物摄入，保持大便通畅，禁用肥皂水灌肠。口服新霉素或甲硝唑抑制大肠埃希菌，以减少游离氨及其他毒素的产生及吸收。严格限制液体入量，每日入量为前日尿量加 500 mL。预防 DIC 和肝肾综合征，用肝素治疗时，注意观察有无全身出血倾向。妊娠末期患重症肝炎者，经积极治疗 24 h 后行以剖宫产结束妊娠。

4）预防产后出血：分娩前 1 周每日肌内注射维生素 K_1 20～40 mg，临产后配备同型新鲜血以预防 DIC，产前 4 h 及产后 12 h 内不宜使用肝素治疗。

（2）分娩期护理

1）密切观察产程进展，正确处理产程，避免产道损伤。第二产程行胎头吸引术或产钳术助产，缩短第二产程。胎肩娩出后立即静脉注射缩宫素，以减少产后出血。若孕妇在使用肝素治疗过程中突然临产或需剖宫产，则应立即停用肝素，4 h 之后才可进行手术。

2）严格执行消毒隔离制度，防止母婴传播。凡病毒性肝炎产妇用过的医疗物品均要用 2 000 mg/L 的含氯消毒液浸泡后按相关规定处理。一次性物品需用双层塑料袋包装后焚烧。

3）注意观察产妇有无出血倾向，准备好新鲜血液，临产时加维生素 K_1 20 mg 静脉注射。做好抢救产妇休克和新生儿窒息的准备。

（3）产褥期护理

1）注意休息和加强营养，避免劳累，继续应用对肝脏损害较小的头孢菌素类或氨苄西林等广谱抗生素预防和控制产褥感染。

2）观察子宫缩复及恶露表现，预防产后出血。

3）指导母乳喂养：对 HBsAg 阳性母亲的新生儿，经过主动及被动免疫后，无论母血 HBsAg 阳性还是阴性，不用检测乳汁中是否有 HBV-DNA，其新生儿均可以母乳喂养。因病情严重不宜母乳喂养者，应及时回乳。不宜用雌激素回乳，可用生麦芽冲剂或芒硝外敷乳房。

4）新生儿护理：HBsAg 阳性母亲的新生儿，应在出生后 24 h 内尽早注射乙型肝炎免疫球蛋白（HBIG），剂量≥100 U，并同时接种 10 μg 重组酵母乙型肝炎疫苗。生后 1 个月、6 个月时接种第 2、第 3 针乙肝疫苗。

Nursing During Pregnancy

For those infected in early pregnancy, if they are mild, they should be treated actively to protect the liver. If the severe condition improves, abortion is performed to terminate pregnancy. Termination of pregnancy is not suitable for patients in the second or third trimester of pregnancy. Termination of pregnancy can be considered if the condition does not improve after active treatment.

● Implement disinfection and isolation system to prevent cross infection: The isolation clinic should be set up for prenatal examination for pregnant women with hepatitis. The used medical materials should be soaked and disinfected with 2,000 mg/L chlorine-containing preparations to prevent cross infection.

● Prevention of causes aggravating hepatitis: When pregnancy is complicated with severe hepatitis, active liver protection treatment should be acted to prevent and treat hepatic encephalopathy. Avoid drugs that damage the liver and prevent infections.

● Prevention of postpartum bleeding: Parturient women need intramuscular injection of vitamin K_1 20 ~ 40 mg daily 1 week before delivery and should be equipped with new blood of the same type after delivery to prevent DIC.

Nursing During Delivery

Closely observe the progress of labor and manage the labor process correctly to avoid damage to the birth canal. The second stage of labor should be shortened by fetal head suction or forceps. Intravenously inject oxytocin immediately after delivery of the fetal shoulder to reduce postpartum bleeding. If a patient suddenly enters labor or requires cesarean section during heparin therapy, heparin should be stopped immediately and surgery should be performed 4 h later.

Strictly implement the disinfection and isolation system to prevent mother-to-child transmission. All the medical articles used by parturients with viral hepatitis should be soaked with 2,000 mg/L chlorine-containing disinfectant and disposed of according to relevant regulations. Disposable goods should be wrapped in double plastic bags and incinerated.

Pay attention to observe whether the maternal bleeding tendency, ready for fresh blood, at the time of delivery with vitamin K_1 20 mg intravenous injection. Be prepared for shock and neonatal asphyxia.

Puerperal Nursing

Patients should pay attention to rest and strengthen nutrition, avoid fatigue, and continue to use cephalosporins or ampicillin and other broad-spectrum antibiotics with little damage to the liver to prevent and control puerperal infection. To observe the manifestations of uterine retraction and lochia and prevent postpartum hemorrhage.

Newborns whose mothers are HBsAg positive should receive HBIG injection as early as possible within 24 h after birth, the dose ≥100 U, and 10 μg recombinant yeast hepatitis B vaccine at the same time. The second and third doses of hepatitis B vaccine were given at 1 month and 6 months after birth.

【健康教育】

①肝炎患者不宜妊娠,应严格避孕,待肝炎痊愈半年,最好2年后再妊娠。夫妻一方患有肝炎者应用避孕套以免交叉感染。②妊娠期加强产前检查,增加营养,增强机体的抵抗力。③及时为新生儿进行乙型肝炎免疫球蛋白和乙肝疫苗预防接种,降低新生儿发病率。④出院后继续保肝治疗,避免过度劳累。

任务四　贫血（Anemia）

工作情景

患者，女，27 岁，G_1P_0，孕 30 周，常觉乏力、腹胀，下午常感头晕、气短、心慌。停经 6 周左右出现恶心、呕吐、不能进食，持续 1 月余。停经 20 周后自觉胎动。平素月经量多。体格检查：面色萎黄，毛发干燥，皮肤干皱。腹围 85 cm，宫高 26 cm，LOA，胎心率 148 次/min。指甲脆薄、扁平、不光整。实验室检查：Hb 70 g/L，RBC $3.0×10^{12}$/L，血清铁 58 μmol/L。骨髓象：幼红细胞增生活跃。

①请明确该患者主要的护理问题。②根据目前的情况对患者进行正确的护理。

任务内容

贫血是指全身循环血液中的红细胞总量或血红蛋白值低于正常值，是妊娠期较常见的一种合并症。贫血有多种类型，如缺铁性贫血、巨幼细胞贫血、再生障碍性贫血等。妊娠期贫血以缺铁性贫血最常见，占妊娠期贫血的 95%。

任务目标

◆ 能叙述妊娠与贫血的相互影响、妊娠合并贫血的表现及处理原则。
◆ 能对妊娠合并贫血进行正确评估及护理。

【概要】

1. 贫血对妊娠的影响

（1）对母体的影响　贫血使血红蛋白减少、血液携氧能力降低，孕妇的抵抗力下降，对分娩、手术和麻醉的耐受能力下降明显，即使贫血程度为轻度或中度，也使孕妇在妊娠和分娩期间的风险增加。重度贫血时，可导致贫血性心脏病、妊娠期高血压疾病或妊娠期高血压疾病性心脏病、失血性休克、产褥感染甚至败血症等并发症，危及孕产妇生命。

（2）对胎儿的影响　铁的受体组织主要是母体的骨髓和胎儿，在竞争摄取母体血清铁的过程中，胎儿组织占优势；而且，铁通过胎盘运向胎儿是单向性运输，不能逆转运输。故一般情况下，胎儿缺铁的程度不会太严重。但母体缺铁严重时，骨髓造血功能低下，导致孕妇重度贫血，胎儿生长发育所需的营养物质及氧缺乏，容易引起胎儿生长受限、胎儿窘迫、早产的发生，使死胎及死产的发生率升高，新生儿窒息及缺血、缺氧性脑病等疾病的发生率和死亡率均升高。

2. 临床表现　轻者无明显症状，重者出现疲劳、头晕、心悸、气短、食欲减退、腹胀、腹泻等症状，容易发生感染而出现相应感染症状。皮肤黏膜苍白，毛发干燥无光泽、脱落，皮肤干燥、皱缩，指（趾）甲扁平、不光整、脆薄易裂。

3. 处理原则　补充铁剂，治疗并发症，预防感染，预防产后出血。

Clinical Signs and Symptoms

Signs and symptoms of iron-deficiency anemia include pallor, fatigue, lethargy, and headache. Clinical findings also may include inflammations of the lips and tongue. Pica (consuming nonfood substances such as clay,dirt,ice,and starch）also is a sign of iron-deficiency anemia.

Principle of Management

Supplement iron,treat complications,prevent infection and postpartum bleeding.

【护理评估】

1．健康史　评估有无不良饮食习惯，如长期偏食或胃肠道功能紊乱导致的营养不良。了解既往有无月经过多等慢性失血性病史。

2．身心状况　孕妇因长期疲倦而容易出现倦怠心理。评估孕妇及家人对缺铁性贫血疾病的认知程度，是否掌握相关的自我保健知识，家庭社会支持系统是否完善。

评估孕妇贫血的程度，是否出现贫血性心脏病、胎儿生长受限、胎儿窘迫、早产、死胎、死产等并发症，有无伴发口腔炎、舌炎等。

3．辅助检查

（1）血常规　外周血象呈典型的小细胞、低色素性贫血。血红蛋白<100 g/L，红细胞计数<3.5×10^{12}/L，血细胞比容<0.30，红细胞平均体积（MCV）<80 fL，血小板及白细胞计数正常。

（2）血清铁测定　反映机体缺铁状况，当孕妇血清铁<6.5 μmol/L（35 μg/dL）时，可确诊。

（3）骨髓象　红系造血增生活跃，以中幼红细胞和晚幼红细胞增生为主。骨髓铁染色可见细胞内外铁均减少，尤其细胞外铁减少明显。

【护理诊断】

1．活动无耐力　与贫血引起的乏力有关。

2．母儿有受伤的危险　与贫血引起的头晕、眼花、胎儿窘迫、胎儿生长受限、早产、死胎、死产等有关。

3．有感染的危险　与血红蛋白低、机体免疫力低下有关。

【护理措施】

1．一般护理　注意休息，适当减轻工作量，血红蛋白在70 g/L以下者应完全休息。加强安全防护，避免因头晕、乏力、晕倒而发生意外。纠正偏食习惯，食物品种应多样化，多摄入含铁丰富的食物，如瘦肉、蛋类、动物肝脏、绿叶蔬菜、红枣、豆制品等。注意科学搭配饮食，避免蔬菜、谷类、茶叶中的磷酸盐、鞣酸等影响铁的吸收。

2．病情观察　监测血常规，观察是否有头晕、疲劳、心悸、气短等症状及表现程度，皮肤黏膜颜色、毛发、指甲等有无改变，密切监测胎儿宫内情况和胎盘功能，密切观察产程进展，产后密切观察子宫收缩及阴道流血情况，是否出现感染征象。

3．心理护理　介绍妊娠合并贫血的相关知识、病情程度和治疗措施，使孕产妇能积极配合治疗。提供心理支持，消除孕产妇及家属的担心、焦虑。促进家庭支持系统发挥作用，加强亲子互动。

4．治疗护理

（1）积极治疗引起慢性失血的疾病。

（2）注意无菌操作，在妊娠、分娩、产褥各期预防感染。

（3）纠正贫血。

1）补充铁剂：妊娠4个月后开始补充铁剂，以口服给药为主。指导孕妇饭后或餐中服用硫酸亚铁0.3 g，3次/d。为促进铁的吸收，可同时服维生素C 0.3 g及10%稀盐酸0.5~2.0 mL；或服用多糖铁复合物每次150 mg，1~2次/d。口服铁剂后胃肠道反应严重者，或妊娠后期重度缺铁性贫血者，可改换剂型，常用有右旋糖酐铁或山梨醇铁注射液，须深部肌内注射。首次给药应从小剂量开始，第1天50 mg，若无不良反应，第2天可增至100 mg。告诉孕妇服用铁剂后大便为黑色属正常现象。产后继续采取措施纠正贫血。

2)输血：当血红蛋白<60 g/L、接近预产期或短期内需行剖宫产术者，应少量多次输血，有条件者可输浓缩红细胞。

(4)临产前按医嘱给产妇应用维生素 K_1、卡巴克洛、维生素 C 等药物，并配血备用。密切观察产程进展，宫口开全后可行阴道助产术缩短第二产程。胎儿前肩娩出后，应及时应用子宫收缩剂预防产后出血。

Client education,nutritional counseling,and possible referrals for supplemental food programs are key elements of nursing care.

A comprehensive 7-day diet history is taken to evaluate the pregnant woman's general nutritional status and the quantity of iron available through nutritional sources. An iron-rich diet is recommended for all pregnant women. The nutritional counselor or nurse should provide instruction about dietary sources of iron. Dietary sources include fortified cereals;liver;beets;raisins;leafy, green vegetables;red meat;eggs; legumes;dried fruits;and whole grains. Ideally,an extra 1,000 mg of iron should be added to the daily diet. Clients should be advised to eat foods rich in vitamin C for optimal absorption of iron. Client also should be informed that iron absorption may be reduced due to phosphates in milk and eggs, bicarbonate,tea,and some food preservatives.

Oral administration of iron is commonly prescribed to prevent or treat iron deficiency. 3-5 mg/d of iron is needed to supply the needs of woman and fetus,with demands for iron increasing in the last 5 months of pregnancy to as much as 3-7 mg/d. A failure to respond to oral iron therapy is the result of failure to take the medication (iron tends to produce gastrointestinal symptoms) or a concurrent folic acid deficiency. It is important to assess the existence of side effects in all pregnant women receiving iron supplementation. The client should be instructed about dietary measures to minimize the gastrointestinal side effects of iron therapy. The nurse also should inform the client that unabsorbed iron is excreted in feces,causing the stool to turn green or black.

【健康教育】

①重度贫血者不宜母乳喂养，指导产妇回奶方法，可口服生麦芽或用芒硝外敷乳房。介绍人工喂养的方法及注意事项。②嘱产妇产后保证休息，加强营养，避免疲劳。

微课　　　　　　　　　　课件　　　　　　　　练习题及参考答案

（王珏辉）

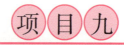

异常分娩妇女的护理
(Nursing of Women with Abnormal Labor)

项目描述

　　异常分娩又称难产,其影响因素包括产力、产道、胎儿及社会心理因素,这些因素既相互影响又互为因果关系。任何1个或1个以上的因素发生异常及4个因素间相互不能适应,而使分娩进程受到阻碍,称为异常分娩。护士的主要任务就是正确地认识影响分娩的4个因素,在产程中提供整体护理,以及时发现和处理异常分娩,获得产妇的配合,维护母儿安全。

　　Dysfunctional labor, or dystocia refers to the abnormal progress of labor. The labor is longer, more painful, or abnormal because of problems with the mechanics of labor, powers, passageway, passenger, or psyche. Any deviation of normal pattern of labor can be designated as dystocia. Overall the incidence of labor disorder is approximately 25% in primigravida and 10% in multigravida. It is one of most common indication for cesarean section.

任务一　产力异常(Abnormal Uterine Action)

工作情景

　　王女士,25岁,G_1P_0,宫内妊娠 38^{+5} 周,阵发性腹痛18 h入院。该孕妇近2 d来一直睡眠差,进食少。查体:BP 124/86 mmHg,心率86次/min,心肺正常。产科检查:宫缩(20~30)s/(5~6)min,胎心率140次/min,先露部S-1,宫口开大1 cm,LOA,胎膜未破。
　　①该患者临产后主要出现了什么问题? ②如何对该患者进行护理?

任务内容

　　子宫收缩力是临产后贯穿于分娩全过程的主要动力,具有节律性、对称性、极性及缩复作用的特点。任何原因引发的子宫收缩的节律性、对称性及极性不正常或收缩力的强度、频率变化均称为子宫收缩力异常,简称产力异常。

任务目标

◆ 能识别产力异常的类型。

◆ 能说出产力异常的处理原则。

◆ 能运用所学的知识对产力异常的妇女进行护理。

临床上,子宫收缩力异常分为子宫收缩乏力(简称宫缩乏力)和子宫收缩过强(简称宫缩过强)两类。每一类又分为协调性子宫收缩异常和不协调性子宫收缩异常(图9-1)。

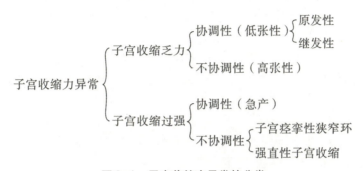

图9-1　子宫收缩力异常的分类

一　子宫收缩乏力

【概要】

1.原因　头盆不称或胎位异常(最常见原因)、子宫局部因素、精神因素、内分泌失调、药物影响等。

2.临床表现

(1)协调性子宫收缩乏力　又称低张性子宫收缩乏力,是指子宫收缩具有正常的节律性、对称性和极性,但收缩力弱,持续时间短,间歇期长,宫缩<2 次/10 min。宫缩高峰期,宫体隆起不明显,按压时有凹陷。此种宫缩乏力多为继发性,对胎儿的影响不大。

(2)不协调性子宫收缩乏力　又称高张性子宫收缩乏力。特点为宫缩失去正常的节律性、对称性,尤其是极性。宫缩的兴奋点来自子宫下段一处或多处,宫缩波自下而上扩散,宫缩时子宫底部较子宫下段弱,宫缩间歇期子宫不能很好地松弛,使宫口扩张受限,胎先露不能如期下降,为无效宫缩。产妇可出现持续性腹痛、腹部拒按、烦躁不安,严重时可出现水及电解质紊乱、尿潴留、肠胀气、胎盘-胎儿循环障碍、静息宫内压升高、胎心异常。此种宫缩乏力多为原发性宫缩乏力。

(3)产程曲线异常

1)潜伏期延长:从临产规律宫缩开始至活跃期起点(子宫颈口扩张 6 cm)称为潜伏期。初产妇>20 h、经产妇>14 h 称为潜伏期延长。

2)活跃期延长:从活跃期起点(子宫颈口扩张 6 cm)至宫口开全称为活跃期。活跃期宫口扩张速度<0.5 cm/h 称为活跃期延长。

3)活跃期停滞:当破膜且子宫颈口扩张≥6 cm 后,若宫缩正常,子宫颈口停止扩张≥4 h,或宫缩欠佳,子宫颈口停止扩张≥6 h 称为活跃期停滞。

4）胎头下降延缓：第二产程初产妇胎头先露部下降速度<1 cm/h，经产妇<2 cm/h，称为胎头下降延缓。

5）胎头下降停滞：第二产程胎头先露部停留在原处不下降>1 h，称为胎头下降停滞。

6）第二产程延长：初产妇>3 h，经产妇>2 h（硬膜外麻醉镇痛分娩时，初产妇>4 h，经产妇>3 h），产程无进展（胎头下降和旋转），称为第二产程延长。

7）滞产：指总产程超过24 h者。

3. 对母儿的影响

（1）对产妇的影响　产程延长产妇休息不好、精神与体力消耗；因呻吟和过度换气、进食减少，可出现精神疲惫、乏力、排尿困难及肠胀气。严重者引起脱水、低钾血症或酸中毒，最终影响子宫收缩，手术产率增加。第二产程延长可因产道受压过久，发生产后尿潴留，受压组织长期缺血，继发水肿、坏死，软产道受损，形成生殖道瘘。同时，易导致产后出血和产褥感染。

（2）对胎儿的影响　不协调性宫缩乏力对子宫胎盘循环影响大，易发生胎儿窘迫；产程延长使胎头及脐带等受压时间过久，手术助产机会增加，易导致新生儿窒息、产伤、颅内出血及吸入性肺炎等。

4. 处理原则

（1）协调性宫缩乏力　查找原因，无头盆不称及胎位异常，估计能从阴道分娩者，可采取措施加强子宫收缩。估计无法经阴道分娩者，行剖宫产。

（2）不协调性宫缩乏力　抑制不协调子宫收缩，使之恢复为协调性宫缩。在未恢复为协调性宫缩之前，禁用缩宫素。

【护理评估】

1. 健康史　了解产妇有无引起宫缩乏力的原因，评估产程进展。

2. 身心状况　测量产妇生命体征，观察产妇神志、皮肤弹性等。注意评估产妇的精神状态、休息、进食及排泄情况。评估产程进展情况，用手触摸孕妇腹部监测宫缩，如出现宫缩乏力，辨别宫缩乏力是协调性还是不协调性。评估产妇及家属的心理状态，因为产程延长，产妇及家属显得焦虑、恐惧，担心母儿的安危。

3. 辅助检查

（1）多普勒胎心听诊仪监测　及时发现胎心异常。

（2）实验室检查　尿酮体阳性，血液生化检查可出现钾离子、钠离子、氯离子及钙离子等电解质的改变，二氧化碳结合力可降低。

【护理诊断】

1. 疲乏　与产程延长、体力过度消耗、进食不足有关。

2. 潜在并发症　产褥感染、产后出血等。

3. 焦虑　与担心母儿安全有关。

【护理措施】

1. 协调性子宫收缩乏力　首先应寻找原因，检查有无头盆不称或胎位异常，若估计不能经阴道分娩者，应及时做好剖宫术前准备。若估计可经阴道分娩者，应做好以下护理。

（1）第一产程

1）一般处理：解除产妇对分娩的心理顾虑与紧张情绪，指导其休息、饮食及大小便，及时补充膳食营养及水分等，必要时可静脉补充营养及水分和给予导尿等措施。对潜伏期出现的宫缩乏力，可用强镇静剂如哌替啶100 mg或吗啡10 mg肌内注射，绝大多数潜伏期宫缩乏力者在充分休息后可自然转入活跃期。

2)加强子宫收缩：①人工破膜：子宫颈口扩张≥3 cm，无头盆不称，胎头已衔接而产程延缓者，可行人工破膜。②缩宫素静脉滴注：适用于协调性宫缩乏力、胎心良好、胎位正常、头盆相称者，原则是以最小浓度获得最佳宫缩。

（2）第二产程　若无头盆不称应静脉滴注缩宫素加强宫缩，同时指导产妇配合宫缩屏气用力。母儿状况良好，胎头下降至≥S+3 水平，可等待自然分娩或行阴道助产分娩；若处理后胎头下降无进展，胎头位置在 S+2 水平以上，应及时行剖宫产术。

（3）第三产程　胎肩娩出后可立即将缩宫素 10～20 U 加入 25% 葡萄糖注射液 20 mL 内静脉注射，预防产后出血。对产程长、破膜时间久及手术产者，应给予抗生素预防感染。

缩宫素使用方法：一般将缩宫素 2.5U 配制于 0.9% 氯化钠注射液 500 mL 中，滴速调节至 4～5 滴/min，根据宫缩强弱进行调整，调整间隔为 15～30 min，通常不超过 60 滴/min。维持宫缩时宫腔内压力达 50～60 mmHg，宫缩间隔 2～3 min，持续 40～60 s。对于不敏感者，可酌情增加缩宫素给药剂量。应用缩宫素时，应有专人监护，严密观察宫缩、胎心、血压和产程进展，若宫缩持续超过 1 min 或胎心异常，应立即停止滴注，通知医生。胎儿未娩出前禁用缩宫素肌内注射。

2. 不协调性子宫收缩乏力　遵医嘱给予哌替啶 100 mg 或吗啡 10 mg 肌内注射，镇静、减轻疼痛，使产妇充分休息。若宫缩仍未恢复，做好剖宫产术前准备。

3. 心理护理　鼓励产妇表达担心和不适，耐心解释，稳定情绪，随时将产程进展及治疗护理计划告知产妇，使其知情同意，增加分娩的信心，并取得良好合作。

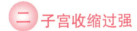

二　子宫收缩过强

【概要】

1. 病因　目前尚不十分明确，但与以下因素有关：经产妇（软产道阻力小），缩宫素应用不当，待产妇精神过度紧张、产程延长、极度疲劳、胎膜早破，以及粗暴的、多次宫腔内操作等。

2. 临床表现

（1）协调性宫缩过强　宫缩的节律性、对称性和极性均正常，但子宫收缩力过强、过频，若产道无梗阻，分娩在短时间内结束，总产程<3 h，称为急产，多见于经产妇。若伴有产道梗阻或瘢痕子宫，可出现病理缩复环，甚至发生子宫破裂。

（2）不协调性宫缩过强

1)强直性子宫收缩：指子宫颈内口以上部分的子宫肌层出现强直性痉挛性收缩，宫缩间歇期短或无间歇。产妇烦躁不安、持续腹痛，胎位、胎心不清，腹部可见一环形凹陷即病理性缩复环，是先兆子宫破裂的征象。

2)子宫痉挛性狭窄环：子宫壁局部肌肉呈痉挛性不协调性收缩，形成环状狭窄，持续不放松。狭窄环可发生在子宫的任何部分，多在子宫上下段交界处或胎体较细部位，如胎儿颈、腰部（图 9-2）。产妇持续腹痛、烦躁不安，胎体被狭窄环卡住，胎先露下降停滞，胎心常不规律。

3. 对母儿的影响

（1）对产妇的影响　宫缩过频过强，产程过快，可致子宫颈、阴道、会阴撕裂伤；接产时来不及消毒而导致感染；有产道梗阻可能发生子宫破裂；胎儿娩出后子宫收缩不良易发生胎盘滞留或产后出血。

（2）对胎儿、新生儿的影响　易发生胎儿窘迫、新生儿窒息、新生儿颅内出血、新生儿感染、骨折及外伤等。

4.治疗原则

（1）协调性宫缩过强　抑制宫缩的同时，尽快做好接生及抢救新生儿窒息的准备。发生急产者，预防产后出血、新生儿颅内出血和感染。

（2）强直性子宫收缩　立即抑制宫缩，如为梗阻性原因，应行剖宫产术结束分娩。

（3）子宫痉挛性狭窄环　消除诱因，给予镇静剂。如狭窄环不能缓解或伴胎儿窘迫者，应立即行剖宫产术。

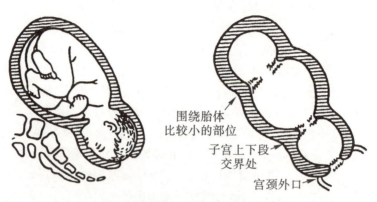

围绕胎体
比较小的部位

子宫上下段
交界处

宫颈外口

图9-2　子宫痉挛性狭窄环

【护理评估】

1.健康史　认真阅读产前检查记录，包括骨盆测量值、胎儿情况及妊娠并发症等有关资料。经产妇需了解有无急产史。重点评估临产时间，宫缩频率、强度，以及胎心、胎动情况。

2.身心状况　密切观察产程进展情况，注意观察宫缩、胎心、血压及产程进展，评估宫缩强度。由于子宫收缩过频、过强，无喘息之机，产程进展很快，产妇毫无思想准备，尤其周围无医护人员及家属的情况下，产妇有恐惧和极度无助感，担心胎儿与自身的安危。

【护理诊断】

1.急性疼痛　与过频、过强的宫缩有关。

2.焦虑　与剧烈腹痛、担心自身及胎儿安危有关。

3.有受伤的危险　与宫缩过强、产程过快有关。

【护理措施】

有急产史的孕妇在预产期前1~2周提前住院待产，以防发生损伤和意外。

1.协调性宫缩过强　剖宫产者做好术前准备，阴道分娩者做好以下护理。

（1）加强产程监护和指导　密切观察宫缩、胎心、产程进展，发现胎儿窘迫、先兆子宫破裂等及时报告医生。产妇有排便感时，要判断宫口及胎先露下降情况，以防在厕所分娩造成意外损伤。提前做好接产和新生儿窒息的抢救准备。宫缩时指导产妇张口哈气，勿向下屏气，减缓分娩速度。

（2）新生儿护理　新生儿娩出后，遵医嘱给予维生素 K_1 肌内注射以预防颅内出血。来不及消毒接生者，遵医嘱注射破伤风抗毒素1 500 U和应用抗生素。

（3）预防产后出血及感染　产后仔细检查软产道，有裂伤及时缝合。未消毒接产者，遵医嘱给予抗生素预防感染。

2.强直性子宫收缩　遵医嘱给予宫缩抑制剂，如25%硫酸镁20 mL加入5%葡萄糖注射液20 mL中缓慢静脉注射（不少于5 min）。对合并产道梗阻或胎儿窘迫者，应立即做好剖宫产准备。

3. 子宫痉挛性狭窄环　停止一切刺激，如阴道内操作和应用缩宫素等，如无胎儿窘迫，给予镇静剂如哌替啶 100 mg 或吗啡 10 mg 肌内注射，多能使宫缩恢复正常。若不能缓解或有胎儿窘迫，应立即做好剖宫产术及新生儿窒息抢救准备。

4. 心理护理　若新生儿出现意外，需协助产妇及家属顺利度过哀伤期，并为产妇提供出院后的避孕指导。

Two types of abnormal uterine activity lead to uterine dystocia. First, there is hypotonic uterine activity, in which the rise in uterine pressure during a contraction is insufficient (less than 25 mmHg) to promote cervical effacement and dilation. The force provided by voluntary contractions of the abdominal musculature, facilitated by the urge to push, may be insufficient to facilitate fetal descent and delivery. Second, there is hypertonic uterine activity, in which the contractions are frequent and painfully strong.

Abnormalities of the Latent Phase of Labor

The normal limits of the latent phase of labor extend up to 20 h for nulliparous patients and up to 14 h for multiparous patients. A latent phase that exceeds these limits is considered prolonged and maybe caused by dysfunctional labor, premature or excessive use of sedatives or analgesics, fetal malposition, or fetal size. A long, closed, firm cervix requires more time to efface and to undergo early dilation than does a soft, partially effaced cervix, but it is doubtful that a cervical factor alone causes a prolonged latent phase. Many patients who appear to be developing a prolonged latent phase are shown eventually to be in false laboror prelabor, with no progressive dilation of the cervix. The outcome of a prolonged latent phase is generally favorable for both the mother and the fetus, provided that no other abnormalities of labor subsequently occur.

A prolonged latent phase caused by premature or excessive use of sedation or analgesia usually resolves spontaneously after the effects of the medication have disappeared. Therapeutic rest with morphine sulfate or an equivalent drug has been shown to be effective in ruling out false labor; women in true labor wakeup in active labor, whereas those in false labor stop contracting.

If a definite diagnosis of prolonged latent phase of labor is made or there are reasons to expedite delivery, augmentation of labor by oxytocin can be performed. This is accomplished by the addition of 2.5 U of oxytocin to 500 mL of intravenous solution for a final concentration of 5 mU of oxytocin to each 1 mL of solution. A number of protocols have been suggested for the infusion of oxytocin. Oxytocin can be given as a low dose, in which the infusion begins at a rate of 1 − 2 mU/min and is increased in 1 − 2 mU/min increments every 15 − 30 min until the desired frequency and intensity are obtained, or a maximum of 20 mU/min is reached.

Amniotomy or artificial rupture of the membranes may be considered as part of the management of the latent phase of labor. An associated risk is an increased incidence of chorioamnionitis.

Abnormalities of the Active Phase of Labor

When the cervix dilates to 6 cm, the rate of dilation progresses more rapidly. Cervical dilation of less than 0.5 cm/h constitutes a protraction disorder of the active phase of labor. During the latter part of the active phase, the fetal presenting part also descends more rapidly through the pelvis and continues to descend through the second stage of labor. A rate of descent of the presenting part of less than 1 cm/h in nulliparous women and 2 cm/h in multiparous women is considered to be a protraction disorder of descent. If a period of 2 h or more elapses during the active phase of labor without progress in cervical dilation, an arrest of dilation has occurred; a period of more than 1 h without a change in station of the fetal presenting part is defined as an arrest of descent. Etiology of active phase abnormalities includes inadequate uterine activity, cephalopelvic disproportion, fetal malposition, or conduction anesthesia. The maternal pelvis should be evaluated, and the presenting fetal part should also be evaluated under these conditions.

The American College of Obstetricians and Gynecologists (ACOG) recommends the use of oxytocin forall protraction and arrest disorders. A patient having four contractions in 10 min, each with an amplitude of 50 mmHg, has adequate labor. Amniotomy should be performed if rupture of membranes has not occurred spontaneously. Before deciding to proceed to cesarean delivery in the first stage of labor for abnormal labor progression, it should be ascertained that at least 4 h of adequate contractions. In a nullipara with dystocia, continuing labor for 6−8 h is still associated with a high likelihood of vaginal delivery provided that the fetal heart rate is reassuring and there is some labor progress. A cesarean delivery is indicated if cephalopelvic disproportion is diagnosed.

Precipitous Labor and Delivery

Labor can be too slow, but it also can be abnormally rapid. Precipitous labor and delivery is extremely rapid labor and delivery. It may result from an abnormally low resistance of the soft parts of the birth canal, from abnormally strong uterine and abdominal contractions, or rarely from the absence of painful sensations and thus a lack of awareness of vigorous labor. Precipitous labor terminates in expulsion of the fetus in less than 3 h. Using this definition, 25, 260 live births—3%—were complicated by precipitous labor in the United States in 2013 (Martin, 2015). Despite this incidence, little published information describes maternal and perinatal outcomes.

For the mother, precipitous labor and delivery seldom are accompanied by serious maternal complications if the cervixis effaced appreciably and compliant, if the vagina has been stretched previously, and if the perineum is relaxed. Conversely, vigorous uterine contractions combined with a long, firm cervix and a noncompliant birth canal may lead to uterine rupture or extensive lacerations of the cervix, vagina, vulva, or perineum (Sheiner, 2004). It is in these latter circumstances that amnionic− fluid embolism most likely develops. Precipitous labor is frequently followed by uterine atony. The uterus that contracts with unusual vigor before delivery is likely to be hypotonic after delivery. In one report of 99 term pregnancies, short labors were more common in multiparas who typically had contractions at intervals less than 2 min. Precipitous labors have been linked to cocaine abuse and associated with placental abruption, meconium, postpartum hemorrhage, and low Apgar scores (Mahon, 1994).

For the neonate, adverse perinatal outcomes from rapid labor may be increased considerably for several reasons. The tumultuous uterine contractions, often with negligible inter. Resistance of the birth canal may rarely cause intracranial trauma. Finally, during an unattended birth, the newborn may fall to the floor and be injured, or it may need resuscitation that is not immediately available.

As treatment, analgesia is unlikely to modify these unusually forceful contractions to a significant degree. The use of tocolytic agents such as magnesium sulfate or terbutaline is unproven in these circumstances. Use of general anesthesia with agents that impair uterine contractibility such as isoflurane is often excessively heroic. Certainly, any oxytocin being administered should be stopped immediately.

【健康教育】

①指导产妇产后保持外阴清洁,注意观察恶露及会阴切口情况,有异常及时就诊。②做好避孕指导,产后42 d复查。

任务实施

缩宫素是由下丘脑分泌的一种激素,其重要作用是选择性兴奋子宫平滑肌,可促进子宫颈成熟、增强子宫收缩力及收缩频率,故临床上广泛应用于妊娠后期引产及产程中加强宫缩,以及在产后促进子宫收缩,减少产后出血发生率。缩宫素应用观察技术见表9-1。

表9-1 缩宫素应用观察技术

项目	内容
用法用量	1. 输液瓶上要做醒目标记,若需使用微量泵控制滴数和用量时,以12 mL/h计算;若无微量泵,以滴管1 mL=15滴计算,调节好滴速后再加入缩宫素,同时摇匀溶液。24 h用药量不超过80 U
	2. 引产或催产时,缩宫素2.5 U加入0.9%氯化钠注射液500 mL中(5 mU/mL)静脉滴注,开始时1 mU/min(滴速约3滴/min),每15~30 min增加1~2 mU,调至有效宫缩,即宫缩间隙2~3 min,每次宫缩持续40 s以上,宫腔压力不超过60 mmHg,通常滴速为8~15滴/min,即2~5 mU/min。缩宫素引产一般在白天进行,一次性用液量不超过1 000 mL,不成功者考虑其他引产方式
	3. 控制产后出血,20~40 mU/min,胎盘娩出后可肌内注射5~10 U
	4. 产前宫缩无力,缩宫素2.5~5.0 U加入0.9%氯化钠注射液500 mL内缓慢静脉滴注(滴速为10~30滴/min)
观察事项	1. 静脉滴注前观察胎心,测血压和脉搏,胎膜早破需观察羊水的色、质、量,确认无胎儿窘迫再进行用药
	2. 专人床旁守护负责观察和调节滴速,静脉滴注5 min应监测胎心,以后每15 min观察1次待产妇的血压、脉搏、胎心率,宫缩的频率、强度和持续时间及主诉等,并记录
	3. 密切观察产妇的产程进展变化及主诉。有条件者可使用胎心监护仪连续监测宫缩、胎心率及胎动反应。若待产妇出现突然破膜现象,应及时通知医生,若发现血压升高,应减慢滴注速度。当胎心持续减速、晚期减速,宫口开全2 cm时,停缩宫素并更换平衡液,同时更换输液器
	4. 注意观察缩宫素的过敏反应及不良反应,向产妇及家属交代缩宫素使用过程中可能出现的意外情况。过敏的临床表现为胸闷、气短、寒战及休克,一旦发现过敏反应及时停用,给予抗休克、抗过敏治疗。不良反应有恶心、呕吐、心率加快或心律失常
结局评价	助产士准确评估产妇状况,安全应用缩宫素并密切观察

任务二 产道异常(Abnormality of Birth Canal)

工作情景

李女士,28岁,初产妇,妊娠39周,规律宫缩20 h入院。查体:髂棘间径24 cm,骶耻外径19 cm,坐骨棘间径10 cm,坐骨结节间径7.5 cm,枕左前位,胎心率140次/min。肛查:宫口开大8 cm,S+1。2 h后产程无进展,产妇呼叫腹痛难忍。检查宫缩1次/min,持续40 s,宫缩时胎心率

116 次/min，子宫下段压痛明显。

①该产妇产程受阻的主要原因是什么？②应给予产妇哪些护理措施？

任务内容

产道包括骨产道和软产道，是胎儿经阴道娩出的必经通道。产道异常可使胎儿娩出受阻，以骨产道异常多见。

任务目标

◆ 能识别产道异常的类型。
◆ 能说出产道异常的处理原则。

一 骨产道异常

骨产道异常即狭窄骨盆，表现为骨盆径线过短或形态异常，可能一个径线也可能多个径线过短，而致一个平面或多个平面狭窄，胎儿在分娩过程中因机械性梗阻而难以娩出。

【概要】

1.分类

（1）骨盆入口平面狭窄　入口平面前后径短，以扁平骨盆为代表。入口平面狭窄分 3 级（表9-2）。常见扁平骨盆有单纯扁平骨盆（图9-3）和佝偻病性扁平骨盆（图9-4）。

表9-2　骨盆3个平面狭窄的分级　　　　　单位:cm

分级	骨盆入口平面狭窄 对角径	中骨盆平面狭窄 坐骨棘间径	骨盆出口平面狭窄		
			坐骨棘间径+中骨盆后矢状径	坐骨结节间径	坐骨结节间径+出口后矢状径
Ⅰ级（临界性）	11.5	10	13.5	7.5	15.0
Ⅱ级（相对性）	10.0～11.0	8.5～9.5	12.0～13.0	6.0～7.0	12.0～14.0
Ⅲ级（绝对性）	≤9.5	≤8.0	≤11.5	≤5.5	≤11.0

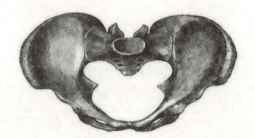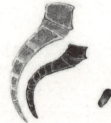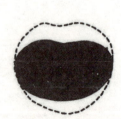

图9-3　单纯扁平骨盆

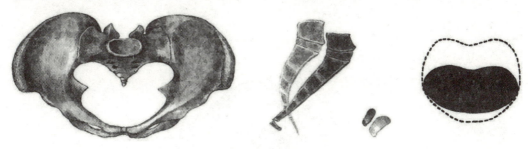

图9-4　佝偻病性扁平骨盆

（2）中骨盆平面狭窄　比骨盆入口平面狭窄更常见，主要见于类人猿型骨盆和男型骨盆，以坐骨棘间径和中骨盆后矢状径狭窄为主，分为3级。

（3）骨盆出口平面狭窄　与中骨盆平面狭窄常并存，主要见于男型骨盆，以坐骨结节间径及骨盆出口后矢状径狭窄为主，分3级。

（4）骨盆3个平面狭窄　骨盆形态正常，但骨盆各平面的径线均比正常值小2 cm或以上，又称均小骨盆。多见于身材矮小、体型匀称的妇女。

（5）畸形骨盆　骨盆失去正常形态与对称性，包括偏斜骨盆（图9-5）、外伤所致的畸形骨盆。

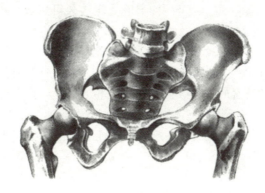

图9-5　偏斜骨盆

2.临床表现

（1）骨盆入口平面狭窄　①导致胎头衔接受阻：于妊娠末期或临产后胎头仍不能入盆，孕妇呈尖腹或悬垂腹（图9-6）。②导致胎位异常：因骨盆入口平面狭窄胎头不易入盆，常导致胎先露异常，如臀先露、肩先露等。

（2）中骨盆平面狭窄　①导致胎方位异常：胎头衔接正常，当胎头下降至中骨盆时，由于内旋转受阻，常出现持续性枕横位或枕后位。②导致产程进展异常：出现继发性宫缩乏力，活跃期后期及第二产程延长，甚至第二产程停滞。

（3）骨盆出口平面狭窄　常与中骨盆平面狭窄并存。易致继发性宫缩乏力和第二产程停滞，胎头双顶径不能通过骨盆出口平面。不宜强行阴道助产，否则会导致严重的软产道裂伤及新生儿产伤。

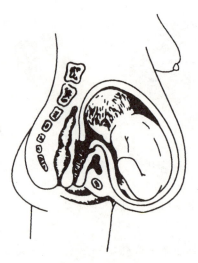

图9-6 悬垂腹

3. 对母儿的影响

（1）对产妇的影响　骨盆狭窄影响胎头衔接和内旋转,容易发生胎位异常、胎膜早破、宫缩乏力和产程延长;胎头下降受阻可能导致子宫破裂;产道受压过久可形成生殖道瘘;产程长、胎膜早破、手术助产等增加产褥感染机会。

（2）对胎儿及新生儿的影响　头盆不称易致胎膜早破、脐带脱垂,导致胎儿窘迫甚至死亡;产程延长胎头受压过久,易致新生儿颅内出血;手术助产,增加新生儿产伤和感染的机会。

4. 处理原则　明确狭窄骨盆的类型、程度,了解胎位、胎儿大小、胎心、宫缩、产程进展情况,结合年龄、产次、既往分娩史等综合判断,决定分娩方式。

（1）试产　骨盆入口平面相对狭窄、胎头跨耻征可疑阳性,可在严密监测下试产2～4 h。

（2）阴道助产　中骨盆平面狭窄,宫口开全,胎头双顶径达坐骨棘水平或以下者,可经阴道助产。

（3）剖宫产　骨盆入口平面绝对狭窄,胎头跨耻征阳性;中骨盆平面狭窄,宫口开全,胎头双顶径在坐骨棘水平以上;坐骨结节间径+后矢状径≤15 cm;严重畸形骨盆等,均应行剖宫产术。

【护理评估】

1. 健康史　了解孕妇有无佝偻病、脊髓灰质炎、脊柱或髋关节的结核及外伤史。若为经产妇,应了解有无难产史及新生儿产伤等。

2. 身心状况　评估本次妊娠经过及身体反应,了解产妇情绪,妊娠早、中、晚期的经过,是否有病理妊娠问题与妊娠并发症的发生,以及产妇的心理状态及社会支持系统等情况。

（1）一般检查　观察腹部形态,尖腹及悬垂腹者应提示可能有盆腔入口平面狭窄。观察产妇的体型、步态,有无脊柱及髋关节畸形,米氏菱形窝是否对称等。身高低于145 cm者,应警惕均小骨盆。

（2）腹部检查　观察腹部形态,初产妇呈尖腹者,可能提示有骨盆入口平面狭窄。测量孕妇宫高、腹围,四步触诊法评估胎先露、胎方位及先露部位是否衔接入盆。临产后应持续观察评估胎头下降情况,有无胎头跨耻征阳性。

检查方法:产妇排空膀胱后仰卧,两腿伸直。检查者将一只手放于产妇耻骨联合上方,另一只手将胎头向盆腔方向推压。

1）胎头跨耻征阴性：胎头低于耻骨联合平面，提示头盆相称（图9-7A）。

2）胎头跨耻征可疑阳性：胎头与耻骨联合在同一平面，表示可疑头盆不称（图9-7B）。

3）胎头跨耻征阳性：胎头高于耻骨联合平面，表示头盆不称（图9-7C）。

对胎头跨耻征阳性的孕妇，应让其取两腿屈曲半卧位，再次检查胎头跨耻征，若转为阴性，提示为骨盆倾斜度异常，而不是头盆不称。

（3）骨盆测量　包括骨盆外测量和内测量。

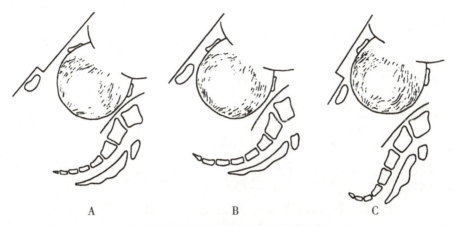

A.头盆相称；B.可疑头盆不称；C.头盆不称。

图9-7　检查头盆相称程度

3.辅助检查　B型超声检查观察胎先露与骨盆的关系，测量胎头双顶径、胸径、腹径、股骨长度，预测胎儿体重，判断胎儿能否通过骨产道。

【护理诊断】

1.潜在并发症　如子宫破裂、胎儿窘迫。

2.有感染的危险　与胎膜早破、产程延长、手术操作有关。

3.焦虑　与担心母儿安危有关。

【护理措施】

1.剖宫产护理　有明显头盆不称、不能从阴道分娩者，做好剖宫产术的围手术期护理。

2.试产护理

（1）安慰产妇，避免紧张，加强休息，注意营养及水分的摄入，必要时静脉补液。

（2）专人守护，注意观察宫缩、胎心及胎头下降情况。

（3）适时人工破膜，试产过程中出现宫缩乏力，可用缩宫素静脉滴注。

（4）试产时间2～4 h，胎头双顶径通过入口平面，即试产成功；若胎头仍未能入盆，宫口扩张缓慢，或出现先兆子宫破裂、胎儿窘迫征象，应做好剖宫产术和新生儿窒息抢救的准备。

3.心理护理　试产过程中，向产妇及家属说明阴道分娩的可能性及优点，给予关爱，增强阴道分娩的信心；使产妇及家属清楚目前产程进展情况及手术产的必要性，取得理解和配合，缓解焦虑心理。

【健康教育】

①骨产道异常为不可逆因素，再次妊娠分娩时应将情况告知医务人员。②注意观察产妇恶露、生命体征，有异常随时就诊。③剖宫产术后，宜避孕2年再妊娠。

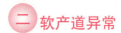
软产道异常

软产道包括子宫下段、子宫颈、阴道及骨盆底软组织,软产道异常所致的难产少见,容易被忽视。软产道异常根据病变程度及对分娩的影响,选择局部治疗、手术或行剖宫产术,护士应积极做好相应的配合工作。

【概要】

1. 外阴异常

(1)外阴坚韧、外阴瘢痕 组织缺乏弹性,使阴道口狭窄,分娩时第二产程易造成严重撕裂伤,应行会阴侧切术或剖宫产术。

(2)外阴水肿 常见于重度妊娠期高血压疾病等引起的全身水肿,临产前及时治疗原发病,局部可用50%硫酸镁湿热敷。临产后可在消毒下多点针刺放液,并行会阴切开术。

2. 阴道异常

(1)阴道横隔、纵隔隔膜较厚 阻碍胎先露下降时,行切开术或剖宫产术。

(2)阴道瘢痕性狭窄 多由产伤、手术感染等所致。若狭窄轻、位置低,可做会阴切开术;若狭窄重、位置高、范围广,应行剖宫产术。

(3)阴道肿瘤 阻碍胎头下降而不能经阴道切除者,应行剖宫产术结束分娩。

3. 子宫颈异常

(1)子宫颈坚韧、水肿 子宫颈坚韧多见于高龄初产妇,子宫颈组织缺乏弹性不易扩张。子宫颈水肿多见于滞产、持续性枕后位、宫口未开全过早用腹压者,影响子宫颈扩张。两者均可在子宫颈两侧注射0.5%利多卡因5~10 mL,处理无效应行剖宫产术。

(2)子宫颈肌瘤 若肌瘤大阻塞骨盆入口,影响胎头入盆,应行剖宫产术;若肌瘤在骨盆入口以上而胎头已入盆,不阻塞产道者,可阴道分娩。

Dystocia Caused by Maternal Pelvic Abnormalities

Cephalopelvic disproportion (CPD) exists if the maternal bony pelvis is not of sufficient size and appropriate shape to allow the passage of the fetal head. This problem may occur as a result of contraction of one of the planes of the pelvis. Relative CPD may exist with a normal pelvis, if the fetal head is excessively large or in an abnormal position. Contraction of the maternal pelvis may occur at the level of the inlet or midpelvis, but contraction of the outlet is extremely unusual unless it is found in association with a midpelvic contraction.

Cephalopelvic disproportion at the level of the pelvic inlet causes a failure of descent and engagement of the head. The finding of an unengaged head in a nulliparous patient at the start of labor indicates anincreased likelihood of CPD at the pelvic inlet, but an unengaged fetal head in a multiparous patient in labor is not an unusual occurrence.

The management of a nulliparous patient with an unengaged fetal head in labor should begin with a careful clinical evaluation of the maternal pelvis. If the pelvis is clinically adequate, expectant management with observation of the labor pattern is appropriate. If uterine contractions are ineffective, oxytocic stimulation of labor may be considered.

The occurrence of CPD at the level of the midpelvis is more frequently than inlet dystocia because the capacity of the midpelvis is smaller than that of the inlet and also because deflection or positional abnormalities of the fetal head are more likely to occur at that level. The occurrence of bony dystocia at the level of the midpelvis is usually indicated by an arrest of descent of the head at a +1 to +2 station. With CPD and arrest of descent, application of the head to the cervix is poor, resulting in the loss of part of the force needed for cervical dilation. Thus, CPD may be associated with a protracted or expected rate of cervical dilation before an arrest of descent is apparent.

任务实施

胎头跨耻征检查流程见表 9-3。

表9-3　胎头跨耻征检查流程

项目	内容
目的	评估头盆关系,判断骨盆入口是否存在狭窄
操作前准备	1.环境准备:关闭门窗,屏风遮挡,注意保护孕妇隐私
	2.护士准备:洗手,戴口罩,温暖双手
	3.孕妇准备:排空膀胱后仰卧,两腿伸直
操作步骤	1.检查者将一只手放于耻骨联合上方,另一只手将胎头向盆腔方向推压。如果胎头低于耻骨联合平面,为胎头跨耻征阴性,提示头盆相称。如果胎头与耻骨联合在同一平面,为胎头跨耻征可疑阳性,表示可疑头盆不称。如果胎头高于耻骨联合平面,为胎头跨耻征阳性,表示头盆不称
	2.对胎头跨耻征阳性的孕妇,让其取两腿屈曲半卧位,再次做胎头跨耻征检查,若转为阴性,提示为骨盆倾斜度异常
整理	1.协助产妇穿好衣物
	2.护士洗手,做记录

任务三　胎儿异常(Fetal Abnormality)

工作情景

李女士,26岁,第1胎,现妊娠30周,最近胎动时感觉肋下胀痛,今日来医院产科门诊做孕检。医生检查后告诉她胎儿为臀位,李女士很担心。

如何指导李女士进行胎位矫正?

任务内容

胎儿异常包括胎位异常、胎儿发育异常和巨大儿等,其中胎位异常是造成难产的常见因素。胎位异常包括胎头位置异常、臀先露及肩先露,其中胎头位置异常居多,又称头位难产,有持续性枕后位或枕横位、面先露、高直位、前不均倾位等。

任务目标

◆ 能识别常见的胎位异常。

◆ 能说出胎位异常的处理原则。

◆ 能运用所学的知识对胎位异常的妇女进行护理。

一 持续性枕后位、枕横位

【概要】

当胎头以枕后位或枕横位衔接,胎头双顶径抵达中骨盆平面时完成内旋转动作,大多数能向前转成枕前位,胎头得以最小径线通过骨盆最窄平面顺利经阴道自然分娩。若经充分试产,胎头枕部不能转向前方,仍位于母体骨盆后方或侧方,致使分娩发生困难者,称为持续性枕后位或持续性枕横位。发生率约占分娩总数的5%。

1. 临床表现　分娩发动后胎头枕后位衔接导致胎头俯屈不良及下降缓慢,子宫颈不能有效扩张及反射性刺激内源性缩宫素释放,易致协调性宫缩乏力,第二产程延长。此外,由于胎儿枕部压迫直肠,产妇自觉肛门坠胀及排便感,宫口尚未开全时过早使用腹压,产妇体力消耗过大,子宫颈前唇水肿,使胎头下降延缓或停滞,产程延长。若在阴道口见到胎发,经过多次宫缩屏气不见胎头继续下降时,应考虑持续性枕后位可能。

2. 对母儿的影响

(1) 对母体的影响　容易导致继发性宫缩乏力,引起产程延长。若胎头长时间压迫软产道,可形成生殖道瘘。邻近脏器受压,如膀胱麻痹可致尿潴留,甚至发生生殖道损伤或瘘。阴道手术助产机会增多,软产道裂伤、产后出血及产褥感染发生率高。

(2) 对胎儿的影响　第二产程延长及手术助产概率增加,易致胎儿窘迫和新生儿窒息等,使围产儿死亡率增高。

3. 处理原则　综合分析骨盆和胎儿大小。头盆不称者行剖宫产术。无骨盆异常、胎儿不大,可以阴道试产。宫口开全后,胎头双顶径在坐骨棘水平或以下者,可手转胎头至枕前位,自然分娩或行阴道助产术,如胎头吸引术或产钳术;若转成枕前位困难,也可转成正枕后位后产钳助产。若胎头双顶径未达坐骨棘水平或出现胎儿窘迫者,行剖宫产术。

胎头吸引术与产钳术

【护理评估】

1. 健康史　评估产妇是否存在影响胎头内旋转的因素,如骨盆狭窄(多见于漏斗骨盆和横径狭窄骨盆)、胎头俯屈不良、宫缩乏力、前置胎盘、膀胱充盈等。

2. 身心状况　产妇因产程延长和身体疲乏失去阴道分娩的信心,产生急躁和焦虑情绪,同时担心自身及胎儿的安危。

腹部检查:胎背偏向母体的后方或侧方不易触及,前腹壁可触及胎儿肢体,胎心在脐下偏外方听得最响亮。阴道检查或肛门检查:枕后位时盆腔后部空虚,胎头矢状缝位于骨盆斜径,大囟门在前,小囟门在后方。若为枕横位,矢状缝与骨盆横径一致,大、小囟门分别在骨盆左、右侧方。

3. 辅助检查　可行 B 型超声检查,根据胎儿颜面及枕部位置,可明确诊断胎方位。

【护理诊断】

1.有母儿受伤的危险　与产妇软产道损伤、新生儿产伤有关。

2.焦虑　与担心自身及胎儿安危有关。

【护理措施】

（1）保证产妇充分的营养和休息，指导产妇朝胎背的对侧方向卧位，以利胎头向前旋转。

（2）密切观察产程进展及胎心，以及时发现和处理异常。若宫缩欠佳，应遵医嘱静脉滴注缩宫素；第一产程指导产妇不要过早屏气用力，以免子宫颈水肿及体力消耗。

（3）需行阴道助产术或剖宫产术时，护士应积极做好术前准备及手术配合，同时做好新生儿抢救准备。

（4）陪伴关心产妇，向产妇及家属解释难产的原因和应对措施，并及时告知产程进展情况，取得理解和配合，增加其安全感和信任感，缓解焦虑。

Persistent Occipitotransverse Position

The fetal head normally enters and engages in the maternal pelvis in an occipitotransverse（OT）position. It subsequently rotates to an OA position or, in a small percentage of cases, to an occipitoposterior position. This rotation occurs because the head flexes as the leading part of the vertex encounters the pelvic floor and then rotates to adjust to the shape of the gynecoid pelvis. In a small number of cases, the head fails to flex and rotate and persists in an OT position. This position may be caused by cephalopelvic disproportion; altered pelvic architecture, such as in a patient with a platypelloid or android pelvis; or a relaxed pelvic floor, brought about by epidural anesthesia or multiparity. The diagnosis of a persistent OT position may be difficult at times, owing to the obscuring of suture lines and fontanelles by the excessive molding and caput formation that often accompany this abnormal position.

A persistent OT position with arrest of descent for a period of 1 h or more is known as transverse arrest. Arrest occurs because of the deflexion that accompanies the persistent OT position, resulting in the larger occipitofrontal diameter（11 cm）becoming the presenting diameter. Until the head undergoes flexion and rotation, further descent cannot take place. Transverse arrest commonly occurs with the vertex at a +1 to +2 station.

The management of transverse arrest at a +1 to +2 station is complex, in part, because at these stations the widest part of the fetal head is at or above the level of the ischial spines. If the midpelvis is compromised, cesarean delivery is indicated. If the pelvis is judged to be of normal size and the fetus is not macrosomic, oxytocic stimulation of labor may be appropriate if uterine contractions are inadequate.

Persistent Occipitoposterior Position

The head generally rotates from OT to OA during the descent through the maternal pelvis. Even if the head initially rotates to an occipitoposterior position, most fetuses will eventually rotate spontaneously during labor to OA, leaving only a small percentage（5%－15%）of fetuses with a persistent OP position. The course of labor in the presence of a persistent OP position is usually normal except for a tendency for the second stage to be prolonged（>2 h）. It is also associated with considerably more discomfort. As with the persistent OT position, the fetal head may become markedly molded with extensive caput formation, which may cause difficulty in diagnosing its correct station and position. Observation of a prolonged second stage of labor is appropriate, provided that labor continues to be progressive, and the fetal heart rate is normal.

Delivery of the head may occur spontaneously in the OP position, but if the perineum provides undue resistance to delivery, a low forceps-assisted delivery may be required (e. g. , using Simpson's forceps). In the past a Kielland forceps rotation was usually performed, but because of a lack of experience and training, fetuses in the OP position are usually now delivered without rotation. Use of a vacuum extractor with a cup designed for a safe and secure posterior application may be performed. Sometimes the head will rotate, but it will usually deliver in the OP position. A wide mediolateral episiotomy may be required to lessen the resistance of the outlet to the delivery of the fetal head.

臀先露

【概要】

臀先露是最常见的异常胎位,占分娩总数的3%~4%。臀先露以骶骨为指示点,有骶左(右)前、骶左(右)横、骶左(右)后6种胎方位。臀先露易导致后出头困难,使围产儿死亡率增高,是枕先露围产儿死亡率的3~8倍。

1. 分类 根据胎儿两下肢的姿势分为3类:①单臀先露或腿直臀先露,最多见,双髋关节屈曲,双膝关节伸直,以臀部为先露部;②完全臀先露或混合臀先露,双髋关节及双膝关节均屈曲,先露部为臀和双足;③不完全臀先露,较少见。以单足或双足、单膝或双膝为先露部(图9-8)。

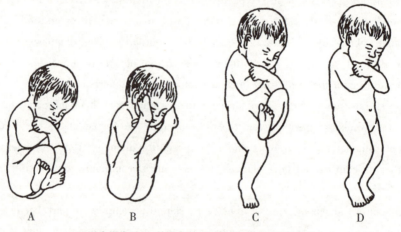

A. 混合臀先露;B. 单臀先露;C. 单足先露;D. 双足先露。

图9-8 臀先露的种类

2. 临床表现 孕妇常感觉肋下或上腹部有圆而硬的胎头,由于胎臀不能紧贴子宫下段及子宫颈,常导致子宫收缩乏力,产程延长,手术产机会增多。胎臀形状不规则,对前羊膜囊压力不均匀,易致胎膜早破。

3. 处理原则 定期产前检查,妊娠30周后矫正胎位。分娩期根据产妇年龄、胎产次、骨盆大小、胎儿大小、臀先露类型等决定分娩方式。如存在狭窄骨盆、软产道异常、胎儿体重估计在3 500 g以上、胎儿窘迫、不完全臀先露、妊娠期合并症、高龄初产、有难产史等,应行剖宫产术。

【护理评估】

1. 健康史 了解产妇有无羊水过多、早产、子宫畸形、胎儿畸形、羊水过少、双胎妊娠、骨盆狭窄、前置胎盘等可导致臀先露的因素。

2.身心状况　产前检查发现臀先露时,孕妇和家属常担心臀先露对母儿的不良影响而焦急。分娩期常需剖宫产或阴道助产,因害怕手术、担心并发症而焦虑不安。

腹部检查:在宫底部触及圆而硬的胎头,耻骨联合上可触到不规则、软而宽的胎臀,胎心音在脐上方听得最清楚。阴道检查:胎膜已破及子宫颈扩张 3 cm 以上可直接触及软而不规则的胎臀或胎足。

3.辅助检查　B 型超声检查可准确判断臀先露类型、胎儿大小、胎头姿势等。

【护理诊断】

1.有母儿受伤的危险　与手术助产、后出胎头困难有关。

2.焦虑　与不了解产程进展及担心分娩结果有关。

3.有感染的危险　与胎膜早破和产程延长有关。

【护理措施】

1.妊娠期　及时发现异常胎位,妊娠 30 周后仍为臀先露者,应指导孕妇纠正胎位,常用方法如下。

(1)胸膝卧位　让孕妇排空膀胱,松解裤带,取胸膝卧位(图9-9),2～3 次/d,每次 15 min,连做 1 周后复查。此法可使胎臀退出盆腔,借助胎儿重心改变,增加转为头先露的机会。

(2)激光照射或艾灸至阴穴(足小趾外侧趾甲角旁0.1 寸)　1～2 次/d,15～30 min/次,1～2 周为 1 个疗程。可促使胎动活跃,配合胸膝卧位使用效果更好。

(3)外倒转术　医生通过向孕妇腹壁施加压力,用手向前或向后旋转胎儿,使其由臀位或横位变成头位的一种操作。虽然存在胎盘早剥、胎儿窘迫、胎膜早破、早产等潜在风险,但发生率低。因此,仍然是一个有价值的相对安全的操作。一般建议妊娠 36～37 周后,排除禁忌证后在超声及电子胎心监护下进行,操作前必须做好紧急剖宫产的准备。

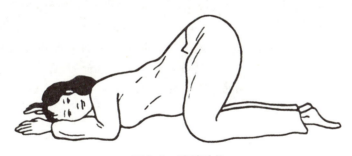

图 9-9　胸膝卧位

2.分娩期　有指征者选择择期剖宫产,做好术前准备。决定阴道分娩者,应行如下处理。

(1)第一产程　尽可能防止胎膜早破,临产后侧卧休息,减少站立走动,不灌肠,少做阴道检查,不用缩宫素引产。一旦破膜,应立即听胎心。若有胎心改变,应及时报告医生,以便及早发现有无脐带脱垂。宫口未开全者,若宫缩时在阴道口见胎足或胎臀,立即通知医生,消毒外阴后,使用"堵"外阴方法。每当宫缩时,以手掌用无菌巾堵住阴道口,待宫口及阴道充分扩张后再让胎臀娩出。在堵的过程中,每隔 10～15 min 听 1 次胎心,并注意宫口是否开全。宫口近开全时,要做好接产和抢救新生儿窒息的准备。

(2)第二产程　导尿排空膀胱,对初产妇协助行会阴侧切后助娩胎儿,一般行臀位助产术。胎臀自然娩出至脐部,胎肩及胎头由接生者协助娩出。从脐部娩出后,一般应在 2～3 min 内娩出胎头,最长不超过 8 min,以免脐带受压过久造成死产。

（3）第三产程　产后检查软产道，如有裂伤及时缝合，遵医嘱用缩宫素与抗生素，预防产后出血和感染。

3.心理护理　耐心解答产妇及家属疑问，对需手术的产妇，讲解手术的必要性，给予鼓励与支持。对阴道分娩者，产程中做好陪护，指导产妇减痛方法及使用腹压等，增强对分娩的信心。

【健康教育】

①指导孕妇加强产前检查，妊娠30周后发现臀先露应及时矫正。②指导矫正胎位的方法，解释孕期矫正胎位的必要性，未能矫正者提前入院待产。③加强卫生宣教，对未能矫正的臀位孕妇嘱其孕晚期减少活动，一旦阴道流液，应立即平卧、臀部抬高，尽快到医院就诊。

Breech presentation

Near term, the fetus typically has spontaneously assumed a cephalic presentation. Conversely, if the fetal buttocks or legs enter the pelvis before the head, the presentation is breech. This fetal lie is more common remote from term, as earlier in pregnancy each fetal pole has similar bulk. At term, breech presentation persists in 3%–5% of singleton deliveries.

• Classification of breech presentation: The categories of frank, complete, and incomplete breech presentations differ in their varying relations between the lower extremities and buttocks. With a frank breech, lower extremities are flexed at the hips and extended at the knees, and thus the feet lie close to the head. With a complete breech, both hips are flexed, and one or both knees are also flexed. With an incomplete breech, one or both hips are extended. As a result, one or both feet or knees lie below the breech, such that a foot or knee is lowermost in the birth canal. A footling breech is an incomplete breech with one or both feet below the breech.

• Route of delivery: Multiple factors aid determination of the best delivery route for a given mother–fetus pair. These include fetal characteristics, maternal pelvic dimensions, coexistent pregnancy complications, provider experience, patient preference, hospital capabilities, and gestational age.

Compared with their term counterparts, preterm breech fetuses have distinct complications related to their small size and immaturity. For example, rates of head entrapment, birth trauma, and perinatal mortality can be greater. Accordingly, separate discussions of term and preterm breech fetuses are more appropriate.

三　巨大儿

胎儿体重≥4 000 g者，称为巨大胎儿。巨大儿与父母身材高大、孕妇患轻型糖尿病、过期妊娠、营养过剩等有关，常引起头盆不称、肩难产、软产道损伤、新生儿产伤、产后出血、生殖道瘘等。产前可根据宫高、腹围、B型超声测胎头双顶径与腹围等，计算胎儿体重。无头盆不称，初产妇可适当试产，但试产不宜过久，如出现异常，应行剖宫产结束分娩。有头盆不称者，择期行剖宫产结束分娩。新生儿娩出后易发生低血糖，应注意观察，及时补充葡萄糖水，以及早开奶。

The ACOG defines macrosomia as a fetus weighing 4,000 g or more. Large for gestational age is defined as birth weight equal to or above the 90th percentile of fetal weight for a given gestational age. Macrosomia is associated with genetic determinants, maternal diabetes, prepregnancy weight, weight gain during pregnancy, multiparity, male sex, gestational age greater than 40 weeks, ethnicity, maternal birth weight, maternal height, and maternal age. Maternal morbidity associated with macrosomia includes labor dystocia, shoulder dystocia, and genital trauma, with a corresponding increase in the cesarean delivery rate.

There is also an increase in postpartum hemorrhage and puerperal infection. There is increased perinatal morbidity resulting from dystocia and birth trauma, especially shoulder dystocia.

The major neonatal complication is the occurrence of Erb's palsy, which can be caused by excessive traction on the brachial plexus by the delivery attendant. This is an important cause of malpractice in obstetrics. Other neonatal complications include Klumpke's palsy, clavicular fracture, humeral fracture, hypoxia, brain injury, and death. Maternal complications include genital tract lacerations and postpartum hemorrhage.

任务实施

臀先露是最常见的异常胎位之一,因后出胎头娩出困难,使围产儿死亡率增加。妊娠30周前臀先露多能转成头先露,但妊娠30周后仍为臀先露者,应积极采取胸膝卧位纠正胎位(表9-4)。其适应证为骨盆测量正常,无胸膝卧位禁忌,单胎,妊娠30周后经检查为胎先露异常的孕妇。

表9-4　产科胸膝卧位指导

项目	内容
目的	使臀先露转为头先露
操作前准备	1. 环境准备:安静、光线适宜、温度24~26 ℃,必要时设置屏风或隔帘遮挡孕妇
	2. 用物准备:胎心监听器(产科听筒、多普勒超声、胎儿电子监护仪)、孕期保健卡、纸、笔
	3. 助产士准备:修剪指甲,洗手、戴口罩
	4. 孕妇准备:产科情况评估,评价孕妇心理及合作程度(有无焦虑、恐惧);解释操作的目的,以取得积极配合;让孕妇排空膀胱,松解裤带
操作步骤	1. 携带用物至孕妇旁边,遮挡、查对,向孕妇解释检查的目的
	2. 助产士站在孕妇右侧,协助孕妇取跪卧姿势。两小腿平放于床上,双腿稍分开,大腿与床面垂直,胸部贴近床面,腹部悬空,背部伸直,臀部抬起,屈肘置于头部两侧,头转向一侧
	3. 指导结束后,协助孕妇缓慢起坐、下床,避免跌伤
注意事项	1. 此操作应在硬板床上进行
	2. 孕妇能复述胸膝卧位的方法和注意事项
	3. 经过矫正仍不能转为头位,由医生指导选择恰当的分娩方式

微课　　　　　　　　课件　　　　　　　练习题及参考答案

（任　美）

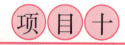

项目十

分娩期并发症妇女的护理
(Nursing of Women with Complication of Labor)

项目描述

分娩过程中有很多不确定因素,可能出现严重威胁母婴生命安全的并发症,如产后出血、羊水栓塞、子宫破裂等,是导致孕产妇死亡的主要原因。

There are many uncertainties during childbirth, some complications will seriously threaten the safety of mother and baby, for example, postpartum hemorrhage, amniotic fluid embolism, rupture of uterus.

任务一 产后出血(Postpartum Hemorrhage)

工作情景

王女士,28岁,G_2P_1,妊娠39^{+5}周,入院待产。入院后第2天经阴道分娩一活婴,胎儿娩出9 min后胎盘娩出。检查发现子宫颈处有一裂伤,缝合修补后仍有阴道出血,呈间歇性,出血量大概600 mL,腹部检查子宫轮廓不清。患者出现眩晕、面色苍白。

①请明确该患者主要的护理问题。②根据目前的情况对患者进行正确的护理。

任务内容

产后出血是分娩期的严重并发症,是我国孕产妇死亡的首要原因。产后出血是指胎儿娩出后24 h内阴道分娩者出血量超过500 mL,剖宫产者超过1 000 mL。国内外文献报道产后出血的发生率占分娩总数的5%~10%,其中80%以上发生在产后2 h之内。

任务目标

◆ 能叙述产后出血的定义、病因、临床表现及处理原则。

◆ 能对产后出血量进行评估。

【概述】

1. 病因　引起产后出血的主要原因有子宫收缩乏力、胎盘因素、软产道损伤及凝血功能障碍。产后出血既可由以上单一因素所致，也可多因素并存，相互影响或互为因果。

（1）子宫收缩乏力　是产后出血最常见的原因，占产后出血总数的70%~80%。引起宫缩乏力的常见因素包括全身因素、产科因素、子宫因素及药物因素。

（2）胎盘因素　根据胎盘剥离情况，胎盘因素所致产后出血的类型包括胎盘滞留、胎盘植入、胎盘部分残留。

（3）软产道裂伤　常见原因有会阴组织弹性差、产力过强、产程进展过快、巨大胎儿、阴道手术助产操作不规范等。软产道裂伤分度按损伤程度分为4度：Ⅰ度裂伤指会阴部皮肤及阴道入口黏膜撕裂，出血不多；Ⅱ度裂伤指裂伤已达会阴体筋膜及肌层，累及阴道后壁黏膜，向阴道后壁两侧沟延伸并向上撕裂，解剖结构不易辨认，出血较多；Ⅲ度裂伤指裂伤向会阴深部扩展，肛门外括约肌已断裂，直肠黏膜尚完整；Ⅳ度裂伤指肛门、直肠和阴道完全贯通，直肠肠腔外露，组织损伤严重，出血量可不多。

（4）凝血功能障碍　妊娠合并凝血功能障碍性疾病或妊娠并发症所致凝血功能障碍均可引起产后出血。

2. 临床表现　产后出血主要表现为胎儿娩出后阴道流血量过多和（或）伴有因失血而引起的相应症状。

（1）阴道流血　胎儿娩出后立即发生阴道流血，持续性，鲜红色，应考虑软产道裂伤。胎儿娩出后数分钟出现阴道流血，间歇性，暗红色，应考虑胎盘因素。胎盘娩出后阴道流血较多，如为间歇性，暗红色，腹部触诊子宫轮廓不清，应考虑子宫收缩乏力；如子宫收缩良好，产后检查胎盘、胎膜不完整应考虑胎盘、胎膜残留。胎儿或胎盘娩出后阴道持续流血，且血液不凝，应考虑凝血功能障碍。失血导致的临床表现明显，伴阴道疼痛而阴道流血不多，应考虑隐匿性软产道损伤，如阴道血肿。

（2）低血压症状　产妇可出现头晕、面色苍白、烦躁、皮肤湿冷、脉搏细数等。

3. 处理原则　针对出血原因，迅速止血；补充血容量，纠正失血性休克；防治感染。

There are four main reasons for postpartum hemorrhage：uterine atony, retained placental fragments, lacerations and coagulation defects.

Etiology

Uterine atony is the most frequent cause of postpartum hemorrhage. It causes 70% ~ 80% of early hemorrhage. The predisposing factors are systemic factors, obstetric factors, uterine factors and drug factors.

Placental factors：retained placenta, placenta implantation and retained placenta fragment.

Trauma to the birth canal is the second most common cause. It includes vaginal, cervical, perineal lacerations as well as hematomas. Cervical lacerations occur frequently when the cervix dilates rapidly during the first stage of labor. Lacerations of the vagina, perineum, and periurethral area usually occur during the second stage of labor, when the fetal head descends rapidly or when assistive devices such as a vacuum extractor or forceps are used to assist in delivery of the fetal heads.

There are two aspects in coagulation defects. One of them is pregnancy with preexisting disease, others are developed during pregnancy.

Clinical Signs and Symptoms

● Vaginal bleeding：The vaginal bleeding immediately after delivery，persistent，bright red，soft canal fracture should be considered. Several minutes after delivery，intermittent，dark red，placental factors should be considered. After the delivery of the placenta，the vaginal bleeding is more，if intermittent，dark red，abdominal touch of the uterine outline is not clear，uterine atony should be considered；if the uterine contraction is good，postpartum examination of the placenta and fetal membrane is incomplete，the residue of placenta and fetal membrane should be considered. Coagulation dysfunction should be considered for vaginal bleeding after delivery of the fetus or placenta and blood does not coagulation. The clinical manifestations caused by blood loss are obvious，with vaginal pain and little vaginal bleeding，and occult soft birth canal injury，such as vaginal hematoma，should be considered.

● Signs of hypotension：If the losing blood affects systemic circulation，the mother will develop signs of shock：an increased，thready，and weak pulse；increased and shallow respirations；decreased blood pressure.

Principle of Management

● Uterine atony：Massage the fundus expell clots from uterus，assist to empty bladder；rapid IV infusion of dilute oxytocin，intravascular；fluids and blood；abdominal hysterectomy if other interventions fail to control bleeding.

● Trauma：When bleeding is caused by trauma of the birth canal，surgical repair often is necessary.

● Retained placental：Fragments manual removal of the placental fragment is necessary to stop bleeding.

● Coagulation deficiency：Original medical disease should be treated.

【护理评估】

1. 健康史　除收集一般健康史外，尤其应注意收集与产后出血病因相关的健康史。

2. 身心状况　注意评估产后出血所致症状和体征的严重程度。发生产后出血后，产妇和家属常常表现出惊慌、焦虑、恐惧，应注意密切观察产妇的表现和倾听其主诉。

（1）评估产后出血量　目前常用的评估出血量的方法有称重法、容积法、面积法、休克指数法。

1）称重法：失血量（mL）=［胎儿娩出后所有敷料湿重（g）−胎儿娩出前所有敷料干重（g）］/1.05（血液比重 g/mL）。

2）容积法：用产后接血容器收集血液后，放入量杯测量。

3）面积法：根据纱布被血液浸湿的面积粗略估计，将血液浸湿的面积按 10 cm×10 cm（4 层纱布）为 10 mL 计算。

4）休克指数法：休克指数（shock index，SI）= 脉率/收缩压（mmHg）。SI = 0.5，血容量正常；SI = 1.0，失血量为 10%～30%（500～1 500 mL）；SI = 1.5，失血量为 30%～50%（1 500～2 500 mL）；SI = 2，失血量为 50%～70%（2 500～3 500 mL）。

（2）评估产后出血的原因　根据阴道流血的表现，初步评估产后出血的原因。

3. 辅助检查　包括血常规，血型，出、凝血时间，纤维蛋白原，凝血酶原时间及中心静脉压测定等。

【护理诊断】

1. 潜在并发症　如失血性休克。

2. 有感染的危险　与失血后抵抗力下降及手术操作有关。

3. 恐惧　与大量失血担心自身安危有关。

【护理措施】

1. 积极预防产后出血

(1)妊娠期　加强孕期保健,以及时治疗高危妊娠,为孕妇提供积极的心理支持。

(2)分娩期

1)第一产程:密切观察产程进展;合理使用子宫收缩药物,防止产程延长;注意水和营养的补充,防止产妇疲劳;消除产妇紧张情绪,必要时给予镇静剂以保证良好的休息。

2)第二产程:对于有高危因素的产妇,应建立静脉通道;正确掌握会阴切开指征并熟练助产;指导产妇正确使用腹压,避免胎儿娩出过急过快;阴道检查及手术助产时动作轻柔、规范;严格执行无菌技术操作。

3)第三产程:胎肩娩出后立即肌内注射或静脉滴注缩宫素,以加强子宫收缩,减少出血;正确处理胎盘娩出,并仔细检查胎盘、胎膜是否完整,检查软产道有无裂伤及血肿;准确收集和测量出血量。

(3)产褥期

1)80%的产后出血发生在产后2 h,所以产妇应留在产房严密观察2 h:观察产妇的子宫收缩、阴道出血及会阴伤口情况,定时测量生命体征,发现异常及时处理。

2)督促产妇及时排空膀胱,以免影响子宫收缩导致产后出血。

3)若无特殊情况,应尽早实施母乳喂养,以刺激子宫收缩,减少阴道流血。

4)对可能发生大出血的高危产妇,注意保持静脉通道,充分做好输血和急救的准备。

2. 出血的处理　针对原因迅速止血,纠正失血性休克,控制感染。

(1)子宫收缩乏力　加强宫缩能快速止血。

1)按摩或按压子宫:包括腹壁按摩宫底(图10-1)和腹壁-阴道双手按摩子宫(图10-2)两种方法。评价按摩有效的标准是子宫轮廓清楚,收缩有皱褶,阴道或子宫切口出血减少。按压时间以子宫恢复正常收缩并能保持收缩状态为止,按摩时配合使用宫缩剂。

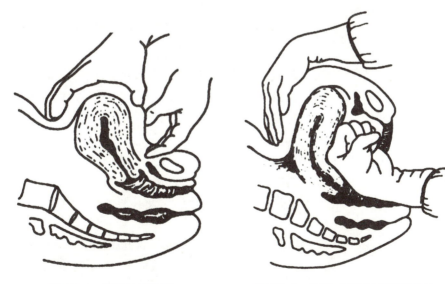

图10-1　腹壁按摩宫底　　　　　图10-2　腹壁-阴道双手按摩子宫

2)应用宫缩剂:①缩宫素,预防和治疗产后出血的一线药物;②麦角新碱,心脏病、妊娠期高血压疾病患者禁用;③前列腺素类药物。

3)宫腔填塞:包括宫腔纱条填塞(图10-3)和宫腔球囊填塞(图10-4)。填塞后24~48 h取出,取出纱条或球囊前遵医嘱先注射宫缩剂,并给予抗生素预防感染。

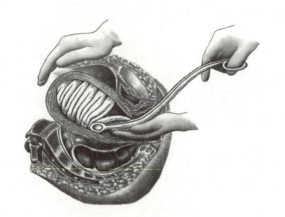
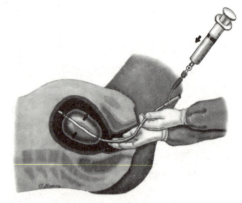

图10-3 宫腔纱条填塞　　　　　　　　　图10-4 宫腔球囊填塞

4)其他:经上述处理无效,还可行子宫压缩缝合术、子宫动脉或髂内动脉结扎术;如患者生命体征平稳,还可以行子宫动脉或髂内动脉栓塞技术介入治疗;如积极抢救无效、危及产妇生命时,应尽早行子宫次全切除术或子宫全切术,以挽救产妇的生命。

(2)胎盘因素　胎儿娩出后疑有胎盘滞留,应立即做宫腔检查。若胎盘已剥离则立即取出胎盘;若胎盘粘连,可试行徒手剥离胎盘后取出;若剥离困难怀疑胎盘植入者,则停止剥离,根据患者出血情况及胎盘剥离面积行保守治疗或子宫切除术;若胎盘、胎膜残留,更换无菌手套,徒手清理宫腔,手取困难者,可用大号刮匙刮取;若为子宫狭窄环所致的胎盘嵌顿,应配合麻醉师使用麻醉剂,待环松解后徒手取出胎盘。

(3)软产道损伤　按解剖关系及时准确地缝合,彻底止血。软产道血肿应切开并清除积血,彻底止血缝合,必要时放置引流条。

(4)凝血功能障碍　应积极止血,治疗原发病。输新鲜血、血小板、纤维蛋白原或凝血因子等,若已发生 DIC,则按 DIC 处理。

(5)失血性休克的护理　保暖,给氧,取平卧位;迅速建立静脉通路,保持输液通畅,做好输血准备,遵医嘱输液、输血;观察并记录血压、脉搏、呼吸及神志变化,留置导尿管,记录出入量;观察、测量出血量,并注意评估产妇的失血表现,如皮肤苍白、发绀、四肢湿冷等;配合医生采取有效的止血措施,如按摩子宫、注射宫缩剂等。

(6)预防感染　抢救过程中,严格无菌操作,遵医嘱给予抗生素预防感染。

3.心理护理　积极做好产妇及家属的安慰、解释工作,避免精神紧张。大量失血后,产妇抵抗力低下,体质虚弱,医护人员应更加主动关心并为其提供帮助,使其增加安全感。

Nursing Intervention

● Preventing hemorrhage:Every nurse should be aware of factors that put the new mother at risk for postpartum hemorrhage. When predisposing factors are present,initiate frequent assessments. The standard of care that calls for assessments every 30 min during the first 2 h after delivery.

● Massage uterus:The emergency measure to contract a uterus with atony is to place one hand on the women's symphysis publis to give good support to the base of the uterus. Grasp the fundus of the uterus with the other hand,and massage gently.

- Keeping the bladder empty：A full bladder pushes an uterus with atomy into an even more uncontracted state. Offer a bedpan at least every 4 h to keep the woman's bladder empty.

- Position：If the mother is experiencing respiratory distress from decreasing blood volume, administer oxygen by facemask is necessary. Keep her flat to allow adequate blood flow to her brain and kidneys.

- Vital signs assessment：If the mother's pulse rate rises rapidly, becomes weak and thready, and the blood pressure drops abruptly, her skin becomes cold and clammy and shows obvious signs of shock. Taking frequent vital signs and monitoring lochia flow, the nurse should be able to detect blood loss before this point is reached.

- Medication：Administer medications and fluids ordered by the doctors and evaluate their effect.

【健康教育】

①指导产妇加强营养,纠正贫血,促进身体康复。②出院后继续观察子宫复旧及恶露的情况,警惕晚期产后出血和产褥感染的发生。③做好产褥期卫生指导及产后避孕指导,产褥期禁止盆浴及性生活。④明确产后复查的时间、目的和意义,使产妇能按时接受检查,以便及时发现问题,及时处理,使其尽快恢复健康。

任务实施

子宫按摩的目的是娩出胎盘、促进子宫收缩、减少出血及排出宫腔内积血,适用于胎盘剥离未娩出、产后子宫收缩乏力及宫腔积血,是产科常用的操作技术(表10-1)。

表10-1　子宫按摩技术操作流程

项目	内容
仪表	仪表端庄,衣帽整洁,洗手,戴口罩
操作前准备	1. 病情评估:产妇生产情况,阴道出血量,子宫收缩强弱
	2. 环境准备:关闭门窗或屏风遮挡,室内温度适宜
	3. 物品准备:无菌包内置治疗巾、孔巾各1块,弯盘、无齿镊或弯血管钳1把;无菌手套1双;清洁大浴巾1条;消毒垫巾1块;碘伏棉球若干;无菌纱布若干
	4. 检查用物:物品完好,在有效期内。将用物按使用顺序放在治疗车上
操作步骤	1. 备齐物品并检查,携带用物至床旁
	2. 核对产妇,解释操作目的,取得配合,嘱其排空膀胱
	3. 遮挡产妇,保护隐私
	4. 洗手
	5. 协助产妇取仰卧膀胱截石位

续表 10-1

项目	内容
操作步骤	6. 按摩子宫 (1)单手按摩:操作者用一只手置于产妇腹部,拇指在子宫前壁,其余4指在子宫后壁,握住子宫底部,均匀而有节奏地按摩子宫,促进子宫收缩,是最常用的方法。 (2)双手按摩:操作者一只手在产妇耻骨联合上缘按压下腹中部,将子宫底向上托起,另一只手握住子宫体,使其高出盆腔,在子宫底部有节律地按摩子宫。同时,双手配合,间断地用力挤压子宫,使积存在子宫腔内的血块及时排出。 (3)腹部-阴道联合按摩:常规消毒产妇会阴部,铺无菌巾,戴无菌手套。操作者一只手进入产妇阴道,握拳置于阴道前穹隆,顶住子宫前壁,另一只手在腹部按压子宫后壁,使宫体前屈,两手相对紧压并均匀有节律地按摩子宫,不仅可刺激子宫收缩,还可以压迫子宫血窦,减少出血。按摩至子宫恢复有效收缩,出血减少时停止
	7. 正确评估阴道流血量、颜色及性状
	8. 协助产妇取舒适体位,整理衣裤
	9. 整理用物
	10. 洗手,记录
注意事项	1. 注意保护产妇隐私
	2. 操作敏捷、细心、准确
	3. 动作轻柔,注意观察产妇的反应

任务二 子宫破裂(Rupture of Uterus)

工作情景

王女士,35 岁,G₁P₀,孕38 周。估计胎儿体重3 800 g,临产15 h。宫口开2 cm,先露部S-1,宫缩弱。以0.9%氯化钠注射液500 mL加催产素5 U静脉滴注。静脉滴注2 h后宫口开3 cm,人工破膜,羊水清。静脉滴注4 h后宫口开大9 cm,但产妇烦躁不安,疼痛难忍。腹部检查,脐下一指处呈环状凹陷,下段有压痛,胎心率170 次/min,导尿呈血性。

①根据上述病史、查体,目前该产妇最可能的诊断是什么? ②作为责任护士,应如何进行护理评估? ③此时应采取哪些紧急护理? ④在该产妇的产程护理中要吸取哪些教训?

任务内容

子宫破裂是指在妊娠晚期或分娩期子宫体或子宫下段发生破裂。它是产科极其严重的并发症,严重威胁母儿生命。子宫破裂的发生率随着剖宫产率增加有上升趋势。

◆ 能识别子宫破裂的先兆。

◆ 能叙述子宫破裂的临床表现、处理原则。

【概述】

1. 病因　梗阻性难产是导致子宫破裂的首位原因，瘢痕子宫是近年来导致子宫破裂的常见原因，子宫收缩药物使用不当、阴道助产手术条件不当或过于粗暴均可引起子宫破裂。

2. 分类　按破裂原因分自然破裂和创伤性破裂；按破裂部位分子宫体破裂和子宫下段破裂；按发生时间分为妊娠期破裂和分娩期破裂；按破裂程度分完全性破裂和不完全性破裂。以破裂程度分类更具有临床意义。

3. 临床特征　子宫破裂多发生于分娩期，部分发生于妊娠晚期。子宫破裂发生通常是渐进的，多数由先兆子宫破裂发展为子宫破裂。

（1）先兆子宫破裂　在分娩过程中，胎儿下降受阻，而子宫呈强直性或痉挛性过强收缩，产妇烦躁不安，下腹剧痛难忍，呼吸急促，脉搏加快；因胎先露部下降受阻，子宫收缩过强，子宫体部肌肉增厚变短，子宫下段肌肉变薄拉长，在两者间形成环状凹陷，称为病理性缩复环（图10-5），该环可逐渐上升达脐平或脐上，压痛明显；由于胎先露部紧压膀胱使之充血，出现排尿困难及血尿；由于子宫收缩过强过频，胎儿供血受阻，表现为胎动频繁、胎心加快或减慢或听不清。病理性缩复环形成、下腹部压痛、胎心改变及出现血尿是先兆子宫破裂的四大主要表现。此时若不及时纠正，子宫将很快在病理性缩复环处及其下方发生破裂。

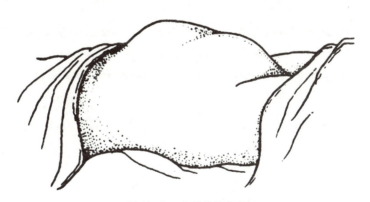

图10-5　病理性缩复环

（2）子宫破裂　产妇继先兆子宫破裂症状后，突感撕裂样剧烈腹痛，随后腹痛稍缓解，但很快出现持续性腹痛。

1）不完全子宫破裂：多见于子宫下段剖宫产切口瘢痕破裂，常缺乏先兆破裂症状，仅在不全破裂处有压痛，体征也不明显。

2）完全性子宫破裂：产妇突感下腹部发生一阵撕裂样的剧痛之后子宫收缩停止，腹部疼痛缓解。稍感舒适后即出现全腹持续性疼痛伴面色苍白、出冷汗、脉搏细数、呼吸急促、血压下降等休克征象。腹壁下可清楚扪及胎体，子宫位于侧方，胎心消失，全腹压痛、反跳痛明显。阴道检查可见鲜血流出，曾扩张的子宫颈口缩小，下降中的胎先露升高甚至消失（胎儿进入腹腔内），部分产妇可扪及子宫颈及子宫下段裂口。子宫体部瘢痕破裂多为完全性破裂,常无先兆破裂典型症状。

4. 治疗原则

(1)先兆子宫破裂　应立即抑制子宫收缩,给予静脉全身麻醉或肌内注射哌替啶 100 mg;同时立即行剖宫产术。

(2)子宫破裂　无论胎儿是否存活,在抢救休克的同时应尽快手术治疗。手术方式应根据产妇的全身情况、破裂的部位及程度、破裂时间及有无严重感染而决定。手术前、后应给予大剂量抗生素控制感染。严重休克者应尽可能就地抢救,若需转院,应输血、输液、包扎腹部后转送。

Uterine rupture may be spontaneous, traumatic, or associated with a prior uterine scar, and it may occur during or before labor or at the time of delivery. A prior uterine scar is associated with 40% of cases. With a prior lower−segment transverse incision, the risk for rupture is less than 1%, whereas the risk with a high vertical (classical) scar is 4%−7%. 60% of uterine ruptures occur in previously unscarred uterine.

Signs and Symptoms

The signs and symptoms of uterine rupture are highly variable. Typically, rupture is characterized by the sudden onset of intense abdominal pain and some vaginal bleeding. Impending rupture may be heralded by hyperventilation, restlessness, agitation, and tachycardia. After the rupture has occurred, the patient may be free of pain momentarily and then complain of diffuse pain thereafter. The most consistent clinical finding is an abnormal fetal heart rate pattern. The patient may or may not have vaginal bleeding, and if it occurs, it can range from spotting to severe hemorrhage. The presenting part may be found to have retracted on pelvic examination, and fetal parts may be more easily palpated abdominally. Abnormal contouring of the abdomen may be seen. Fetal distress develops commonly, and fetal death or long−term neurologic sequelae may occur in 10% of cases.

Management

A high index of suspicion is required, and immediate laparotomy is essential. In most cases, total abdominal hysterectomy is the treatment of choice, although debridement of the rupture site and primary closure may be considered in women of low parity who desire more children.

【护理评估】

1. 健康史　评估与子宫破裂相关的既往病史、现病史,如胎产次、有无子宫手术史;本次分娩过程中有无头盆不称、胎位异常、缩宫素滥用、阴道助产术操作史等。

2. 身心状况　评估产妇宫缩强度、持续时间、间隔时间,腹部疼痛的部位、性质、程度;有无排尿困难、血尿;有无出现病理性缩复环;监测胎心、胎动情况,评估有无胎儿宫内窘迫表现;产妇有无烦躁不安、疼痛难忍、恐惧、焦虑等。腹部检查可发现子宫破裂不同阶段相应的临床症状和体征。

3. 辅助检查

(1)实验室检查　血常规检查可见血红蛋白下降,白细胞计数增加。尿常规检查可见红细胞或肉眼血尿。

(2)其他　B 型超声检查可协助确定子宫破裂的部位及胎儿与子宫的关系;腹腔穿刺可证实腹腔内出血。

【护理诊断】

1. 疼痛　与强直性子宫收缩、病理性缩复环、子宫破裂后血液刺激腹膜有关。

2. 潜在并发症　失血性休克。

3. 有感染的危险　与多次阴道检查、宫腔内损伤、大量出血等有关。

4.预感性悲哀　与切除子宫及胎儿死亡有关。

【护理措施】

1.预防子宫破裂　做好产前检查,有瘢痕子宫、产道异常等高危因素者,应在预产期前2周住院待产。严格掌握缩宫素、前列腺素等子宫收缩剂的使用指征和方法。严密观察产程进展,以及时发现先兆子宫破裂征象并立即处理。正确掌握产科手术助产的指征及操作常规,阴道助产术后应仔细检查子宫颈及宫腔,以及时发现损伤给予修补。

2.先兆子宫破裂产妇的护理

(1)密切观察产程进展,以及时发现导致难产的诱因,注意胎心变化。

(2)待产过程中,出现宫缩过强及下腹部压痛或腹部出现病理性缩复环时,应立即报告医生并停止使用缩宫素和一切操作,同时密切监测产妇生命体征,按医嘱给予抑制宫缩、吸氧并做好剖宫产的术前准备。

3.子宫破裂产妇的护理

(1)遵医嘱迅速给予输液、输血、吸氧等处理,短时间内补足血容量;同时补充电解质及碱性药物,纠正酸中毒;积极进行抗休克处理。

(2)快速做好术前准备。

(3)术中、术后按医嘱应用大剂量抗生素以防感染。

(4)严密观察并记录生命体征、出入量。

4.心理护理　手术前、后向产妇及家属解释子宫破裂的治疗计划和对未来妊娠的影响。如胎儿已死亡,应提供机会使产妇表达悲伤情绪,陪伴并倾听产妇的感受,表示理解和同情。为产妇及其家属提供舒适的环境和全面的产褥期的休养计划,帮助产妇尽快调整情绪,适应现实生活。

【健康教育】

①加强营养,纠正贫血;注意卫生,预防感染。②对子宫破裂行子宫修补术的患者,若无子女应指导其避孕2年后再受孕,避孕方法可选用药物避孕或避孕套。子宫切除者应劝其调整心态,转移生活重心,增加生活情趣,提高生活质量。③若再次妊娠,应定期去产科高危门诊检查。

任务实施

子宫破裂应急预案及抢救程序

1.应急预案

(1)立即通知医生,建立两路以上静脉通道,面罩吸氧,快速补液,维持血容量并联系输血,积极抗休克治疗。

(2)密切监护孕产妇生命体征,观察孕产妇意识、尿量变化,注意记录病情。

(3)在抢救孕产妇的同时,及时与孕产妇家属沟通,下病危通知单,交代病情,签字。

(4)先兆子宫破裂:立即采取措施抑制子宫收缩;肌内注射哌替啶100 mg,或静脉全身麻醉,立即行剖宫产术。

(5)子宫破裂:一旦发生就地抢救,启动危重孕产妇抢救预案。下病危通知单,准备手术,专人取血、抢救休克的同时,无论胎儿是否存活,均尽快手术治疗;如胎儿存活,则抢救成员应包括新生儿科医生。若破口整齐、距离破裂时间短、无明显感染者或全身情况差不能耐受大手术者,可行修补术;若破口大、不整齐,有明显感染者应行子宫次全切除术;若破口大、撕裂伤超过子宫颈者,应行子宫全切术。

（6）手术前、后应给予大量广谱抗生素预防感染。

（7）术后密切监护病情变化，记录病情，及时完成抢救记录。

2. 程序　发生子宫破裂→立即通知医生，启动危重孕产妇抢救预案→抢救休克、吸氧、建立静脉通道→同时手术准备→下病危通知单，及时交代病情，签字→尽快手术→预防感染→术后密切监护→病情记录。

任务三　羊水栓塞（Amniotic Fluid Embolism）

工作情景

张女士，31 岁，G_1P_1，孕 40 周，自然分娩一活女婴，产程顺利。胎儿娩出时明显感觉胸闷、气促，6 min 后缓解，胎盘、胎膜自娩完整，会阴轻度裂伤，阴道一直持续出血，无凝血块，经用缩宫素、卡孕栓加强宫缩等措施仍出血不止。该孕妇既往无肝炎、血液病等病史。查体：P 110 次/min，R 30 次/min，BP 90/60 mmHg。产科情况：宫底平脐，轮廓尚清、质硬，外阴可见活动性出血，色暗红，无凝血块。实验室检查：Hb 9.7 g/L，WBC $13.2×10^9$/L。床旁心电图检查：窦性心动过速，右心房、右心室扩大。

①目前该产妇最可能的诊断是什么？②作为责任护士，该如何进行护理评估？③此时应采取哪些紧急护理？还需协助做哪些实验室检查？

任务内容

羊水栓塞是由于羊水进入母体血液循环，而引起的肺动脉高压、低氧血症、循环衰竭、弥散性血管内凝血（DIC）及多器官功能衰竭等一系列病理生理变化的过程。以起病急骤、病情凶险、难以预测、病死率高为临床特点，是极其严重的分娩并发症。发病率为（1.9～7.7）/10 万，死亡率为19%～86%。

任务目标

◆能叙述羊水栓塞的病因和预防措施。

◆能早期识别羊水栓塞。

◆能配合羊水栓塞的抢救。

【概述】

1. 病因　高龄初产、经产妇、子宫颈裂伤、子宫破裂、羊水过多、多胎妊娠、子宫收缩过强、急产、胎膜早破、前置胎盘、子宫破裂、剖宫产和刮宫术等可能是羊水栓塞的诱发因素。具体原因不明，可能与羊膜腔内压力过高、血窦开放、胎膜破裂等有关。

羊水栓塞的病理生理变化

2.病理生理　羊水成分进入母体循环是羊水栓塞发生的先决条件,可能发生的病理生理变化见图10-6。

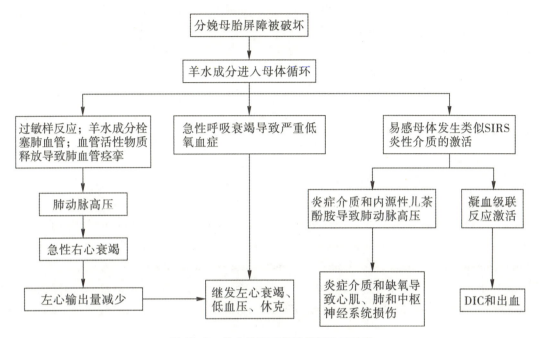

图 10-6　羊水栓塞可能的病理生理变化

3.临床表现　羊水栓塞通常起病急骤、来势凶险。70%发生在阴道分娩时,19%发生在剖宫产时。大多发生在分娩前2 h至产后30 min之间。极少发生在中孕引产、羊膜腔穿刺术中和外伤时。典型羊水栓塞以骤然出现的低氧血症、低血压(血压与失血量不符合)和凝血功能障碍为特征,也称羊水栓塞三联征。

(1)前驱症状　30%～40%的患者会出现非特异性的前驱症状,如呼吸急促、胸痛、憋气、寒战、呛咳、头晕、乏力、心慌、恶心、呕吐、麻木、针刺样感觉、焦虑、烦躁和濒死感,胎心减速,胎心基线变异消失等。重视前驱症状有助于及时识别羊水栓塞。

(2)心肺功能衰竭和休克　出现突发呼吸困难和(或)发绀、心动过速、低血压、抽搐、意识丧失或昏迷、突发血氧饱和度下降、心电图 ST 段改变及右心受损和肺底部湿啰音等。严重者,产妇于数分钟内猝死。

(3)凝血功能障碍　出现以子宫出血为主的全身出血倾向,如切口渗血、全身皮肤黏膜出血、针眼渗血、血尿、消化道大出血等。

(4)急性肾衰竭等脏器受损　全身脏器均可受损,除心肺功能衰竭及凝血功能障碍外,中枢神经系统和肾脏是最常见受损的器官。

羊水栓塞以上临床表现有时按顺序出现,有时也可不按顺序出现,表现具有多样性和复杂性。

4.处理原则　一旦怀疑或确诊羊水栓塞,应立即抢救。主要原则是抗过敏、纠正呼吸循环功能衰竭、改善低氧血症、抗休克、防止 DIC 和肾衰竭。

Cause

Amniotic fluid enters the circulation as a result of a breach in the physiological barrier that normally exists between maternal and fetal compartments. There may be maternal exposure to various fetal elements during pregnancy termination, following amniocentesis or trauma, or more commonly during labor or delivery as small lacerations develop in the lower uterine segment or cervix. Other predisposing factors associated with amniotic fluid embolism include multiparity, advanced maternal age, large fetus, intrauterine fetal death, and meconium in the amniotic fluid.

Pathophysiology

Amniotic fluid invariably contains small particles of matter, such as vernix caseosa, lanugo, and sometimes meconium. These form multiple tiny emboli, causing occlusion of the pulmonary capillaries when reaching the lungs, subsequently develop an anaphylactic reaction to fetal debris, coagulopathy. The lethality of intravenously infused amniotic fluid varies depending on the particular matter it contains.

Manifestation

This is a complex disorder classically characterized by the abrupt onset of hypotension, hypoxia, and consumptive coagulopathy.

Classically, a woman in the late stages of labor or immediately postpartum begins gasping for air, and then rapidly suffers seizure or cardiorespiratory arrest complicated by disseminated intravascular coagulation, massive hemorrhage, and death. Classically there are three phases.

Initially, there is a transient phase of intense pulmonary vasospasm leading to acute right heart failure and hypoxemia. There also may be an anaphylactic reaction to fetal debris, acting as matter foreign to the woman's body.

Hemorrhage is another major concern, with thromboplastic materials in the amniotic fluid triggering a sequence of events leading to disseminated intravascular coagulation.

Acute renal failure: the patient develops anuria and oliguria in the late phase of amniotic fluid embolism.

There is great individual variation in its clinical manifestation.

Management

Although an initial period of systemic and pulmonary hypertension appears to be involved in amniotic fluid embolism, this phase is transient. Women who survive long enough to receive any treatment other than cardiopulmonary resuscitation should receive therapy directed at oxygenation and support of the failing myocardium. Circulatory support and blood and component replacement are paramount. Treatment may include intubation and mechanical ventilation with 100% oxygen if the client is unconscious. Central venous pressure monitoring and blood transfusions may be used as appropriate. IV fluids in normotensive clients should be restricted to avoid pulmonary edema.

【护理评估】

1. 健康史　评估发生羊水栓塞的各种诱因,如高龄初产妇、多产妇、前置胎盘、胎盘早剥、胎膜早破、子宫收缩过强、子宫颈裂伤、子宫不完全破裂、是否中期妊娠引产或钳刮术、有无羊膜腔穿刺术等病史。

2. 身心状况　评估患者生命体征、发病时期,有无呼吸循环衰竭表现,有无全身性出血尤其是阴道流血表现,血液能否凝固,有无少尿、无尿情况。观察宫缩强度、宫口开大、先露部下降及胎心音等产程进展情况。

3.辅助检查

(1)血涂片查找羊水成分　采集下腔静脉血,查找羊水有形物质。

(2)床旁胸部 X 射线摄片　约90%的患者可见双侧肺部弥漫性点状、片状浸润影,沿肺门周围分布,伴轻度肺不张及心脏扩大。

(3)床旁心电图或心脏彩色多普勒超声检查　提示 ST 段下降,右心房、右心室扩大。

(4)DIC 有关的实验室检查　提示凝血功能障碍。

(5)尸检　可见肺水肿、肺泡出血,主要脏器如肺、胃、心、脑等血管及组织中或心内血液经离心处理后,镜检找到羊水有形物质。

【护理诊断】

1.气体交换受损　与肺动脉高压致肺血管阻力增加及肺水肿有关。

2.组织灌注量改变　与 DIC 及失血有关。

3.有胎儿窘迫的危险　与羊水栓塞、母体呼吸循环功能衰竭有关。

4.恐惧　与病情危重、濒死感有关。

5.潜在并发症　休克、肾衰竭、DIC。

【护理措施】

1.羊水栓塞的预防　密切观察产程进展,严格掌握子宫收缩药物的使用指征及方法,防止宫缩过强;不在宫缩时行人工破膜,人工破膜时不进行剥膜,以减少子宫颈管部位的小血管破损;剖宫产术中刺破羊膜前保护好子宫切口,避免羊水进入切口处开放性血管;及时发现前置胎盘、胎盘早剥等并发症并及时处理,对死胎、胎盘早剥的孕产妇,应密切观察出凝血等情况;中期妊娠引产者,羊膜穿刺次数不应超过 3 次,穿刺时避开胎盘;行钳刮术时应先刺破胎膜,待羊水流尽后再钳夹胎块。

2.羊水栓塞患者的处理与配合　一旦出现羊水栓塞的临床表现,应及时识别并立即给予紧急处理。

(1)增加氧合　应立即保持气道通畅,尽早实施面罩吸氧、气管插管或人工辅助呼吸,维持氧供以避免呼吸和心搏骤停。

(2)配合治疗　配合医生进行抗过敏、解痉挛、抗休克、纠正酸中毒、纠正心力衰竭、纠正凝血功能障碍的治疗。

(3)产科处理　密切观察产程进展、宫缩强度与胎儿情况。如羊水栓塞发生在胎儿娩出前,抢救的同时应及时终止妊娠,阴道助产或短时间内剖宫产终止妊娠。密切观察产妇出血量、血凝情况,若子宫出血不止,应及时报告医生做好子宫切除术的术前准备。

3.心理护理　对于神志清醒患者,应给予安慰和鼓励,使其放松心情,配合治疗和护理。对于家属的恐惧情绪表示理解和安慰,适当的时候允许家属陪伴患者,向家属介绍患者病情的严重性,以取得配合。如患者死亡,尽量做好家属的解释工作,帮助其度过悲伤阶段。

The nurse's role in the event of amniotic fluid embolism includes responsibility for monitoring client responses, anticipating possible therapies, and providing supportive care for the client and her family. The client should be placed in Fowler's position. Oxygen, medication, and blood products should be administered as ordered. Intake and output should be monitored closely. The client should not be left alone. If the fetus is undelivered, monitoring the fetal heart rate pattern and preparing for emergency delivery are additional nursing activities. Because there is such a high incidence of maternal death with this condition, the nurse also may need to help the family through the grieving process.

【健康教育】

①指导产妇加强营养,提高机体抵抗力。②指导产妇保持会阴清洁,特别是阴道助产术后,避免感染。③向患者解释此次发病可能的原因,进行创伤后应激障碍心理辅导。

微课　　　　　　　　　课件　　　　　　　练习题及参考答案

（史利锋）

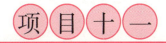

项目十一

产褥期疾病妇女的护理
（Nursing of Women with Postpartum Disease）

项目描述

　　产褥期为女性一生生理及心理发生急剧变化的时期之一，多数产妇恢复良好，少数可能发生产褥期疾病，如产褥感染、晚期产后出血等。

　　The period of menstruation is one of those periods in which the physiology and psychology of women undergo a violent change. Most postpartum women recover well, and a few may develop postpartum diseases such as infection of the perineum and postpartum hemorrhage.

任务一　产褥感染（Puerperal Infection）

工作情景

　　29 岁产妇，足月妊娠，胎膜早破。自然分娩后第 4 天，体温 39.1 ℃，下腹痛，恶露血性、浑浊、有臭味，宫底平脐，子宫压痛。白细胞计数 $16.5×10^9$/L，中性粒细胞百分比 85%。

　　①目前该产妇最可能的诊断是什么？②作为责任护士，该如何进行护理评估？③此时应采取哪些护理措施？

任务内容

　　产褥感染是指分娩及产褥期生殖道受病原体侵袭，引起局部或全身感染。产褥病是指分娩24 h以后的 10 d 内，用口表每日测量体温 4 次，每次间隔 4 h，有 2 次体温≥38 ℃。引起产褥病的原因以产褥感染为主，但也包括生殖道以外的乳腺炎、上呼吸道感染、尿路感染等。产褥感染、产后出血、妊娠合并心脏病及严重的妊娠期高血压疾病仍是目前导致孕产妇死亡的四大原因。

任务目标

◆ 能区别产褥感染和产褥病。

◆ 能根据产妇的临床表现识别产褥感染。

◆ 能对产褥感染的患者进行护理。

【概述】

1. 病因

(1)诱因　正常女性生殖道对外界致病因子有一定的防御功能。正常妊娠和分娩通常不会增加感染的机会。只有在机体免疫力、细菌毒力、细菌数量三者平衡失调时，才会增加感染的机会，导致感染发生。产褥感染的诱因有胎膜早破、羊膜腔感染、产程延长、产前产后出血、产科手术操作、慢性疾病、孕期贫血、营养不良、体质虚弱及妊娠晚期性生活等。

(2)感染途径

1)内源性感染：正常孕产妇生殖道或其他部位寄生的病原体，多数并不致病，当抵抗力降低等感染诱因出现时可致病。研究表明，内源性感染更重要。

2)外源性感染：指外界病原体进入产道所致感染。

(3)病原体　正常女性生殖道内寄生大量的微生物，包括需氧菌、厌氧菌、假丝酵母菌、衣原体、支原体，可分为致病性微生物和非致病性微生物两类。有些非致病的微生物在一定条件下可以致病，称为机会致病菌。产褥感染常见病原体有需氧性链球菌、厌氧革兰氏阳性球菌、大肠埃希菌属、葡萄球菌、类杆菌属、厌氧芽孢梭菌、支原体、衣原体、淋病奈瑟球菌等。

2. 临床表现　产褥感染的三大主要症状是发热、疼痛、异常恶露。

(1)急性外阴、阴道、子宫颈炎　分娩时会阴损伤或手术导致感染，表现为会阴部疼痛，坐位困难。局部伤口红肿、发硬，伤口裂开，有脓性分泌物流出，压痛明显，较重时可伴有低热。阴道裂伤及挫伤感染表现为阴道黏膜充血、水肿、溃疡，脓性分泌物增多。感染部位较深时，可以引起阴道旁结缔组织炎。子宫颈裂伤向深部蔓延达宫旁组织，引起盆腔结缔组织炎。

(2)子宫感染　子宫感染包括急性子宫内膜炎、子宫肌炎。病原体经胎盘剥离面侵入，扩散至子宫蜕膜层称为子宫内膜炎，侵入子宫肌层称为子宫肌炎，两者常伴发。若为子宫内膜炎，子宫内膜充血、坏死，阴道内有大量脓性分泌物且有臭味。若为子宫肌炎，恶露量多、脓性，子宫压痛明显、复旧不良，可以伴有高热、寒战、头痛、心率增快、白细胞增多等全身感染的症状。

(3)急性盆腔结缔组织炎、急性输卵管炎　病原体沿宫旁淋巴和血行达宫旁组织引起盆腔结缔组织炎，形成炎性包块，同时累及输卵管时可引起输卵管炎。表现为下腹痛伴肛门坠胀，伴有持续高热、寒战、脉速、头痛等全身症状。体征有下腹明显压痛、反跳痛、肌紧张，子宫复旧差，宫旁一侧或两侧结缔组织增厚、触及炎性包块，严重者累及整个盆腔形成"冰冻骨盆"。

(4)急性盆腔腹膜炎及弥漫性腹膜炎　炎症进一步扩散至子宫浆膜层形成盆腔腹膜炎；继而发展成弥漫性腹膜炎。全身中毒症状明显，如高热、恶心、呕吐、腹胀等，检查腹部有压痛、反跳痛、肌紧张。腹膜面分泌大量渗出液，纤维蛋白覆盖引起肠粘连，可以在直肠子宫陷凹形成局限性脓肿，若脓肿波及肠管及膀胱，可有腹泻、里急后重和排尿困难。

(5)血栓性静脉炎　来自胎盘剥离处的感染性栓子，经血行播散可引起盆腔血栓性静脉炎，可以累及子宫静脉、卵巢静脉、髂内静脉、髂总静脉及阴道静脉。病变单侧居多，产后1~2周多见。表现为寒战、高热，症状可持续数周或反复发作。病变多在股静脉、腘静脉及大隐静脉处，当髂总静或股静脉栓塞时影响下肢静脉回流,出现下肢水肿、皮肤发白和疼痛(称股白肿)。小腿深静脉栓塞时可出现腓肠肌及足底部疼痛和压痛。

(6)脓毒血症及败血症 当感染血栓脱落进入血液循环可引起脓毒血症,出现肺、脑、肾脓肿或肺栓塞。当侵入血液循环的细菌大量繁殖引起败血症时,可出现严重全身症状及感染性休克症状,如寒战、高热、脉搏细数、血压下降、呼吸急促、尿量减少等,可危及生命。

3.处理原则 一旦诊断产褥感染,原则上应给予广谱、足量、有效抗生素,并根据感染的病原体调整抗生素治疗方案。中毒症状严重者短期选用肾上腺皮质激素,提高机体应激能力。对脓肿形成或宫内残留感染组织者,应积极进行感染灶的处理。腹部或外阴切口感染及时切开引流;盆腔脓肿者可经腹或阴道后穹隆切开引流;宫腔内有胎盘、胎膜残留者,应控制感染后清除宫腔内残留物;子宫感染严重,经积极治疗无效者,应及时行子宫切除术。血栓性静脉炎应在应用大量抗生素同时,加用肝素、双香豆素、阿司匹林等药物进行抗凝、溶栓治疗。

Etiology

Every part of the reproductive tract is connected to every other part, and organisms can move from the vagina, through the cervix, into the uterus, up the fallopian tubes, and out the tubes to infect the ovaries and the peritoneal cavity. The normal physiologic changes of childbirth increase the risk of infection. During labor and postpartum, the acidity of the vagina is reduced by amniotic fluid, blood, and lochia, which are alkaline. The alkaline environment encourages growth of bacteria.

Clinical Signs and Symptoms

● Infection of the perineum: Infection of the perineum generally remains localized and manifested the symptoms of any suture line infection: pain, heat, and a feeling of pressure. The mother may have an elevated temperature.

● Metritis: The mother with severe metritis looks sick. The major signs and symptoms of metritis are fever, chills, malaise, lethargy, anorexia, abdominal pain and cramping, and purulent, foul-smelling lochia.

● Thrombophlebitis: Thrombophlebitis is the least common of the puerperal infections. It usually is not seen until 2 weeks after childbirth. It occurs when infection spreads along the venous system and thrombophlebitis develops. It occurs more often in women with wound infection and usually involves the ovarian, uterine, or hypogastric veins. The primary symptom is pain in the groin, abdomen, or flank. The others, such as tachycardia, gastrointestinal distress, and decreased bowel sounds may be present. Fever that does not respond to antibiotics may be the only sign.

Management

● Antibiotics use: The goal of this therapy is to confine the infectious process to the local sites and to prevent spread of the infection throughout the body. IV administration of antibiotics is the initial treatment for infections. The best use of antibiotics should accord a report of the antibiotic-sensitive organism. Broad-spectrum antibiotics, such as ampicillin and cephalosporins, are rapidly effective for mild to moderate infection after vaginal birth. For some cases, a combination of clindamycin plus gentamicin or cephalosporins may be necessary.

● Release the symptoms: Drug includes antibiotics for fever and reducing pain; to increase drainage of lochia and promote involution. Inflammations of episiotomy site can be warm compresses or/and sitz bath, because they can provide comfort and promote healing by increasing circulation to the area.

【护理评估】

1.健康史 评估患者有无妊娠期、分娩期及产后引起感染的诱因。了解有无贫血、泌尿生殖系统感染的病史。

2. 身心状况　评估患者生命体征,了解有无高热、腹痛、外阴或下肢疼痛等症状,了解恶露的量、色、味。评估腹部有无压痛、反跳痛及肌紧张,会阴局部有无红肿、硬块、脓性渗出,阴道有无脓性分泌物,评估子宫复旧情况,了解子宫大小、硬度,有无压痛,双附件区有无压痛及包块,有无下肢局部静脉压痛及水肿。评估患者是否存在心理沮丧与焦虑情绪,家庭支持系统是否健全。

3. 实验室及其他检查

(1)超声检查、CT、磁共振等检测手段能够对感染形成的炎性包块、脓肿做出定位及定性诊断。

(2)血清 C 反应蛋白升高,有助于早期诊断感染。

(3)取宫腔分泌物、脓肿穿刺物、阴道后穹隆穿刺物做细菌培养及药敏试验;病原体抗原和特异抗体检测可以作为快速确定病原体的方法。

【护理诊断】

1. 体温过高　与感染有关。

2. 急性疼痛　与感染有关。

3. 焦虑恐惧　与母子分离及疾病严重性有关。

【护理措施】

1. 一般护理　保证患者休息,取半卧位以利恶露引流和炎症局限。加强营养,鼓励患者多饮水,必要时静脉输液。患者出现高热、疼痛、呕吐时做好症状护理。

2. 治疗配合　严格床边隔离及无菌操作,避免院内感染。会阴侧切口感染者取健侧卧位;下肢血栓性静脉炎者,抬高患肢,局部保暖、湿热敷,促进血液循环,减轻肿胀。配合做好脓肿引流术、清宫术、阴道后穹隆穿刺术、子宫切除术的术前准备及护理。遵医嘱应用抗生素及肝素。

3. 心理护理　耐心解答家属及患者的疑虑,向其讲解疾病的知识,让其了解病情和治疗护理情况,增加治疗信心,缓解疑虑情绪。

Nursing Interventions

- Observation: Measure the vital signs every 4 h. Observe the surgical incision for redness, tenderness, edema, drainage, approximation and note the odor of lochia every 4 h. The mother may be medicated as needed for abdominal pain or cramping, which may be severe. The nurse should give the medications as directed and observe the mother for signs of improvement or new symptoms, such as nausea and vomiting, abdominal distention, absent bowel sounds, and severe abdominal pain.

- Position: The mother should be placed in a Fowler's position to promote drainage of lochia, prevent the inflammation spread.

- Instruct mother in hygienic practices to prevent infection: Careful hand washing before and after perineal care; perineal cleansing after elimination; wiping the perineum from front to back.

- Nutrition: Encourage mother to eat well-balanced meals when she progresses to a regular diet. Emphasize the importance of a diet high in protein and vitamin C.

- Touch with infant: Encourage maximum mother-newborn contact, and provide continuous information of newborn to enhance the bonding and attachment process.

【健康教育】

①加强孕期卫生宣教,临产前 2 个月避免性生活及盆浴,加强营养,增强体质。②产褥期注意外阴清洁,产后 1 周内不坐浴,严禁性生活,对有感染可能者及早应用抗生素预防感染。③指导暂停哺乳者定时挤奶,以维持泌乳,感染控制后可继续哺乳。

任务实施

会阴湿热敷可以促进局部血液循环及组织再生,具有消炎、消肿、镇痛、利于外阴伤口愈合和陈旧性血肿局限等作用。会阴湿热敷适用于会阴部水肿、血肿吸收期、会阴伤口硬结、早期感染等患者,其操作流程见表11-1。

表11-1　会阴湿热敷操作流程

项目	内容
操作前准备	1. 操作者准备:衣帽整洁,修剪指甲,洗手,戴口罩
	2. 环境准备:温暖,隐蔽性好,必要时用屏风遮挡
	3. 物品准备:治疗车、治疗盘、消毒弯盘(或换药碗)、无菌长镊子2把、无菌纱布、医用凡士林、沸水、热源袋(热水袋或电热宝)、红外线灯、煮沸的50%硫酸镁溶液、棉垫1块、橡胶单和治疗巾或一次性垫单、一次性手套、洗手液等
操作步骤	1. 核对、解释:携用物至床旁,核对患者姓名、床号、医嘱,评估病情;解释会阴湿热敷的目的及方法,可能出现的不适,以取得配合
	2. 安置体位:屏风遮挡,协助患者取屈膝仰卧位,双腿屈曲向外分开,充分暴露会阴部。放好橡胶单,先行外阴擦洗,清除外阴局部污垢
	3. 湿热敷:热敷部位先涂一薄层凡士林,盖上纱布,轻轻敷上浸有热敷溶液的温纱布,外面盖上棉布垫保温。一般3~5 min更换1次热敷垫,热敷时间为15~30 min,也可用热源袋放在棉垫外或用红外线灯照射,以延长更换敷料的时间
	4. 热敷完毕移去敷料,观察热敷部位皮肤,用干纱布拭净皮肤
操作后	1. 撤去橡胶单及一次性垫单,协助患者整理衣裤及床单位
	2. 整理用物,处理污物
	3. 洗手,记录
注意事项	1. 会阴湿热敷应在会阴擦洗、清洁外阴局部伤口的污垢后进行
	2. 动作轻柔,避免牵扯伤口引起疼痛。保护患者隐私,避免受凉
	3. 会阴湿热敷的温度一般为41~48 ℃
	4. 湿热敷的面积应是病损范围的2倍
	5. 定期检查热源袋的完好性,防止烫伤,对休克、虚脱、昏迷及术后感觉不灵敏的患者应特别注意

任务二 晚期产后出血（Late Postpartum Hemorrhage）

工作情景

孙女士,8 d 前顺产一男婴。今早突感阴道流血量增多。查体:体温 37.9 ℃,脉搏 120 次/min,呼吸 24 次/min,血压 80/50 mmHg。妇科检查:子宫大而软,宫口松弛,有残留组织堵塞。B 型超声示宫腔内有残留物。诊断为晚期产后出血。

①该患者发生晚期产后出血的原因是什么? ②目前该患者最主要的护理诊断是什么? ③护士针对上述护理诊断应为患者实施哪些护理措施?

任务内容

分娩 24 h 后,在产褥期内发生的子宫大量出血,称为晚期产后出血。产后 1~2 周发病最常见,亦有迟至产后 2 月余发病者。

任务目标

◆ 能叙述晚期产后出血的临床表现及处理原则。
◆ 能对晚期产后出血的患者实施整体护理。

【概述】

1.病因　晚期产后出血最常见的原因是胎盘、胎膜残留,多发生于产后 10 d 左右。其他还有蜕膜残留,子宫胎盘附着面复旧不全,感染(以子宫内膜炎多见),剖宫产术后子宫切口裂开,产后子宫滋养细胞肿瘤、子宫黏膜下肌瘤等。

2.临床表现

(1)症状

1)阴道流血:胎盘、胎膜残留,蜕膜残留引起的阴道流血多在产后 10 d 左右发生。子宫胎盘附着部位复旧不良引起的出血多发生在产后 2 周左右,可以反复多次阴道流血,也可突然大量阴道流血。剖宫产子宫切口裂开或愈合不良所致的阴道流血,多在术后 2~3 周发生,常为子宫突然大量出血,可导致失血性休克。

2)腹痛和发热:常合并感染,伴恶露增多、恶臭。

3)全身症状:继发性贫血,严重者因失血性休克危及生命。

(2)体征　可有面色苍白、脉细弱及血压下降。子宫复旧不佳可扪及子宫大而软,宫口松弛,有时可触及残留组织和血块,伴有感染者子宫明显压痛。

3.处理原则　治疗原则是抗感染,加强子宫收缩,针对原因行刮宫或剖腹探查手术。

【护理评估】

1.健康史　若为阴道分娩,应注意产程进展及产后恶露变化,有无反复或突然阴道流血病史;若为剖宫产,应了解手术指征、术式及术后恢复情况。

2.身心评估　注意评估患者子宫复旧情况,评估恶露量的多少,有无臭味,有无腹痛、发热、贫血。患者因反复阴道流血、发热、腹痛、母子分离等,出现紧张、恐惧、焦虑、不安、内疚等不良情绪。

3.辅助检查

(1)血常规　了解贫血和感染情况。

(2)B 型超声　了解子宫大小、宫腔有无残留物及子宫切口愈合情况。

(3)病原体确定和药敏试验　可进行宫腔分泌物培养或发热时行血培养,以便选择有效的广谱抗生素。

(4)血 hCG 测定　有助于排除胎盘残留及绒毛膜癌。

(5)病理检查　宫腔刮出物或切除子宫标本,应送病理检查。

【护理诊断】

1.外周组织灌注无效　与子宫大量流血有关。

2.焦虑　与担心自身安危和婴儿喂养有关。

3.潜在并发症　失血性休克。

【护理措施】

1.治疗配合　密切配合医生进行相关检查,积极查找出血原因,并给予相应处理。

(1)少量或中等量阴道出血,遵医嘱用止血剂、宫缩剂及广谱抗生素。

(2)发现大块胎盘、胎膜残留者,应在输液、输血的同时行清宫术,将刮出物送病理检查,以明确诊断。

(3)疑为剖宫产子宫切口裂开,即使少量阴道流血也应收住院,遵医嘱静脉补液、药物治疗;阴道流血多者,做好剖腹探查术准备。

(4)保持静脉输液通畅,严密观察病情变化,注意生命体征、子宫复旧、阴道出血情况,若阴道出血量增多,应立即报告医生。

2.心理护理　向患者及家属解释病因及治疗措施,使其树立信心。鼓励患者说出担忧、焦虑,消除不良情绪。关心、安慰患者,帮助护理新生儿,使其情绪稳定,配合治疗和护理。

【健康教育】

指导产妇注意休息,保持会阴清洁,摄入高蛋白、高维生素、富含铁剂、易消化食物。指导产妇早期下床活动,利于恶露排出,促进子宫复旧,恶露异常及时就诊。产褥期禁止性生活,避免感染。

产后抑郁症

微课　　　　　　　　　课件　　　　　　　　练习题及参考答案

（李海燕　张　爽）

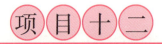

项目十二

女性生殖系统炎症患者的护理（Nursing of Women with Inflammation of Reproductive System）

项目描述

　　女性生殖系统炎症是妇科常见病、多发病，发病年龄段广泛，炎症部位涉及外阴、阴道、子宫颈、内生殖器及周围结缔组织等，临床上以阴道炎、慢性子宫颈炎最常见。

　　Inflammation of the female reproductive system is a common and widespread gynecological condition that affects a wide range of age groups. The sites of inflammation involve the vulva, vagina, cervix, internal genitalia and surrounding connective tissue, among others. In clinical practice, vaginitis and chronic cervicitis are the most common.

女性生殖器官的
自然防御功能

任务一　　外阴炎（Vulvitis）

工作情景

　　患者，女，32岁，以外阴部肿胀疼痛2 d为主诉就诊。患者于2 d前出现外阴部右侧肿胀疼痛，逐渐加重，行走受到影响。既往体健，无手术、外伤史。体格检查：T 36.8 ℃，P 80 次/min，R 20 次/min，BP 120/80 mmHg，心肺肝脾未查到异常。妇科检查：外阴已产式，右侧大阴唇处见一囊肿，表面红肿，压痛明显，有明显波动感。阴道通畅，子宫及附件无异常。

　　①请明确该患者主要的护理问题。②根据目前的情况对患者进行正确的护理。

任务内容

　　外阴炎是指发生在外阴皮肤与黏膜的炎症，包括非特异性外阴炎和前庭大腺炎。

◆ 能叙述非特异性外阴炎和前庭大腺炎的病因、临床表现及处理原则。

◆ 能对非特异性外阴炎和前庭大腺炎进行正确评估和护理。

【概要】

1. 病因

（1）非特异性外阴炎　外阴与尿道、肛门邻近，容易受到阴道分泌物、经血、尿液、粪便的刺激引起炎症。此外，糖尿病患者的糖尿刺激、穿着紧身化纤内裤，或经期使用卫生巾等使局部透气性差、潮湿，也可引起炎症发生。

（2）前庭大腺炎　即病原体侵入前庭大腺引起的炎症。前庭大腺位于大阴唇后 1/3 深部，腺管开口于小阴唇与处女膜间沟的中、下 1/3 处，在性交、分娩或外阴卫生不良时容易发生炎症，多见于生育期妇女。

2. 临床表现

（1）非特异性外阴炎　外阴瘙痒、疼痛、灼热感，在活动、排便、性交时可加重。妇科检查可见外阴皮肤、黏膜充血、水肿、糜烂、抓痕，重者出现溃疡、湿疹等。

（2）前庭大腺炎　单侧发病多见。初起时局部疼痛、肿胀、烧灼感、压痛明显，患者行走不便、发热等。脓肿（图 12-1）多发于一侧，脓肿形成时可呈鸡蛋大小，表面发红，有波动感。前庭大腺囊肿直径>6 cm 时，外阴有坠胀感或性交不适。

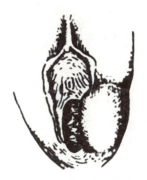

图 12-1　前庭大腺脓肿

3. 处理原则

（1）非特异性外阴炎　积极去除病因，局部清洁消炎，如坐浴、涂抹抗生素软膏。

（2）前庭大腺炎　形成前庭大腺脓肿时，选择针对性抗生素治疗，并切开引流；前庭大腺囊肿者，常行前庭大腺造口术。

Etiology

● Vulvitis：Vulvitis can be caused by systemic conditions, direct contact with irritants and extension of infections from the vagina. Main causes include vaginal discharge, menstrual flow, lochia, urine and feces. Other causes of vulvitis include diabetic women's urine.

● Bartholinitis：Bacteria, mycoplasmas, and protozoa are transmitted from the gastrointestinal tract, vulva, or vagina to the Bartholin's gland duct while sex intercourse, abortion, and delivery.

Clinical Signs and Symptoms

- Vulvitis：Adult women describe the vulva symptoms using a variety of terms such as itching, pain, swelling, discharge, discomfort, burning, external dysuria, soreness, pain with intercourse or sexual activity.

- Bartholinitis：Perineal pain is the symptom that most commonly motivates the woman to seek medical assistance. Additional presenting symptoms include fever, labial edema, chills, malaise, and purulent discharge.

Principle of Management

- Vulvitis：Medical treatment of clients with vulvitis depends on the cause. If infection is the underlying cause of diabetics, the physician treats the diabetics.

- Bartholinitis：Rest is necessary to the acute woman. If there is exudate, a specimen may be processed for culture and sensitivity testing. Conservative treatment consists of oral analgesics and moist heat in the form of frequent sitz baths or hot wet packs. The moist heat relieves pain and facilitates spontaneous rupture and drainage of the abscess. Surgical incision and drainage of the abscess may be done by the physician. More aggressive treatment with broad-spectrum antibiotics is indicated if symptoms of systemic infection are present.

【护理评估】

1. 健康史　询问个人卫生情况、衣着习惯，饮食、药物等有无过敏史，有无糖尿病、尿瘘、粪瘘等疾病，外阴不适的程度和发病时间。

2. 身心状况　检查外阴局部有无红肿、渗出、湿疹、溃疡、脓性分泌物等炎症表现。了解患者病程长短及对外阴不适的心理反应。

3. 辅助检查　脓性分泌物培养，可培养出病原体。

【护理诊断】

1. 舒适度的改变　与外阴瘙痒、疼痛、分泌物多有关。
2. 皮肤、黏膜完整性受损　与局部炎症所致的抓伤、湿疹、溃疡有关。
3. 疼痛　与炎症刺激外阴红肿、化脓有关。
4. 焦虑　与外阴瘙痒、疼痛不适有关。

【护理措施】

1. 一般护理　保持外阴清洁，促进伤口愈合。前庭大腺炎急性期卧床休息，及时给予热敷、理疗，增加舒服感。

2. 心理护理　解释炎症发生的原因，增强患者治疗信心，缓解其焦虑情绪。

3. 治疗护理　前庭大腺脓肿或囊肿切开后，局部放置引流条，每日更换。外阴用消毒液擦洗，2 次/d，伤口愈合后改为坐浴。前庭大腺炎者，必要时可在其开口处取分泌物进行细菌培养和药敏试验，遵医嘱应用抗生素。

教会患者坐浴方法，包括坐浴液的配制、温度、时间等。常用的坐浴液有 1：5 000 的高锰酸钾或 0.1% 的聚维酮碘液。坐浴时要使会阴部浸没于溶液中，每天 2 次，每次 15 ~ 20 min，7 ~ 10 次为 1 个疗程。

Nursing Intervention

- Direct treatment：Teach the patient to confect the treatment water, including the temperature, the time, etc.

- Rest in bed：Basic practices include soap-and-water cleansing at least once daily and wiping the perineal area with a clean tissue from front to back following urination or defecation.
- Obey the order of the physician：Antibiotics and analgetic are needed.

【健康教育】

①注意个人卫生，勤洗、勤换内衣，保持外阴干燥、清洁，穿着棉质内衣裤。②勿使用刺激性药物或肥皂清洗会阴部。③经期、孕期和产褥期注意卫生保健，指导患者注意性卫生，经期、产褥期禁止性交。

任务实施

坐浴护理技术见表12-1。

表12-1　坐浴护理技术

操作项目	操作内容
操作目的	可以促进局部组织的血液循环，减轻外阴局部的炎症及不适，使创面清洁，有利于组织的恢复。适用于治疗或辅助治疗外阴炎、阴道炎、子宫脱垂、会阴切口愈合不良，以及外阴阴道术前的准备等。此方法简便易行，患者可于家中使用
评估要点	1.评估患者的年龄、病情、意识、心理状态、自理能力、合作程度
	2.评估会阴部的皮肤情况
	3.向患者解释坐浴的目的及注意事项，以取得配合
操作准备	1.护士准备：着装整洁规范，仪表端庄大方
	2.操作用物 (1)治疗车上：坐浴盆、干毛巾、高锰酸钾、水壶(内盛35～37 ℃的温水，热水浴41～43 ℃，冷水浴14～15 ℃) (2)其他：医嘱单、治疗卡、快速手消毒剂、医用垃圾桶、生活垃圾桶
操作步骤	1.核对医嘱
	2.核对床号、姓名、住院号，评估患者
	3.洗手，戴口罩
	4.携用物至患者床旁，再次核对
	5.协助患者穿宽松的裤子，必要时用屏风遮挡，注意保暖
	6.将准备好的温水倒入坐浴盆，根据水量加入高锰酸钾，浓度要适宜
	7.协助患者将裤子脱至膝盖下，缓慢坐入盆中，使患者臀部及全部外阴浸入药液中持续20 min
	8.协助患者用干毛巾擦干会阴部，穿好裤子
	9.协助患者取舒适体位，整理床单位。询问患者的需要
	10.处理用物
	11.洗手，取口罩
	12.记录
	13.操作速度：完成时间在10 min以内

续表 12-1

操作项目	操作内容
指导要点	1.告知患者坐浴时的注意事项,操作前嘱患者排空膀胱,经期、阴道流血、孕妇及产后7 d内的产妇禁止坐浴
	2.告知患者穿防滑的鞋子,避免滑倒
注意事项	1.坐浴溶液浓度按比例配制,浓度过高易造成黏膜损伤,浓度太低则影响治疗效果
	2.水温适中,不能过高,以免烫伤皮肤
	3.坐浴前先将外阴及肛门周围擦洗干净
	4.坐浴时需将臀部及全部外阴浸入药液中
	5.注意保暖,以防受凉

任务二　阴道炎(Vaginitis)

工作情景

患者,女,34 岁,G_3P_1,因外阴瘙痒、白带增多伴尿急、尿痛3 d来院就诊。无明显发病诱因,阴道分泌物有腥臭味、呈灰黄色,既往体健。妇科检查:外阴潮红,阴道黏膜红肿,阴道穹隆部有多量分泌物,呈泡沫状、灰黄色,阴道壁上分布较多散在出血点。

①请明确该患者主要的护理问题。②根据目前的情况对患者进行正确的护理。

任务内容

阴道炎是常见的妇科炎症。临床常见的炎症类型有滴虫性阴道炎、外阴阴道假丝酵母菌病、细菌性阴道病和萎缩性阴道炎。

任务目标

◆能叙述各种阴道炎的病因、临床表现及处理原则。
◆能对各种阴道炎正确评估及护理。

【概要】

1.滴虫性阴道炎

(1)病因　由阴道毛滴虫感染引起。阴道毛滴虫(图 12-2)适宜在温度为 25～40 ℃、pH 为 5.2～6.6 的潮湿环境中生长,如果生活环境的 pH<5 或 pH>7 则不能存活。在月经周期中,月经后阴道酸度减弱,pH 接近中性,隐藏在腺体及阴道皱褶中的滴虫大量繁殖,导致炎症易在月经后复发。阴道毛滴虫除寄生在阴道外,还可寄生在尿道、尿道旁腺、膀胱、肾盂及男性的包皮褶、尿道、前列腺中。

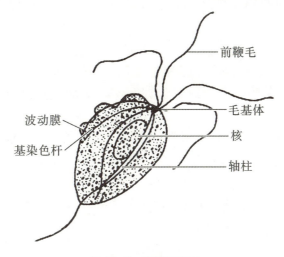

图 12-2　阴道毛滴虫

（2）传播途径

1）直接传播：经性交传播。男性感染阴道毛滴虫后常成为带虫者而成为传染源。

2）间接传播：通过被污染的游泳池、公共浴池、浴盆、浴巾、坐便器、衣物及污染的医疗器械和敷料等感染。

（3）临床表现　感染后一般有 4～28 d 的潜伏期。

1）症状：主要症状是出现大量的稀薄、泡沫状白带及外阴瘙痒，如合并其他细菌感染，白带可呈黄绿色、脓性、泡沫状，且有臭味。瘙痒部位主要在阴道口及外阴，可伴有灼热感、疼痛、性交痛等。如感染累及泌尿系统，可有尿频、尿急、尿痛或血尿表现。

2）体征：妇科检查可见阴道及子宫颈黏膜充血，有散在的出血点，以阴道穹隆部明显，阴道内有稀薄泡沫状或脓性泡沫状分泌物，子宫颈呈现"草莓样"改变。

（4）处理原则　切断传播途径，全身应用抗滴虫药物，避免阴道冲洗，性伴侣同时治疗，防止复发。

2. 外阴阴道假丝酵母菌病

（1）病因　病原体为假丝酵母菌，80%～90% 的病原体为白假丝酵母菌，10%～20% 为光滑假丝酵母菌、近平滑假丝酵母菌、热带假丝酵母菌等。此菌适宜在 pH 为 4.0～4.7 的酸性环境中生长。白假丝酵母菌为机会致病菌，平时可在阴道、口腔、肠道内寄生不引起症状，当机体抵抗力低下或阴道局部环境适宜时，假丝酵母菌大量繁殖致病。在月经周期中，月经前阴道酸度增加，因而炎症易在月经前复发。

（2）传播途径

1）内源性传播：寄生在阴道、口腔、肠道内的假丝酵母菌为机会致病菌，当条件适合时大量繁殖致病，不同部位间还可互相传染。

2）直接传播：经性交传播。

3）间接传播：极少数通过接触被污染的衣物传染。

（3）临床表现

1）症状：主要症状为白带增多、外阴瘙痒明显。白带呈现白色稠厚豆渣状或凝乳状特点，量多少不定。瘙痒部位多从小阴唇内侧开始,并蔓延到外阴部,严重者影响工作和睡眠,可伴有外阴灼热痛、尿频、性交痛等。

2)体征:妇科检查见外阴、阴道红肿,小阴唇内侧、阴道壁黏膜上附有一层白色膜状物,附着紧密不易擦除,擦除后露出红肿黏膜,急性期还能见到糜烂及浅表溃疡。

(4)处理原则　改善阴道环境,局部或全身应用抗真菌药物,消除致病诱因。

3. 细菌性阴道病

(1)病因　细菌性阴道病是指阴道内菌群失调(正常菌群减少,厌氧菌群数量增加)所致的一种混合感染。妊娠期患病可导致绒毛膜羊膜炎、胎膜早破、早产;非孕妇女可导致子宫内膜炎、盆腔炎、子宫切除术后阴道残端感染。由于阴道内乳酸杆菌减少,厌氧菌增多,产生胺类物质(尸胺、腐胺、三甲胺),致使阴道分泌物增多并有臭味。阴道菌群紊乱的原因尚不清楚,可能与多个性伴侣、频繁性交或阴道冲洗致阴道环境碱性化有关。

(2)临床表现

1)症状:部分患者无症状,有症状者主要表现为阴道分泌物增多,有鱼腥臭味,尤其性交后加重,可伴有轻度外阴瘙痒或烧灼感。

2)体征:阴道黏膜无充血红肿的炎症表现,可见灰白色、均匀一致、稀薄的分泌物黏附于阴道壁,黏度低,容易将分泌物从阴道壁拭去。

(3)处理原则　酸性溶液冲洗阴道,局部使用或口服抗厌氧菌药物。

4. 萎缩性阴道炎

(1)病因　常见于绝经后妇女,由于卵巢功能衰竭,雌激素水平降低,阴道上皮萎缩,上皮细胞内糖原减少,阴道酸度减弱,阴道的自净作用降低,局部抵抗力下降,致病菌侵入、繁殖引起阴道炎。或者见于因病行盆腔放疗或卵巢切除术后的妇女。

(2)临床表现

1)症状:主要症状为白带增多及外阴瘙痒、灼痛,或伴有尿频、尿痛等。白带为黄色水样、血性及脓性白带。

2)体征:妇科检查可见阴道黏膜呈萎缩性改变,上皮皱褶消失、菲薄,阴道黏膜潮红,有散在的出血斑点,有时见表浅溃疡,严重时溃疡可导致阴道壁粘连、狭窄进而发生阴道积脓、子宫腔积脓。

(3)处理原则　用抗生素抑制细菌生长,适当补充雌激素,增加阴道防御能力。

Trichomonal Vaginitis

• Etiology: The pH of the vagina is usually in the range of 5 – 7. Before menstruation and after menstruation the pH of the vagina changed. The parasite is an anaerobe that has the ability to generate hydrogen to combine with oxygen to create an anaerobic environment. Besides, pregnancy stage and postpartum the pH of the vagina changed also and deduce inflammation.

• Spread modes: There are three transmission modes. Sexual activity is a major route of spread for it. It is a direct contact. Transmission by shared bath facilities, wet towels, or wet swimsuits may also be possible. Nosocomial infections is the third threat to the women.

• Clinical manifestation: Latent period is 4–28 days.

Symptoms: The usual symptoms of trichomoniasis are vaginal pruritus, superficial dyspareunia, frequency, dysuria, and a malodorous, yellow – green, frothy vaginal discharge. Moderate to severe itching is common. Infertility and frequent urine, urgent urine is induced.

Signs：The vaginal mucosa is typically erythematous, and punctate hemorrhages may be present on the cervix.

● Principles of treatment：Cut off the pass of spread. Medical treatment for trichomonas vaginitis consists of metronidazole, 2 g orally in a single dose or 400 mg tid for 7 days. The woman's sexual partner should be treated simultaneously.

Vulvovaginal Candidiasis

● Etiology：Candidiasis albicans is the fungus. Candidiasis is not usually a sexually transmitted disease. Yeast is part of the normal vaginal flora in many women, and symptoms develop only when overgrowth of these organisms occurs. Candida albicans is widely distributed in nature and often found on the skin and mucous membranes. It occurs more frequently in women who are pregnant, have diabetes, and take higher dose estrogen oral contraceptives because of its ability to thrive in well – estrogenized, high-glycogenic vaginal tissue. Women taking systemic antibiotics are more susceptible to Candida due to suppression of normal vaginal flora and changes in pH and enzymes. Stress decreases resistance to Candida vaginitis, as do some hygiene practices, such as douching, using perfumed or medicated sprays and soaps, or wearing nylon underwear. Several conditions predispose to symptomatic moniliasis, including recent antibiotic or corticosteroid therapy, diabetes, use of oral contraceptives, pregnancy, and immunodeficiency states. Serious systemic infections are uncommon unless the patient is receiving hyperalimentation or is immunocompromised.

● Spread modes：Candidal infections may also be present at other body sites, such as the oral cavity or a wet moist area such as the umbilicus.

● Clinical manifestation.

Symptoms：Infected patients usually report vaginal and vulvar pruritus and a cheesy-white, curd-like vaginal discharge. Urine pain, urine frequency and sex intercourse pain are also the main symptoms.

Signs：The vaginal mucosa and vulva may be erythematous and edematous, punctate, erythematous lesions may be present to the lateral aspect of the vulva and medial aspect of the thighs. The vagina sometimes shows white "patches" on the walls that are adherent and cannot be scraped away without bleeding.

● Principles of Treatment.

Eliminate risk factors：Treat diabetes mellitus actively. Do not use estrogen and antibiotic (which destroys normal vaginal flora and lets fungal organisms grow more readily).

Vaginal tablets or creams：For uncomplicated Candida infections, topical therapy for 3–7 d with agents such as miconazole, terconazole, clotrimazole, mycostatin and butoconazole is usually highly effective.

Oral antifungal medications：Persistent or chronic Candida vaginitis may be treated with oral antifungal medications, such as mycostatin, ketoconazole, or fluconazole.

Bacterial Vaginosis

Bacterial vaginosis(BV) is the most common cause of vaginal discharge, but is often without other symptoms. BV occurs subsequent to a significant disruption of "healthy" vaginal microflora (typically Lactobacillus jensenii and Lactobacillus crispatus) by a characteristic set of BV complex microorganisms：Gardnerella vaginalis, genital mycoplasmas (Mycoplasma hominis, Ureaplasma urealyticum) and vaginal anaerobic bacteria, including Prevotella, Bacteroides, and Mobiluncus species.

Classic features of BV discharge include a profuse, milky, nonadherent discharge that demonstrates anamine or fishy odor after alkalization with a drop of KOH (positive whiff test).

The treatment principle is to use anti-anaerobic agents. Metronidazole (400 mg) twice a day for 7 d is the first choice of oral medications. Local application of metronidazole suppositories has similar efficacy, with cure rates about 80%. Partner treatment is generally not recommended.

Atrophic Vaginitis

Atrophic vaginitis is the most common cause of vaginal irritation among climacteric patients. As the term indicates, the atrophy of the vaginal epithelium results in secondary infection. The vulva and introitus quickly become involved because of the associated discharge, and the situation may be exacerbated by a foreign ody (such as a pessary). Patients complain of vulvar irritation and discharge, which may be clear or purulent and yellow but occasionally will be blood tinged. Associated symptoms of frequency, urgency, and stress incontinence may occur.

The treatment of choice is topical estrogen available in vaginal creams, suppositories, or rings. If systemic hormonal treatment is desirable, oral tablets, transdermal patches, sprays, and gels are available. Aerobic cultures for predominant microorganisms should be obtained in refractory cases and when infection is suspected.

【护理评估】

1. 健康史　了解疾病发生与月经周期的关系,是否伴有排尿异常。既往有无阴道炎,治疗的经过及效果。有无糖尿病病史,有无大量使用抗生素或免疫抑制剂的用药史,目前是否妊娠,个人卫生习惯如何。询问患者年龄、是否绝经、发病诱因,有无卵巢手术史或盆腔放疗史。

2. 身心状况　患者常因外阴瘙痒影响生活、工作和睡眠而烦躁,因疾病反复发作而情绪低落、焦虑。

评估患者外阴瘙痒的程度,阴道分泌物的量、颜色、气味等性状,如为血性白带应注意与生殖器官肿瘤进行鉴别。询问是否有其他不适症状,是否有不孕现象。评估阴道黏膜有无充血红肿、出血点、糜烂、溃疡等。评估生殖器官是否呈现老年性改变。

3. 辅助检查

(1)悬滴法　为最常用的辅助检查方法。取阴道分泌物混合于0.9%氯化钠注射液中,在低倍镜下检查,如找到活动的阴道毛滴虫可确诊滴虫性阴道炎;部分滴虫感染者没有表现出症状但实验室检查阳性称为带虫者。取阴道分泌物混合于10%氢氧化钾溶液中,镜下找到白假丝酵母菌的芽孢或者假菌丝均可确诊外阴阴道假丝酵母菌病。

(2)培养法　临床症状可疑而多次悬滴法阴性者,可做培养法,准确率可达98%。

(3)细菌性阴道病的诊断方法　线索细胞阳性、胺臭味试验阳性、阴道分泌物 pH>4.5、鱼腥臭味匀质稀薄白带,其中4项中有3项符合即可诊断细菌性阴道病。

(4)防癌检查　患者有血性分泌物或白带带血时,应行子宫颈刮片细胞学检查或分段诊刮等,以排除生殖器官恶性肿瘤。

【护理诊断】

1. 舒适度的改变　与外阴及阴道口瘙痒、局部灼痛、白带增多有关。

2.皮肤黏膜完整性受损　与炎性分泌物刺激引起黏膜损害、外阴瘙痒致搔抓皮肤有关。

3.睡眠型态紊乱　与外阴瘙痒影响睡眠有关。

4.焦虑　与瘙痒困扰、担心疾病传给配偶和子女或疾病反复发作有关。

【护理措施】

1.一般护理　保持局部清洁,避免交叉感染。勤换内裤,用过的内裤、盆及毛巾均用开水烫洗。

2.观察病情　观察白带的量、性状、有无特殊气味,了解外阴瘙痒程度,是否伴有灼热和疼痛感,有无合并尿路感染。检查局部皮肤有无抓痕、糜烂和溃疡,生殖器官是否萎缩性改变,阴道壁上附着分泌物的特征,有无其他部位(口腔、肠道)白假丝酵母菌的感染。

3.心理护理　解释阴道炎是临床妇科常见的炎症,正规治疗有好的疗效,减轻其思想压力和紧张焦虑的情绪。鼓励患者及配偶积极配合并坚持治疗。

4.用药护理

(1)滴虫性阴道炎　主要药物为甲硝唑或替硝唑。指导患者正确用药,并告知治疗中注意事项和可能发生的药物不良反应。

1)局部用药:先用酸性溶液进行坐浴或阴道冲洗,改善阴道环境,增强局部酸度。教会患者和家属配制药液、阴道灌洗和上药的方法,并介绍注意事项。坐浴或阴道冲洗后,把200 mg甲硝唑塞入阴道深部,1次/d,7~10 d为1个疗程。常用酸性溶液有1%乳酸、0.5%醋酸、1:5 000高锰酸钾。

2)全身用药:患者及配偶有泌尿系、前庭大腺感染者可全身用药。顿服甲硝唑或替硝唑2 g,或甲硝唑400 mg,2次/d,连服7 d。服用甲硝唑可能发生胃肠道反应,如食欲减退、恶心、呕吐,也可引起头痛、皮疹、白细胞减少等,必要时就诊。在应用甲硝唑过程中及停药24 h内,应用替硝唑期间及停药72 h内禁止饮酒。服用甲硝唑者,服药后12~24 h内避免哺乳;服用替硝唑者,服药后72 h内避免哺乳。

(2)外阴阴道假丝酵母菌病

1)局部用药:先用碱性溶液进行坐浴或阴道冲洗,降低局部酸度。1次/d,7~10 d为1个疗程。常用药液为2%~4%的碳酸氢钠。之后选用抗真菌药物(克霉唑栓、咪康唑栓、制霉菌素栓)塞入阴道深部。指导患者正确操作,注意水温不超过40 ℃以免烫伤,掌握药液的配制方法和治疗时间。

2)全身用药:对局部治疗效果差或顽固病例、合并肠道感染者,可口服用药(伊曲康唑、氟康唑、制霉菌素)。嘱患者按时按量服用,及时复查。

3)特殊用药:阴道黏膜有溃疡者,局部涂擦1%甲紫,每周3次,连用2周。注意保护正常阴道组织避免损伤。妊娠合并外阴阴道假丝酵母菌病,应注意药物对胎儿的影响,以局部治疗为主,可重复多个疗程治疗。

(3)细菌性阴道病　遵医嘱应用抗厌氧菌药物,常用甲硝唑、替硝唑、克林霉素,可口服应用,或用酸性溶液冲洗阴道后行局部上药。教会患者和家属配制药液、阴道灌洗和上药的方法,并介绍注意事项。常用酸性溶液有1%乳酸、0.5%醋酸、1:5 000高锰酸钾。

(4)萎缩性阴道炎

1)局部用药:坐浴或阴道冲洗方法同滴虫性阴道炎,擦干后局部应用抗生素及雌激素。如甲硝唑200 mg或诺氟沙星100 mg,己烯雌酚0.25 mg,1次/d,连用7~10 d。

2)全身用药:适当补充雌激素,提高阴道的抵抗力。常用尼尔雌醇首次口服4 mg,以后每2~4周服用1次,2 mg/次,连用2~3个月;也可用雌激素软膏局部涂抹,1~2次/d,14 d为1个疗程。

Nursing Interventions

● General nursing care: The nurse should ask the patient to have enough rest, avoid tiring. Direct the patient intake appropriate nutrition and diet. The patient need drink more water while she has fever. Pay attention to personal hygiene, such as wearing cotton underwear and change it timely. The nurse may direct the woman to take care of her nutrition. The women also need to do pelvic examination timely to prevent the illness recrudesce.

● Observe the state of an illness and recording: The nurse should observe signs, vaginal discharge, reaction of medicine and record.

● Psychological nursing: The woman who contracts inflammations often feels anxious or fearful about the outcome for herself and if pregnant, her fetus. The nurse can be especially helpful in encouraging the woman to explore and discuss her feelings about the diagnosis. A nonjudgmental, accepting attitude and an empathic manner are important.

● Direct drug regimen: The nurse teaches the client to insert creams or tablets at bedtime to maximize the effectiveness of the medication. A minipad can be advised during the day to absorb drainage. Women should not use tampons during treatment because they absorb the medication. Douching should be avoided, and intercourse is preferably stopped.

If treatment includes medications, the nurse stresses the importance of taking medications as directed, completing the course of treatment, and following other directions, such as refraining from alcohol or dairy products when taking certain medications. The nurse can facilitate compliance with medication regimens by reviewing expected minor side effects, such as diarrhea and gastric upset, and advising remedies to ease these. Women must be clearly informed of potential allergic reactions, such as hives and respiratory distress. Contacting and treatment of sexual partners are important adjuncts to treatment.

【健康教育】

①加强自身保健意识,避免性行为不洁和紊乱;积极治疗糖尿病,合理使用抗生素、糖皮质激素及雌激素。不用肥皂等刺激性物品清洗外阴,避免搔抓外阴部。治疗期间禁止无保护性性交,所用盆具、毛巾和更换的内裤每日煮沸消毒5～10 min,避免交叉感染。②萎缩性阴道炎应用雌激素治疗须谨慎,在排除与雌激素有关的肿瘤后遵医嘱用药。③滴虫性阴道炎易在月经后复发,若连续3个月在月经后复查白带,均为阴性说明治愈。④外阴阴道假丝酵母菌病易在月经前复发,其治愈标准为连续3个月在月经前复查白带,均为阴性说明治愈。

任务实施

阴道灌洗具有清洁、收敛与热疗的作用,能促进阴道血液循环、减少阴道分泌物、缓解局部充血、控制和治疗炎症。阴道灌洗适用于各种阴道炎、子宫颈炎的治疗,经腹子宫全切术或阴道手术的术前准备,腔内放疗后常规清洁冲洗等(图12-3)。

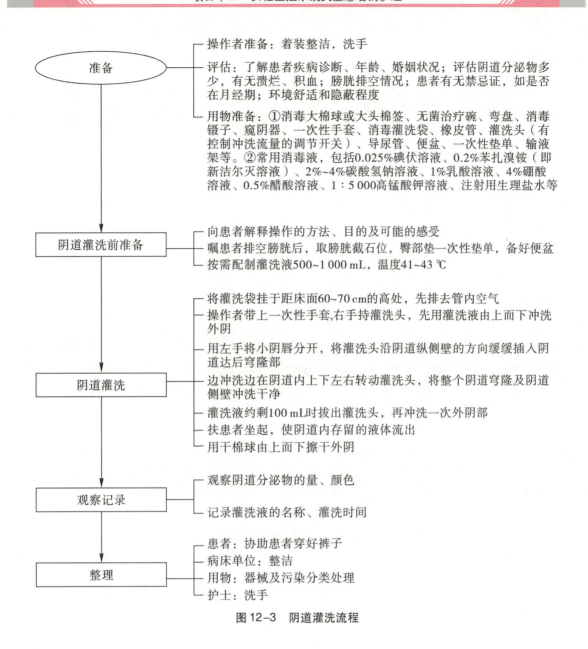

图12-3　阴道灌洗流程

流程图文字内容：

准备
- 操作者准备：着装整洁，洗手
- 评估：了解患者疾病诊断、年龄、婚姻状况；评估阴道分泌物多少，有无溃烂、积血；膀胱排空情况；患者有无禁忌证，如是否在月经期；环境舒适和隐蔽程度
- 用物准备：①消毒大棉球或大头棉签、无菌治疗碗、弯盘、消毒镊子、窥阴器、一次性手套、消毒灌洗袋、橡皮管、灌洗头（有控制冲洗流量的调节开关）、导尿管、便盆、一次性垫单、输液架等。②常用消毒液，包括0.025%碘伏溶液、0.2%苯扎溴铵（即新洁尔灭溶液）、2%~4%碳酸氢钠溶液、1%乳酸溶液、4%硼酸溶液、0.5%醋酸溶液、1：5 000高锰酸钾溶液、注射用生理盐水等

阴道灌洗前准备
- 向患者解释操作的方法、目的及可能的感受
- 嘱患者排空膀胱后，取膀胱截石位，臀部垫一次性垫单，备好便盆
- 按需配制灌洗液500~1 000 mL，温度41~43 ℃

阴道灌洗
- 将灌洗袋挂于距床面60~70 cm的高处，先排去管内空气
- 操作者带上一次性手套，右手持灌洗头，先用灌洗液由上而下冲洗外阴
- 用左手将小阴唇分开，将灌洗头沿阴道纵侧壁的方向缓缓插入阴道达后穹隆部
- 边冲洗边在阴道内上下左右转动灌洗头，将整个阴道穹隆及阴道侧壁冲洗干净
- 灌洗液约剩100 mL时拔出灌洗头，再冲洗一次外阴部
- 扶患者坐起，使阴道内存留的液体流出
- 用干棉球由上而下擦干外阴

观察记录
- 观察阴道分泌物的量、颜色
- 记录灌洗液的名称、灌洗时间

整理
- 患者：协助患者穿好裤子
- 病床单位：整洁
- 用物：器械及污染分类处理
- 护士：洗手

任务三　子宫颈炎（Cervicitis）

工作情景

患者，31岁，主诉"腰骶部疼痛，伴白带增多20余天"。20余天前曾行清宫术，术后感觉分泌物增多并伴有腰酸、腹部下坠感，以为是术后正常反应未就医诊治。近几天感觉阴道分泌物明显增多，腰骶部不适加重，即来院检查。查体：子宫颈充血、水肿，子宫颈口可见脓性分泌物流出。

①请明确该患者主要的护理问题。②根据目前的情况对患者进行正确的护理。

任务内容

子宫颈炎是育龄期妇女常见的妇科疾病，有急性和慢性两种。急性子宫颈炎常见的是急性子宫颈管黏膜炎，若急性炎症得不到及时治疗或病原体持续存在，可导致慢性子宫颈炎。慢性子宫颈炎是指子宫颈间质内有大量淋巴细胞、浆细胞等慢性炎症细胞浸润，可伴有子宫颈腺上皮及间质的增生和鳞状上皮化生。

任务目标

◆ 能叙述子宫颈炎的病因、临床表现及处理原则。
◆ 能对急、慢性子宫颈炎正确评估和护理。

【概要】

1. 急性子宫颈炎

（1）病因　多与子宫颈局部损伤有关，如分娩、清宫术后、人工流产术后及子宫颈手术扩张子宫颈时损伤，使病原体侵入而发生感染。病原体包括性传播疾病病原体（如淋病奈瑟球菌、沙眼衣原体等）及内源性病原体，部分患者病原体不明。内源性病原体与持续阴道菌群异常、细菌性阴道病、支原体感染、阴道灌洗等有关。

（2）临床表现　阴道分泌物增多、性交后出血、经间期出血等，可伴外阴瘙痒、灼热感，或尿急、尿频、尿痛等症状。妇科检查见子宫颈充血、水肿，有时可见黏液脓性分泌物从子、宫颈管流出。淋病奈瑟球菌感染者除上述表现外，还可见尿道口、阴道口黏膜充血、水肿及多量脓性分泌物。

（3）处理原则　治疗以抗生素为主，遵循及时、足量、规范、彻底、有效的原则。

2. 慢性子宫颈炎

（1）病因　可由急性子宫颈炎迁延而来，也可见于各种物理、化学因素的影响，或病原体持续感染所致，病原体与急性子宫颈炎相似。

（2）病理

1）慢性宫颈管黏膜炎：子宫颈管黏膜皱襞较多，感染后容易形成持续性宫颈管黏膜炎，以反复发作的子宫颈黏液及脓性分泌物增多为主要表现。

2）子宫颈柱状上皮异位：子宫颈柱状上皮异位会使子宫颈外口表现出糜烂样的红色改变，子宫颈上皮内瘤变、早期子宫颈癌也会呈现出糜烂样改变，需对患者进行相关检查进行鉴别。

3）子宫颈息肉：由于炎症长期刺激，子宫颈管黏膜局限性增生，并突出于子宫颈口外，形成息肉（图12-4）。息肉呈舌状，有细蒂与子宫颈相连，单一或多发性，鲜红色，质脆，易出血。摘除息肉后如炎症未消除，仍易复发，极少恶变。

4）子宫颈肥大：因慢性炎症的长期刺激，子宫颈组织充血、水肿，腺体与间质增生，使子宫颈体积肥大，质地变硬，但表面光滑。

（3）临床表现　慢性子宫颈炎症多无症状。部分患者出现白带增多，多为乳白色黏液样，也可呈淡黄色、脓性或血性，可有外阴瘙痒或不适。一些患者有下腹部坠胀、腰骶部酸痛，尤其

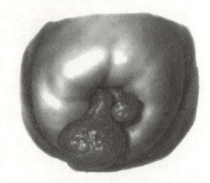

图12-4　子宫颈息肉

在月经前和性生活时明显。妇科检查可发现子宫颈呈糜烂样改变,或子宫颈肥大、息肉,或有分泌物从子宫颈口流出等征象。

(4)处理原则　慢性子宫颈炎以局部治疗为主,不同的病变类型采用不同的治疗方法。

Chronic Cervicitis

● Etiology：Cervicitis is caused by a variety of agents：infectious organisms, scraping of cells for diagnostic tests, cryosurgery, use of vaginal tampons or medications, childbirth, postmenopausally decreased estrogen levels, and use of oral contraceptives.

● Clinical manifestation.

Symptoms：The main symptom is visible mucopurulent discharge flow from endocervix. If the causative agent is an infection, the infection may ascend through the reproductive trace and cause pelvic inflammatory disease. Pelvic pain and infertility are the symptoms of the diffused infection.

Signs：On inspection via a speculum, the cervix appears swollen and reddened, bleeding may be precipitated by gentle touch alone.

● Principles of treatment.

Treatment depends on the causative agent（s）：Infections are treatment by systemic or topical medications appropriate to the identified organisms.

Physical treatment：Laser treatment is the use in common to cure cervicitis.

Medication treatment：Chinese tradition medication is efficient to cervicitis.

Operation：Treatment extirpate polypus or cervical taper excision could be taken to treat cervicitis.

【护理评估】

1. 健康史　评估有无致病因素存在。了解患者婚育史、阴道分娩史,有无子宫颈损伤史、妇科手术史、流产后感染、产褥感染病史,个人卫生习惯如何。

2. 身心状况　患者常因性交后出血或发现血性白带怀疑恶变,而表现出紧张甚至恐惧心理。了解患者是否不孕,有无下腹部及腰骶部疼痛不适、接触性出血,白带的性状。尿道口、子宫颈有无充血、红肿表现。评估患者慢性子宫颈炎的病理类型。

3. 辅助检查

(1)急性子宫颈炎

1)阴道分泌物涂片:白细胞>10/高倍视野(排除阴道炎引起的白细胞增多)。

2)子宫颈管脓性分泌物检查:中性粒细胞>30/高倍视野。

3)病原体检测:行淋病奈瑟球菌培养诊断淋病、核酸检测诊断沙眼衣原体。

(2)慢性子宫颈炎　子宫颈刮片细胞学检查可鉴别炎症与肿瘤。目前多选用子宫颈液基薄层细胞检查(TCT),可早期发现子宫颈癌细胞,还能检测微生物如假丝酵母菌、滴虫、病毒、衣原体等。必要时采用子宫颈活组织检查,进一步明确诊断。

【护理诊断】

1. 舒适度的改变　与炎性分泌物多引起局部瘙痒、灼痛,或炎症刺激引起腰骶部酸痛、下腹坠痛等有关。

2. 组织完整性受损　与子宫颈慢性炎症和分泌物刺激导致子宫颈柱状上皮异位及鳞状上皮脱落有关。

3. 焦虑　与担心治疗效果不佳或担心子宫颈炎癌变有关。

【护理措施】

1. 一般护理　保持外阴部清洁、干燥,减少局部刺激。

2. 心理护理　解释慢性子宫颈炎与子宫颈癌虽有关联性但不是必然会癌变,消除患者的恐癌心理,能积极配合治疗。

3. 急性子宫颈炎治疗护理　遵医嘱及时、足量、规范应用抗生素。

(1)经验性抗生素治疗　未获得病原体检测结果之前,常用阿奇霉素 1 g 单次顿服,或多西环素 100 mg 口服,2 次/d,连用 7 d。

(2)针对病原体的抗生素治疗　对于检测出病原体的,选择针对性治疗。

1)急性淋病奈瑟球菌性子宫颈炎:多采取大剂量单次给药。常用头孢菌素类药物,如头孢曲松钠 250 mg,单次肌内注射;头孢克肟 400 mg,单次口服;或头孢唑肟 500 mg,肌内注射等;或应用氨基糖苷类的大观霉素 4 g,单次肌内注射。

2)沙眼衣原体感染所致子宫颈炎:常用四环素类、红霉素类、喹诺酮类药物进行治疗,如多西环素 100 mg,2 次/d,连服 7 d;红霉素 500 mg,4 次/d,连服 7 d;氧氟沙星 300 mg,2 次/d,连服 7 d。

(3)合并症治疗　合并细菌性阴道病者应同时治疗,避免子宫颈炎持续存在。

4. 慢性子宫颈炎治疗护理

(1)慢性子宫颈管黏膜炎　需了解有无沙眼衣原体及淋病奈瑟球菌感染,有无细菌性阴道病及其性伴侣治疗情况,针对病因给予治疗。病原体不清者,可试行物理治疗。

(2)子宫颈柱状上皮异位　无症状的生理性柱状上皮异位无须治疗。有炎症表现的"糜烂样"改变,如分泌物增多或接触性出血等,可给予局部物理治疗,包括激光、冷冻、微波等,治疗前需常规行子宫颈细胞学检查,排除子宫颈上皮内瘤变和子宫颈癌。

子宫颈柱状上皮异位的物理治疗常用方法有激光、冷冻、红外线凝结及微波等,其治疗原理是使病变处的柱状上皮坏死、脱落,生长出新的鳞状上皮。接受物理治疗者,术前应常规做子宫颈刮片细胞学检查,排除宫颈癌方可进行治疗。手术时间安排在月经干净后 3~7 d 内进行。

物理治疗后阴道分泌物增多,甚至有大量黄水样白带流出,术后 1~2 周脱痂时可有少量出血,若出血多需及时就诊处理。创口愈合需 4~8 周。术后嘱患者保持外阴清洁、干燥,勤换会阴垫,每日 2 次清洗外阴,术后 2 个月内禁止盆浴、阴道冲洗和性生活。2 次月经干净后复查,治疗效果欠佳者可行第 2 次治疗。

(3)子宫颈息肉　应摘除息肉并送病理组织学检查。

(4)子宫颈肥大　一般无须治疗。

Nursing Points

- Post-operational care:Keep the vulva clean after operation twice a day. Sexual intercourse and tubbing are forbidden.

- Illness prevention:Avoid cervix trauma during delivery. Surgical repair trauma timely after delivery is important.

【健康教育】

①定期进行妇科普查,发现子宫颈炎及时治疗。②注意个人卫生,特别是经期、妊娠期、产褥期卫生,避免发生感染。③避免不安全或不洁性行为,由淋病奈瑟球菌及沙眼衣原体引起的子宫颈炎患者,其性伴侣应同时进行检查及治疗。④物理治疗后注意观察阴道流液的性状,如有流血、臭味等及时来院检查。

任务实施 //

　　阴道或子宫颈上药是将治疗性药物涂抹到阴道壁或子宫颈黏膜上,达到局部治疗的作用,适用于各种阴道炎、子宫颈炎及术后阴道残端炎症的治疗。由于阴道或子宫颈上药操作简单,既可在医院由护士操作,也可教会患者在家进行局部上药(表12-2)。

表12-2　阴道或子宫颈上药操作步骤

项目	内容
操作前准备	1.用物准备:阴道灌洗用物1套,阴道扩张器1个,无菌长镊2把,带尾线的大棉球,消毒长棉签,橡胶单和治疗巾或一次性垫单,一次性手套等。药品:①阴道后穹隆塞药,常用甲硝唑、制霉菌素等药片、丸剂或栓剂;②局部非腐蚀性药物上药,常用1%甲紫、大蒜液、新霉素或氯霉素等;③局部腐蚀性药物上药,常用20%~50%硝酸银溶液、20%或100%铬酸溶液;④子宫颈棉球上药,有止血药、消炎止血粉或抗生素等;⑤喷雾器上药,常用土霉素、磺胺嘧啶、呋喃西林、己烯雌酚等
	2.环境准备:温暖,隐蔽性好,必要时用屏风遮挡
	3.患者准备:排空膀胱,脱下近侧裤腿
	4.护生准备:衣帽整洁,修剪指甲,洗手,戴口罩
操作步骤	1.核对、解释:核对患者,做到准确无误;向患者说明阴道或子宫颈上药的目的及方法,可能出现的不适,以取得患者的配合
	2.安置体位:屏风遮挡,协助患者取膀胱截石位,充分暴露会阴部
	3.阴道灌洗:上药前先阴道灌洗,再用阴道扩张器暴露子宫颈,用消毒干棉球拭去子宫颈黏液或炎性分泌物
	4.上药:根据病情和药物的不同剂型选用不同的上药方法 (1)阴道后穹隆塞药:常用于治疗各种阴道炎及慢性子宫颈炎等。用阴道扩张器暴露子宫颈,用长镊子夹取药片放置于阴道后穹隆部。取下阴道扩张器、镊子,避免药栓移位。也可指导患者自行放置,于临睡前戴指套,用一手示指将药片或栓剂向阴道后壁推进直至示指完全伸入。为保证药物疗效,宜睡前用药 (2)局部腐蚀性药物上药:用于治疗慢性子宫颈炎颗粒增生型患者。上药前先将纱布或干纱球垫于阴道后壁及阴道后穹隆,预防药液下流灼伤正常组织。用长棉签蘸药液(如20%铬酸溶液)涂于子宫颈糜烂面,使局部呈黄褐色,顺序为先涂抹子宫颈上唇,再涂抹子宫颈下唇,然后涂抹子宫颈内口,再插入子宫颈管内约0.5 cm,保留约1 min,最后用干棉球吸干残留药液。每周1次,2~4次为1个疗程 (3)局部非腐蚀性药物上药:用于治疗阴道假丝酵母菌病及亚急性或急性子宫颈炎患者。用棉球或长棉签蘸药液涂擦阴道壁或子宫颈,注意旋转阴道扩张器,使药物均匀分布 (4)子宫颈棉球上药:适用于伴有出血者。用阴道扩张器充分暴露子宫颈,用长镊子夹持带尾线的子宫颈棉球浸蘸药液后塞至子宫颈处,同时将阴道扩张器轻轻退出阴道,取出镊子,防止棉球被带出或移位,将线露于阴道口外,并用胶布固定于阴阜侧上方。嘱患者于放药12~24 h后牵引棉球尾线自行取出 (5)喷雾器上药:适用于非特异性阴道炎及萎缩性阴道炎患者。将药粉放置于喷雾器内,对准患处,挤压喷雾器,使药粉均匀散布于炎性组织表面上

续表 12-2

项目	内容
操作后处理	1.撤去橡胶单及一次性垫单,协助患者整理衣裤,下妇科检查床
	2.整理用物,处理污物
	3.洗手,记录
注意事项	1.上腐蚀性药物时,注意保护阴道壁及周围正常组织;上非腐蚀性药物时,应转动阴道扩张器,使阴道四壁均能涂布药物
	2.阴道栓剂或片剂最好在晚间临睡前上药,以免脱出,影响治疗效果
	3.用药期间禁止性生活
	4.经期或子宫出血者不宜阴道上药
	5.无性生活史者上药时禁止使用阴道扩张器,可用长棉签涂抹或用手指将药片轻轻推入阴道
	6.上药完毕,切记嘱患者按时取出阴道内的棉球或纱布

任务四　盆腔炎性疾病(Pelvic Inflammatory Disease)

工作情景

患者,32 岁,G_3P_1。以白带增多、下腹坠感伴腰骶部酸痛半年为主诉就诊。1 年前曾行人工流产术,近半年来经量增多,经期腹痛、腰骶部酸痛明显。查体:发育营养中等,一般情况良好,心肺无异常,腹软,肝脾未触及。妇科检查:外阴已产型,阴道通畅,有少量分泌物,子宫颈表面光滑,子宫后位,大小正常,活动稍受限,双附件区增粗变厚呈条索状,质地较硬,有压痛。

①请明确该患者主要的护理问题。②根据目前的情况对患者进行正确的护理。

任务内容

盆腔炎性疾病(简称盆腔炎)是指女性上生殖道及其周围组织的炎症,包括子宫内膜炎、输卵管炎、输卵管卵巢炎、输卵管卵巢脓肿、盆腔腹膜炎。多发生在性活跃期的妇女。病变可局限于一个部位,也可同时累及几个部位,最常见的是输卵管炎、输卵管卵巢炎。急性盆腔炎若未能得到及时治愈,可迁延形成慢性盆腔炎,导致不孕、输卵管妊娠、慢性盆腔痛。慢性盆腔炎病程长,顽固难愈,机体抵抗力下降时反复发作,严重影响患者的身心健康。

任务目标

◆ 能叙述盆腔炎的病因、临床表现及处理原则。

◆ 能对急、慢性盆腔炎正确评估和护理。

【概要】

1. 急性盆腔炎

（1）病因　女性生殖系统在解剖和生理上具有自然的防御功能，但由于阴道口与尿道、肛门毗邻，女性内生殖器官又与外界直接相通，病原体容易入侵；女性在特殊生理时期如月经期、妊娠期、分娩期和产褥期，生殖系统的防御功能受到破坏，机体免疫力下降，容易发生感染。

1）感染来源：①内源性感染。各种原因引起阴道内正常菌群的生态平衡被破坏（如体内雌激素水平低、频繁性交、阴道灌洗、长期应用广谱抗生素等），或机体抵抗力低下使致病菌大量繁殖引起炎症。②外源性感染。病原体通过检查器械、手术操作、盆浴等途径进入生殖系统导致炎症，如流产或分娩后感染、宫腔手术无菌操作不严、经期及性卫生不良等。

2）感染途径：①沿黏膜上行性蔓延。常见于葡萄球菌、淋病奈瑟球菌、衣原体等感染。②淋巴系统传播。这是产褥感染、流产后感染的主要途径，多见于链球菌、葡萄球菌等。③血液循环传播。这是结核分枝杆菌的主要传播途径。④直接蔓延。邻近器官炎症直接蔓延到内生殖器，如阑尾炎时感染可蔓延至右侧子宫附件区引起炎症、肠结核可蔓延到盆腔等。

（2）病理

1）急性子宫内膜炎及子宫肌炎：子宫内膜充血、水肿，有炎性渗出物，炎症侵及子宫肌层则形成子宫肌炎。

2）急性输卵管炎、输卵管积脓、输卵管卵巢脓肿：输卵管充血、肿胀、增粗、弯曲，黏膜粘连可使管腔及伞端闭锁，若有脓液积聚则形成输卵管积脓。卵巢与输卵管伞端发生粘连可形成卵巢周围炎，若形成卵巢脓肿，脓肿壁可与输卵管积脓粘连并贯通，形成输卵管卵巢脓肿。

3）急性盆腔结缔组织炎：常见宫旁结缔组织炎，局部充血、增厚或形成肿块，以后向盆壁两侧浸润，若组织化脓形成盆腔腹膜外脓肿，可自发破入直肠或阴道。

4）急性盆腔腹膜炎：严重感染者容易蔓延至盆腔腹膜，引起盆腔腹膜炎，导致盆腔脏器粘连；脓性渗出液积聚可形成盆腔脓肿，若脓肿破溃脓液流入腹腔引起弥漫性腹膜炎。

5）败血症及脓毒血症：当抵抗力降低而病原体毒力强、数量多时，可形成败血症危及生命。若患者身体其他部位发现多处炎症病灶或脓肿，应考虑有脓毒血症。

6）肝周围炎：肝周围炎是指无肝实质损害的肝包膜炎症。5%～10%输卵管炎可出现肝周围炎，与淋病奈瑟球菌及衣原体感染有关。

（3）临床表现

1）症状：主要症状为下腹痛，于活动、月经期或性交后加重，并向双侧大腿放射。阴道分泌物增多，呈黄白色或脓性，偶有恶臭味。轻者无症状或症状轻微，严重者可出现发热甚至高热、寒战、头痛、食欲减退症状。如有输卵管炎的症状及体征，并同时有右上腹疼痛者，应怀疑有肝周围炎。

2）体征：轻者无明显异常，或妇科检查仅有子宫颈举痛或宫体压痛或附件区压痛。重者则呈急性病容，体温升高，心率加快，腹膜炎征象明显。妇科检查因病理不同则征象不同：急性子宫内膜炎及子宫肌炎者，可见阴道有脓性臭味分泌物，或子宫颈充血、水肿，有脓性分泌物从子宫颈口流出，阴道穹隆触痛明显，子宫颈举痛，子宫体稍大、有压痛、活动受限；急性输卵管炎者，可触及输卵管增粗，压痛明显；输卵管积脓或输卵管卵巢脓肿者，附件区可触及压痛明显的不活动包块；位置较低的盆腔脓肿，可在阴道后穹隆或侧穹隆扪及有波动感肿块；急性盆腔结缔组织炎者，患侧可触及片状增厚，或子宫骶韧带增粗、压痛明显。

（4）处理原则　抗生素治疗为主，遵循经验性、广谱、及时、个体化的治疗原则，必要时手术治疗。

2.慢性盆腔炎

(1)病因 常因急性盆腔炎未能及时治疗或治疗不彻底或患者体质较弱、病程迁延而致,但也有无急性感染史者,如沙眼衣原体感染引起的输卵管炎。

(2)病理

1)慢性子宫内膜炎:发生于流产后、产后或剖宫产后,也可见绝经后的老年妇女。子宫内膜充血、水肿,间质有大量淋巴细胞或浆细胞浸润。

2)慢性输卵管炎与输卵管积水:慢性输卵管炎最常见,多为双侧性,呈轻度或中度肿大。若炎症使输卵管峡部及伞端粘连闭锁,浆液性渗出物积聚于管腔而形成输卵管积水,其表面光滑,管壁薄,形状如腊肠。

3)输卵管卵巢炎及输卵管卵巢囊肿:如果输卵管炎症波及卵巢,甚至伞端与卵巢粘连贯通,可形成输卵管卵巢炎或输卵管卵巢囊肿。

4)慢性盆腔结缔组织炎:多见于慢性子宫颈炎蔓延而致。炎症蔓延至子宫旁结缔组织及子宫骶韧带,导致纤维组织增生、变硬,子宫与周围组织粘连、活动度下降。病情严重者,子宫颈旁组织增厚变硬、向外呈扇形扩散直达骨盆壁,子宫固定,形成"冰冻骨盆"。

(3)临床表现

1)症状:①慢性盆腔痛。约20%急性盆腔炎发作后遗留慢性盆腔痛。慢性盆腔痛常发生在盆腔炎急性发作后的4~8周。患者表现为下腹部坠胀、疼痛及腰骶部酸痛,常在劳累、性交后及月经前后加剧。②不孕。输卵管粘连阻塞可致不孕,发生率为20%~30%。③异位妊娠。盆腔炎后异位妊娠发生率是正常妇女的8~10倍。④盆腔炎反复发作。盆腔炎造成的输卵管组织结构的破坏,局部防御功能减退,若患者仍处于同样的高危因素,可造成再次感染导致盆腔炎反复发作。

2)体征:子宫内膜炎常使子宫增大、压痛;若是输卵管炎,在一侧或两侧子宫附件区可触摸到增粗的条索状管状物,有压痛;如为输卵管积水或输卵管卵巢囊肿,常触及腊肠样囊性肿物,活动受限;盆腔结缔组织炎时,子宫常呈后位,活动受限,子宫一侧或两侧区域及宫骶韧带增生变厚、压痛。

(4)处理原则 根据不同情况选择治疗方案,如急性发作时可选用抗菌药治疗;不孕者多需要辅助生育技术协助受孕;慢性期多采取中西医结合的综合治疗;输卵管积水或形成囊肿者需行手术治疗。

【护理评估】

1.健康史 了解患者有无宫腔手术操作史,经期、流产及产后卫生习惯;有无急性盆腔炎病史,治疗方法及效果;询问此次发病的诱因,以前有无类似情况、治疗经过,平素身体健康状况等。

2.身心状况 由于病程长、反复发作甚至不孕,影响患者的正常生活,常表现出烦躁、焦虑等。了解患者的精神状态、睡眠状况,下腹部及腰骶部疼痛的性质、程度,是否在月经期、劳累和性交后加重,阴道分泌物是否增多,有无发热等全身症状,月经是否正常,是否不孕。评估病变部位及程度。子宫颈是否充血,有无脓性分泌物从子宫颈口流出,阴道后穹隆是否触痛,能否触到有波动感肿块,有无子宫颈举痛;了解子宫的位置、活动度,有无增大、压痛;附件区是否触及压痛明显的包块,或触到增粗的条索状或腊肠状物,子宫一侧或两侧区域有无片状增生、变厚及压痛。

3.辅助检查 子宫颈管分泌物及阴道后穹隆穿刺液涂片、培养及核酸扩增检测病原体,为急性盆腔炎患者选择抗生素提供依据。B型超声、腹腔镜检查可了解子宫、附件及盆腔病变情况。

【护理诊断】

1.体温过高 与急性盆腔炎有关。

2.急性疼痛 与生殖系统急性感染有关。

3.慢性疼痛　与慢性盆腔炎引起的增生、粘连有关。

4.睡眠型态紊乱　与长期心理压力有关。

5.焦虑　与病程长、疗效不佳或不孕有关。

【护理措施】

1.一般护理　注意休息,疼痛时可采取按摩、热敷局部缓解症状。睡眠不佳者,在睡前用热水泡脚,保持室内安静,必要时适当服用镇静药物。体温过高者及时给予物理降温,必要时采取药物降温。

2.病情观察　观察患者精神、营养状态,了解腹痛程度,白带性状和量,月经正常与否,有无焦虑、烦躁、失眠等。

3.心理护理　解释盆腔炎的病因、发展过程和治疗特点,鼓励患者增强信心,坚持按疗程治疗。

4.治疗护理

(1)急性盆腔炎　半卧位休息,加强会阴部护理。遵医嘱应用抗生素,观察药物的不良反应。盆腔脓肿形成者应切开引流,注意脓液的量及性状。

(2)慢性盆腔炎

1)局部物理治疗的护理:物理治疗可改善盆腔血液循环,提高新陈代谢,有利于炎症的吸收和消退,常用方法有红外线、短波、超短波、蜡疗、离子透入、激光等,或用食盐炒热放袋中热敷下腹部。注意观察患者有无不适反应。

2)中药治疗的护理:多用具有清热利湿、活血化瘀的中药。遵医嘱帮助患者不同途径用药,可服用、腹部外敷或保留灌肠。中药灌肠者嘱患者灌肠后俯卧休息 30 min 以上。

3)其他药物治疗的护理:除急性发作外,一般不用抗生素。应用抗生素时,可同时使用 α 糜蛋白酶 5 mg 或透明质酸酶 1 500 U 肌内注射,隔日 1 次,5~10 次为 1 个疗程,也可同用地塞米松,利于炎症和粘连的吸收。嘱患者坚持按时用药,注意 α 糜蛋白酶在应用之前须先做皮试。

4)手术治疗的护理:适于输卵管积水、输卵管卵巢囊肿等盆腔包块,做好术前准备和术后护理工作。

【健康教育】

①养成良好卫生习惯,注意经期卫生和性生活卫生,减少感染概率。选择适宜的运动方式增强体质。②采取有效的避孕措施,流产、放置或取出宫内节育器、分娩等到正规医院。③有下生殖道炎症时,应及时就诊治疗,避免感染扩散。

Clinical Manifestation

● Symptoms：Women with symptomatic PID commonly have lower abdominal pain and tenderness (especially when walking or during coitus), abnormal vaginal discharge, chills, and fever. Less common symptoms include irregular vaginal bleeding, dysuria, nausea, and vomiting. No specific combination of symptoms is consistently associated with PID. Some women are asymptomatic.

● Signs：Clinical signs in women with laparoscopically confirmed PID most frequently include lower abdominal tenderness, with or without rebound tenderness; uterine and adnexal tenderness to palpation and motion; and findings of mucopurulent cervicitis. Fever is the least common finding. A pregnancy test should be performed when symptoms or signs of pregnancy are present.

Complications

The sequelae of PID are much more common, morbid, and costly than previously recognized. A previous study indicates women with clinical PID were 6 times more likely to have an ectopic pregnancy and 14 times more likely to have tubal factor infertility than women without PID. Women with a history of PID were 6 – 10 times more likely than healthy controls to have the diagnosis of endometritis, suffer from chronic pelvic pain, or require a hysterectomy. Women with prior salpingitis are at increased risk for premature labor. Fitz−Hugh−Curtis syndrome is a rare complication of PID characterized by perihepatic inflammation. The most common symptom is an acute onset of right upper abdominal pain aggravated by inhaling. There are also unique "violin−string" adhesions between the liver and the abdominal wall in the late stage.

Treament

The rapeutic goals for treating PID are elimination of reproductive tract infection and inflammation, improvement of symptoms and physical findings, prevention or minimization of long−term sequelae, and eradication of causal agents from the patient and her sexual partner. Empiric antibiotic regimens should be aimed at treating likely causative agents, that is, N. gonorrhoeae, C. trachomatis, genital mycoplasmas, and BV−associated endogenous microflora. The latter include anaerobic (Bacteroides and Prevotella species and anaerobic streptococci) as well as aerobic organisms (G. vaginalis, E. coli, and facultative streptococci).

The need for hospitalization is an important treatment decision. Women with severe infections or an inability to take and absorb oral antibiotics (nausea, vomiting, possible peritonitis, and ileus) should be hospitalized and treated until clinical improvement is evident. Similarly, women with a questionable diagnosis, pregnancy, or unreliability, should be admitted initially and treated with parenteral agents to ensure compliance and treatment efficacy, as should those who fail to respond to outpatient therapy. In the face of clinical deterioration or the absence of obvious clinical improvement after 48 – 72 h of antibiotic treatment for TOAs or pelvic abscesses, other modalities should be used. Aspiration using vaginal, abdominal, or rectal ultrasonic guidance should be considered initially. When uterine and ovarian preservation is agoal, drainage of the abscess, possibly combined with salpingectomy, may be required. Total abdominal hysterectomy and bilateral salpingo−oophorectomy may be necessary in refractory cases, usually by a laparotomy.

Outpatient treatments may be selected for most women, who will return promptly if no improvement is seen within 24−48 h and who are likely to be compliant. Direct observation of initial oral treatment is preferred.

Patients should be reevaluated 3−4 weeks after treatment. Pelvic examination should be done at that time to ensure adequacy of treatment. Counseling regarding preventative strategies for STIs and HIV infection, as well as contraceptive advice, should be repeated at the follow−up visit.

微课

课件

练习题及参考答案

（王珏辉）

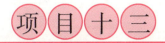

项目十三

妇产科手术患者的护理（Nursing of Obstetrics and Gynecology Surgery Patients）

项目描述

　　妇产科手术是妇产科疾病特别的、主要的治疗手段之一。妇产科手术按手术途径可分为腹部手术和外阴阴道手术两种。手术本身既是治疗的过程，又是创伤的过程。要保证手术顺利进行，患者术后如期康复，必须做好充分的术前准备和精心的术后护理。

　　Obstetrics and gynecology operation is one of the special and main therapeutic means for gynecological diseases. Obstetrics and gynecology surgery according to the surgical route can be divided into abdominal surgery and vulvovaginal surgery two kinds. The operation itself is both a healing process and a traumatic process. In order to ensure the smooth operation, the patient postoperative rehabilitation as scheduled, we must do a good job of preoperative preparation and careful postoperative nursing.

任务一　腹部手术（Abdominal Surgery）

工作情景

　　王女士，43岁，已有2个孩子，近半年不明原因出现月经过多。原来经期每次用一包半卫生巾，现在需要2包，在门诊行B型超声检查发现子宫肌瘤近拳头大小，医生建议入院手术治疗。明天患者将经腹行子宫全切术，因担心手术效果患者非常焦虑，心情沉重而哭泣。

　　①如何对王女士进行心理护理？②如何为王女士进行正确的术前准备？

任务内容

　　妇科腹部手术按手术范围区分主要有剖腹探查术、附件切除术、子宫次全切除术或子宫全切术、子宫及附件次全切除术、子宫及附件全切除术、子宫根治术、肿瘤细胞减灭术等；按手术急缓程度又分为择期手术、限期手术和急诊手术3种。

任务目标

◆ 能叙述妇科腹部手术前、后患者的护理措施。
◆ 能运用护理程序为妇科腹部手术前、后患者进行护理评估、护理诊断。

一 腹部手术的术前准备及护理配合

【护理评估】

1.健康史　了解患者的一般情况、月经史、性生活史、婚育史、既往病史、手术史、过敏史、饮食及生活习惯。

2.身体评估

（1）症状　根据疾病种类、疾病部位、疾病的发展评估患者出现的症状。如子宫肌瘤可有月经过多、下腹部包块、继发性贫血等症状,卵巢肿瘤可有包块、压迫症状等。

（2）体征　评估患者的生命体征,一般情况,心、肺、肝、脾、肾等重要器官的功能,检查子宫及子宫附件情况,评估子宫颈有无肥大、子宫有无结节、附件区有无包块等改变。

3.辅助检查　术前应行血、尿、便三大常规,血型鉴定及交叉配血试验,B型超声,心电图,胸部X射线片,肝肾功能,血生化检查等检查,了解患者有无贫血及各重要脏器如心、肺、肝、肾、脑等的功能状态,以判断患者术前身体状况和对手术的耐受力。

4.心理-社会支持状况　由于患者对生殖器官和疾病的认识不足,常常会担心手术引起疼痛,恐惧疾病的性质和手术对生命的威胁,想了解手术的过程、效果,担心切除子宫后会失去女性特征、影响夫妻关系,担心术后并发症等,从而产生焦虑、恐惧、紧张、悲观等各种不良的心理状态,并因此而影响患者术后的康复。

【护理诊断】

1.焦虑　与担心手术是否顺利及手术预后有关。

2.知识缺乏　缺乏疾病有关知识及手术配合知识。

【护理措施】

1.提供心理支持　护士应主动与患者及家属沟通,了解患者的心理动态,对患者及家属的疑问做出比较科学又满意的解释。向患者及家属讲解疾病知识,更重要的是用浅显易懂的语言或资料向患者及家属说明手术目的、麻醉方式、手术过程、手术过程中可能出现的情况,手术前、后的注意事项及护理配合,使患者和家属有心理准备,消除其思想顾虑和紧张情绪,增强战胜疾病的信心,积极配合手术。

2.提供相关信息　结合患者的年龄、文化水平,给予相应的健康教育。

（1）讲解疾病有关知识,如子宫切除术后丧失了生育功能,但不会丧失女性的第二性征;卵巢切除后会出现雌激素减少所致的一系列症候群,但可通过雌激素治疗缓解症状。

（2）介绍术前准备的内容与术前常规检查的目的,协助患者主动配合术前准备和术前各项检查。用通俗易懂的语言向患者介绍手术名称、范围、过程及麻醉方法等。简单讲解术后可能出现的问题及注意事项。

（3）指导患者进行预防术后并发症的锻炼,如教会患者在床上使用便器,避免术后发生排尿困难;训练患者胸式深呼吸、咳嗽、咳痰的方法,可指导患者双手按压切口两侧,先深吸气再用力咳嗽;

教会患者在别人的协助下进行翻身、收缩和放松四肢肌肉的运动等。患者要重复训练至掌握为止。

3. 做好术前准备

（1）术前一般准备

1）术前观察生命体征，测量体温、脉搏、呼吸，3 次/d，测血压，1 次/d。若患者有发热、血压升高等异常均应配合医生积极寻找原因，以及时处理。对于生命体征异常或有月经来潮需推迟手术时间者，应向患者及家属做好解释。

2）遵医嘱进一步完善必要的术前辅助检查。

3）术前指导患者合理饮食，进食高蛋白、高热量、高维生素食物，以保证机体术前处于最佳的营养状况，为手术成功和术后康复创造条件。

4）认真做好术前合并症的处理，如贫血、糖尿病等内科合并症的治疗，调整患者的身心状况，为手术成功创造条件。

（2）手术前日准备

1）协助医生给患者家属讲明术中、术后可能的并发症，得到家属的理解并签手术同意书。将手术通知单和麻醉通知单送往手术室。

2）皮肤准备：指导患者沐浴、更衣、修剪指（趾）甲，然后进行手术区皮肤准备。经腹部手术备皮范围上自剑突下，两侧至腋中线，下至两大腿上 1/3 处及外阴部，注意脐窝的清洁。阴部手术备皮范围上至耻骨联合上 10 cm，下至大腿上 1/3 的前、内、后侧，会阴、臀部和肛周。备皮完毕用温水洗净、拭干。

3）消化道准备：一般手术前日灌肠 1~2 次，或口服缓泻剂，使患者排便 3 次以上；术前 1 d 晚餐减量，术前 8 h 禁食，4 h 禁饮；预计手术可能涉及肠道时，如妇科恶性肿瘤有肠道转移者，术前 3 d 进无渣半流质饮食，并遵医嘱给予肠道抗生素；术前 1 d 晚灌肠，至排出的灌肠液中无大便残渣。阴部手术者术前 3 d 开始进无渣半流质饮食 2 d，流质饮食 1 d 并按医嘱给予肠道抗生素；手术前日晚餐后 2~3 h 和手术日晨给予清洁灌肠。

4）休息与睡眠：为保证患者在术前得到充分的休息，于术前 1 d 晚，给患者适量的镇静剂，以减轻患者的焦虑程度，保证充足的睡眠。

（3）手术当日护理

1）手术日晨，护士应尽早看望患者，核查生命体征，评估患者的情况。取下患者的义齿、发卡、首饰及贵重物品交给家属或护士长保管。常规留置导尿管，排空膀胱。经阴道手术一般不需留置尿管，带导尿包于手术室备用。

2）根据患者手术种类和麻醉方式，铺好麻醉床，准备好床旁监护仪、负压吸引器及吸引管、输液装置及各种急救用物。

3）遵医嘱术前 30 min 肌内注射苯巴比妥、阿托品。

（4）阴道准备　行子宫切除术的患者，术前 3 d 开始进行阴道准备，常用 1∶5 000 高锰酸钾溶液、0.05% 碘伏溶液、1∶1 000 新洁尔灭溶液等行阴道冲洗或坐浴，1 次/d；手术当日晨用消毒液行阴道（尤其是穹隆处）、子宫颈消毒，用棉球擦干子宫颈、阴道后，在子宫颈和穹隆处涂 1% 甲紫。阴部手术者术前 3 d 行阴道冲洗，冲洗后放入甲硝唑片 0.2 g，1 次/d，连用 3 d。术日早晨用消毒液行阴道消毒，应特别注意消毒阴道后穹隆，消毒后用大棉签拭干。

Preoperative Psychosocial Nursing

Preoparation informational interventions have generally proved effective to relieve mood disrupt. So first, provide explanations and printed information about the disease and the scheduled surgery. The patient should have a complete idea of what the preoperative, intraoperative, and postoperative course entails.

Especially for some women, who are more concerned that the procedure will result in a loss of femininity, a decrease in sexual satisfaction, or and increase in interpersonal problems with their spouses, to minimize the possibility that the patient has a poor outcome, preoperative counseling and preparation are essential.

Preoperative Instructions

The medical staff should explain what type of surgery will be done and what approach will be used. And should also anticipate the woman's questions about her sexual function and indicate when she will be able to resume sexual relations, whether she will have a surgical menopause, and whether she will be able to have children. Many women are unfamiliar with the reproductive anatomy and may wonder just what is going to happen to them. When the physician has explained the surgery, the nurse can reinforce the explanation and answer questions that the woman might have.

Preparation for Surgical Intervention

● Skin preparation: To reduce the colony count of skin bacteria, the patient is asked to shower and change clothes in the day before surgery. Then hair surrounding the incision area may be removed. Pay more attention to the cleaning of the umbilical region.

● Bowel preparation: Preparation of the lower gastrointestinal tract prior to elective gynecologic surgery has several goals. In most gynecologic surgery, when the gastrointestinal tract is not entered, mechanical preparation of the bowel reduces gastrointestinal contents and thus allows more room in the abdomen and pelvis, facilitating the surgical procedure; if a rectosigmoid colon enterotomy occurs, the mechanical bowel preparation eliminates formed stool and reduces the risk of bacterial contamination, thus reducing infectious complications. For general operations such as hysterectomy or adnexectomy, enema may be administered twice or oral laxatives are taken the day before operation, no further preparation is needed. If the patient is likely to sustain bowel damage or if the bowel is to be opened, such as cytoreductive surgery to treat ovarian cancer, the patient should be on a non-residue semi-soft diet and be given oral prophylactic antibiotics for three days before surgery, such as neomycin lgm, qid, PO or gentamycin 80,000 U, tid, PO. The day before surgery, the patient is usually given a clear liquid diet to further reduce the accumulation of fecal wastes and slow intestinal peristalsis. Enemas are administered at the evening before surgery until the rectal effluent is clear. Begin the status of nothing by mouth from midnight of operative day. If the surgeon anticipates excessive manipulation of the intestines, a nasogastric tube may be inserted before surgery to prevent abdominal distention.

● Vaginal preparation: For a patient to be performed total hysterectomy, antiseptic vaginal douche is needed the day before operation to decrease transvaginal microbial invasion of the surgical site. Then the morning of operative day, the cervix and vagina, especially the vaginal fornix should be sterilized and dried in operational room.

● Bladder preparation: The bladder must be decompressed to prevent pressure on the surgical site and to protect it from trauma during surgery. An indwelling catheter is inserted in the bladder before surgery and will usually remain in place for several days after surgery.

● Others: To prepare for possible peri-operative blood transfusion and medication administration, the cross matching test and drug sensitivity test is necessary. Pre-operative medication, such as diazepam 5 mg, PO, the night before operation, is to decrease anxiety experienced by the patient and to ensure adequate sleep and rest. Hairpin, metal ornaments, dental prostheses and contact lenses and make-up should be removed before transference of the patient to the operating room.

二　腹部手术的术后护理

术后的精心护理是患者术后恢复良好的关键,能促使患者尽快康复,又能及早发现和防止术后并发症的发生。术后护理中还要鼓励患者和家属积极地参与到护理活动中,发挥患者的主观能动性,提高患者的自护能力,促进康复。

【护理评估】

1.术中情况　患者术后由麻醉医师和参加手术的护士一起送回病房,责任护士应与其进行床边交接班并记录,了解患者术中情况。

2.身体评估

(1)一般评估　评估患者基本生命体征,观察患者是否清醒;了解导尿管及引流管位置是否正常、引流是否通畅,评估引流液的量、性状及颜色;评估手术部位伤口敷料有无渗血、渗液;评估阴道出血情况。

(2)疼痛　麻醉作用消失后,一般患者术后4～6 h开始感觉切口疼痛,24 h内最剧烈,凡是增加切口张力的动作(如咳嗽、翻身等)都会加剧疼痛的程度。2～3 d后疼痛明显减轻。

(3)发热　是术后常见症状。术后1～3 d由于机体对手术创伤的反应可出现体温升高,但一般不超过38 ℃,属于正常现象;若术后3～6 d发热或体温持续升高或正常后又升高,应考虑有感染的可能。

(4)恶心、呕吐　其最常见的原因是麻醉反应,待麻醉作用消失后,即可停止。

(5)腹胀　由于手术刺激肠管、麻醉药物作用等,肠蠕动减慢,患者在术后可出现腹胀,通常在术后24～48 h肛门排气,肠蠕动恢复,腹胀随即缓解。如术后数日发生腹胀,可能由腹膜炎、肠麻痹、早期肠梗阻引起。

(6)尿潴留　由于不习惯床上排尿、留置尿管的机械性刺激、麻醉作用及切口疼痛抑制排尿反射等因素的影响,术后容易发生尿潴留。

3.辅助检查　复查血常规以了解有无贫血及感染,根据患者术后具体情况做相应辅助检查。

4.心理-社会支持状况　术后患者对手术是否成功表现出极大的关注,担心术后并发症;术后的疼痛和其他不适也让患者感到紧张、焦虑、不安、困惑。患者及家属对术后体力的恢复、性生活的恢复等也表示担忧。

【护理诊断】

1.疼痛　与手术创伤有关。

2.自理能力缺陷　与切口疼痛、持续留置导尿管及引流管、术后输液等有关。

3.有感染的危险　与术后机体抵抗力降低及手术创伤有关。

4.自我形象紊乱　与手术切除部分生殖器官有关。

5.焦虑　与担心手术效果及术后康复有关。

【护理措施】

1.一般护理

(1)体位　按手术及麻醉方式决定术后体位。全身麻醉患者清醒前应有专人守护,去枕平卧,头侧向一旁,清醒后根据需要选择体位:蛛网膜下腔麻醉者,去枕平卧12 h;硬膜外麻醉者,去枕平卧6～8 h。如果患者情况稳定,术后次晨可取半卧位。阴部术后根据不同的手术选择不同的体位,如子宫脱垂术后采取平卧位为宜;生殖道瘘修补术后采取健侧卧位;外阴癌根治术后采取平卧位,双腿屈膝外展。

(2)监测生命体征　术后要认真观察并记录生命体征的变化。术后一般 15~30 min 监测 1 次血压、呼吸、脉搏,平稳后改为每 4~6 h 1 次,24 h 后每日测量 4 次,直至正常后 3 d。若有异常则应增加监测次数。

(3)切口护理　保持切口敷料清洁、干燥,观察切口有无渗血、渗液,敷料是否脱落,切口有无感染征象,发现异常应立即报告医生。阴部术后阴道内留置纱条压迫止血者应于术后 12~24 h 取出。

(4)饮食　妇科腹部手术当日禁食,术后 1~2 d 进流食,忌牛奶与糖类等产气食物,以免肠胀气。肛管排气后逐渐改为半流质和普通饮食。术后饮食要注意营养丰富、易消化,高热量、高蛋白、富含维生素,以促进机体恢复。阴部手术、会阴Ⅲ度裂伤修补术后 5 d 内进少渣半流质饮食,术后按医嘱服用抗生素和复方樟脑酊,抑制肠蠕动,控制 5 d 内不解大便。

(5)活动与休息　镇痛的前提下,让患者安静休息,有充足的睡眠。同时鼓励患者活动肢体,每 15 min 进行 1 次腿部运动,每 2 h 翻身、咳嗽、做深呼吸 1 次。尽早活动有助于改善循环,防止下肢静脉血栓形成,促进肺部和肠道功能的恢复。阴部术后尽量避免使腹压增加的动作,如下蹲、用力排便等,以免增加局部切口的张力,影响切口的愈合。

(6)留置管的护理　注意保持留置管的固定、引流通畅,保持留置管周围皮肤的清洁和干燥,观察并记录引流液的量、颜色。

1)一般术后留置尿管 24~48 h;子宫颈癌根治术后留置导尿管 10~14 d,阴部手术需留置导尿管 2~10 d。长期留置导尿管者应给予膀胱冲洗,注意保持外阴清洁,拔出导尿管前 1 天应进行夹管,每 2~4 h 开放 1 次,以锻炼膀胱逼尿肌的舒缩功能,次晨拔出导尿管。导尿管拔出后应嘱咐患者多饮水,尽早排尿。

2)留置的腹腔或盆腔引流管,根据具体情况决定留置时间。一般在 24 h 内负压引流液不应该超过 200 mL。

(7)外阴护理　阴部术后常规使用 0.05% 碘伏溶液擦洗外阴,2 次/d,禁止做外阴冲洗。外阴擦洗的范围要广,擦洗时应注意观察阴道分泌物的量、性质、气味及阴道有无流血,如有异常情况及时报告医生给予处理。

2. 预防感染　术后有发生切口感染、肺部感染等多种感染的可能,要注意保持切口敷料的清洁、干燥、无污染;注意口腔护理;要指导患者改善营养状况,增强机体抵抗力;遵医嘱正确合理应用抗生素。

3. 术后不适的应对和护理

(1)腹胀　术后询问肛门排气的时间,观察排气后腹胀是否减轻。术后 48 h 仍未恢复正常肠蠕动,可采用热敷下腹部、0.9% 氯化钠注射液低位灌肠、注射新斯的明等方法刺激肠蠕动,缓解腹胀。必要时还可行肛管排气。术后协助患者尽早下床活动,可预防或减轻腹胀。

(2)尿潴留　首先安定患者情绪,焦虑、紧张会加重尿道括约肌痉挛;在床边遮挡屏风,鼓励患者定期坐起排尿;拔出导尿管前应进行夹管,定时开放,以锻炼膀胱逼尿肌的舒缩功能;热敷、轻柔按摩下腹部,必要时遵医嘱给膀胱肌收缩剂;如以上措施无效,可在无菌操作下导尿。

(3)疼痛　指导患者正确使用自控镇痛泵,协助患者取舒适的体位,护理操作轻柔,遵医嘱应用镇痛剂如哌替啶等,以缓解或减轻患者的疼痛。

(4)发热　严密观察体温变化,体温超过 39 ℃者,可采取物理降温,如头部冷敷、温水或酒精擦浴,必要时遵医嘱用解热镇痛药。

4. 提供心理支持　护士应仔细了解患者的心理状态,耐心听取患者的疑问,并对患者的疑问给予细致的解释,消除其思想顾虑。采取积极的措施,减轻疼痛,解除不适。给患者讲解手术的情况及术后注意事项,提高患者的自理能力。

【健康教育】

要为术后患者提供详细的术后康复计划,包括患者的自我护理能力训练,如何适应术后生活形态的改变,术后及出院后的饮食、休息与活动、用药、可能的异常症状等,还要指导患者定期门诊随访。

After surgery the nurse should assess the vital signs and dressings to detect bleeding. Immediate hemorrhage or continuing hemorrhage is always declared by a rising pulse rate or a decreasing blood pressure. The woman who has had an abdominal surgery will have an abdominal dressing and a perineal dressing, whereas the woman who has had a vaginal hysterectomy will have only the perineal dressing. The nurse assesses all the dressings each time vital signs are taken. When inspecting the dressing, the nurse checks for drainage and notes the amount, color, consistency and odor of the drainage fluid.

In general, anesthetic effect will disappear 6 hours after cessation of anesthetics. Conscious recovery should be closely observed for patients undergoing general anesthesia until the patient comes to be fully conscious. Post lumbar puncture headache is due to decreased cerebrospinal pressure and vasodilatation, which result from extra flowing out of spinal fluid into the peridural space via puncture hole. It lasts 5 d and then disappears. So supine bed rest for at least 6 h is required for patients undergoing epidural anesthesia to prevent the headache. For patients undergoing spinal anesthesia, supine bed rest for at least 6 h is also preferred because accidental entry to spinal cavity of puncture needle is possible. Sometimes analgesic is needed to relieve the headache.

For patients undergoing pelvic exenteration or debulking surgery, transvaginal suction drainage of each side of the groin is often used to provide an outlet for fluid that would otherwise accumulate and be a medium for infection or cause pressure on the surgical site. The nurse should ensure the tubes are attached to suction as ordered and drain freely, and at the same time observe and record the amount, color and appearance of drainage fluid. Generally the amount is less than 200 mL and the color gradually become clear. When nothing drains out, the drain tube can be removed.

Post-operative bladder drainage should be employed after any procedure in which spontaneous, complete voiding is not anticipated. A Foley catheter is often used. The nurse should observe the catheter for patency and record the output, color and consistency of the urine for early detection of possible injury to ureter or bladder during major surgery. The catheter is usually removed on the first or second postoperative day. For major surgery, such as radical hysterectomy and debulking surgery, the catheter is often remain for seven days or longer for bladder to resume its function. After removal of bladder catheter, the nurse should note the time and amount of the first voiding. Some physicians may order a catheterized specimen for residual urine after the first voiding. If over 100 mL of residual urine is obtained at this time, the catheter may be reinserted. When the catheter is removed? The woman is encouraged to drink fluids to promote urinary drainage and encourage early spontaneous voiding so that she will not need to be catheterized again.

Pain medication may be given as needed. Although satisfactory analgesia is easily achievable with currently available methods, patients continue to suffer unnecessarily from postoperative pain. There are several reasons for the existing inadequacies in pain management. First, patient expectations of pain relief are low and they are not aware of the extent of analgesia that they should expect. Second, attitudes continue to be influenced by the common misconception that the use of narcotics in the post-operative period can result in opioid dependance. So nurses should be equipped with pain control knowledge. The patients and their relatives should be informed that pain could be controlled to a level acceptable to them and there is no need to suffer from post-operative pain, provided with their cooperation to report experiencing pain correctly. At the same time, nurses should assess patients' pain continually and regulate the pain control regimen timely according to the intensity of pain experienced by patients.

To maintain circulation and prevent circulatory and respiratory complications, the woman is encouraged to turn, cough, and deeply breathe. The patient is usually permitted to be out of bed on the second postoperative day, but the nurse should encourage the patient to dangle her legs and sit on the side of the bed before standing and walking to prevent the effects of postural hypotension. Elastic stocking or elastic bandages may be used to prevent thrombus or embolus formation, and the legs should be exercised frequently when the woman is in bed to prevent pooling of venous blood.

任务二　外阴、阴道手术(Vulvar and Vagina Surgery)

工作情景

王阿姨,64 岁,外阴癌根治术后 1 d,神志清醒,有合作能力。她因伤口疼痛让家属找护士给予处理。

请对王阿姨的会阴切口进行评估,并对王阿姨进行正确的疼痛护理。

任务内容

外阴、阴道手术主要有外阴癌根治术、处女膜切开术、会阴Ⅲ度裂伤修补术、阴道前后壁修补术、经阴道子宫切除术、阴道成形术等。外阴、阴道手术与腹部手术的不同在于其手术部位的神经、血管较为丰富,与尿道、肛门邻近,导致患者容易出现与疼痛、感染、出血等相关的护理问题。由于手术涉及患者隐私部位,故对患者的心理问题也应予重视。

任务目标

◆ 能叙述妇科外阴、阴道手术前和手术后患者的护理措施。
◆ 能运用护理程序为妇科外阴、阴道手术前和手术后患者进行护理评估、护理诊断。

一 外阴、阴道手术的术前准备及护理

【护理评估】

1. 健康史　了解患者的一般情况,月经史、性生活史、婚育史、既往病史、手术产史及其他手术史、过敏史等,饮食习惯及有无吸烟或酗酒等;评估患病的部位,拟施行的麻醉方法、手术方式、手术范围及手术时间等。

2.身体评估　评估内容同腹部手术。

3.辅助检查　血、尿常规,肝、肾功能测定,血型鉴定及交叉配血试验,B型超声,心电图,X射线检查等。

4.心理-社会支持状况　手术区域神经、血管丰富且为隐私部位,患者可能因为暴露身体的隐私部位、担心手术顺利与否及术后疼痛而产生紧张、害羞、焦虑心理。其家属也可能对手术康复及性生活的恢复表示担忧。

【常见护理诊断】

1.恐惧/焦虑　与担心手术是否顺利及预后有关。

2.知识缺乏　缺乏疾病有关知识及手术配合知识。

【护理措施】

1.心理护理　护士应理解患者对保护隐私的要求,尽可能提供有利于保护患者隐私的环境,在进行术前准备检查和手术时注意用屏风遮挡,尽量减少暴露部位,减轻患者羞怯感。做好家属特别是丈夫的心理疏导工作,让其充分理解患者,给患者提供心理支持,积极配合治疗和护理。可通过个别谈话和开展讲座等方式向患者讲解疾病的有关知识,说明手术的必要性和重要性,介绍手术方式、麻醉方式、手术过程、手术中可能遇到的情况、术前术后的注意事项和护理配合。让患者在术前心理上做好充分的准备,消除其紧张情绪。

2.术前准备

(1)皮肤准备　保持外阴部皮肤清洁、干燥,每日清洗外阴。若皮肤有破溃,炎症者应治愈后再行手术。术前1 d备皮,范围为上自耻骨联合上10 cm,下至会阴部、肛门周围、腹股沟和大腿上1/3处。剃去阴毛并清洁皮肤。

(2)肠道准备　术前3 d开始进食无渣饮食,并按医嘱口服抗生素。手术前日晚或手术当天清洁灌肠,术前8 h禁食,4 h禁饮。

(3)阴道准备　术前3 d开始阴道准备,一般行阴道冲洗或坐浴,每天2次。常用1∶5000高锰酸钾、0.2‰的碘伏溶液和1∶1 000苯扎溴铵。手术当天用消毒液行阴道消毒,特别注意消毒阴道穹隆部。

(4)膀胱准备　患者术前一般不留置尿管,嘱其术前排空膀胱。带无菌导尿管备用。

Preoperative Preparation

● Skin preparation:Keep the skin of the vulva clean and dry,and wash the vulva daily. If the skin is ulcerated,the inflammation should be cured before surgery. The skin was prepared 1 d before the operation,ranging from 10 cm above the pubic symphysis,down to the perineum,around the anus,groin and upper 1/3 of the thigh. Shave the pubic hair and clean the skin.

● Intestinal preparation:3 d before the operation,start eating a scum-free diet,and take antibiotics orally as directed by the doctor. Clean the enema the night before the operation or the day of the operation,fast for 8 h before the operation,and drink for 4 h.

● Vaginal preparation:Start vaginal preparation 3 d before the operation,usually vaginal douche or sitz bath,2 times a day. Commonly used 1∶5,000 potassium permanganate,0.2‰ iodophor and 1∶1,000 benzalkonium bromide. Disinfect the vagina with a disinfectant on the day of the operation,and pay special attention to disinfecting the vaginal vault.

● Bladder preparation:patients generally do not indwell a urinary tube before surgery,and ask them to empty their bladder before surgery. Bring a sterile urinary catheter for use.

二 外阴、阴道手术的术后护理

【护理评估】

同妇科腹部手术患者的评估。

【护理诊断】

1.急性疼痛 与手术创伤有关。

2.有感染的危险 与伤口部位特殊及留置导尿等有关。

3.焦虑 与担心手术效果及术后康复有关。

4.自我形象紊乱 与对外阴和阴道手术的认识不足有关。

【护理措施】

1.术后体位 术后根据不同手术采取不同的体位,处女膜闭锁及先天性无阴道患者,术后应采取半卧位;外阴癌根治术的患者术后采取平卧位,双腿外展屈膝,膝下垫软枕,减少腹股沟及外阴部的张力,有利于伤口愈合;尿瘘修补术的患者采取健侧卧位,使瘘孔居于高位,以减少尿液对伤口的浸泡。

2.防止感染 注意保持外阴部清洁,每天擦洗外阴2次,便后清洁外阴。手术时阴道内填塞止血纱条,术后12~24 h内取出,核对纱条数目,并观察有无出血。严密观察切口的情况,有无渗血、红肿、化脓的炎症反应,注意阴道分泌物的量、颜色和气味。

3.伤口的护理 外阴、阴道手术由于切口位置邻近肛门,术后排便易污染伤口,因此需控制首次排便的时间。尿瘘及会阴Ⅲ度裂伤修补术后,5 d内进少渣半流质饮食,一般控制5~7 d内不解大便。患者肛门排气后遵医嘱口服复方樟脑酊,抑制肠蠕动控制排便。术后第5天,可给患者使用液态石蜡,软化大便,避免排便困难。

4.导尿管的护理 外阴、阴道术后一般需留置导尿管,应注意保持导尿管通畅,观察并记录尿量,特别是尿瘘修补术患者,注意有无阴道漏尿。拔出导尿管前帮助患者训练膀胱功能,如有排尿困难者给予诱导、热敷等措施帮助其排尿,必要时可重新留置导尿管。

Nursing Measures

● Postoperative position:After operation, different positions are adopted according to different operations. Patients with hymen atresia and congenital absence of vagina should be in semi–recumbent position after surgery;while patients undergoing radical vulvar cancer surgery should be in supine position with both legs abducted. Bend your knees and cushion your knees with soft pillows to reduce tension in the groin and vulva,which is beneficial to wound healing. Patients undergoing urinary fistula repair should be placed on the contralateral side to keep the fistula in a high position to reduce urine soaking to the wound.

● Prevent infection:Pay attention to keep the vulva clean,scrub the vulva twice a day,and clean the vulva after defecation. The hemostatic gauze was packed in the vagina during the operation,and the gauze was taken out within 12–24 h after the operation. The number of gauze was checked and observed for bleeding. Observe closely the condition of the incision,whether there is any inflammatory reaction such as bleeding,redness,and suppuration. Pay attention to the amount,color and smell of vaginal secretions.

● Wound care:Vulvar and vaginal surgery. Since the incision is located close to the anus,it is easy to contaminate the wound after defecation. Therefore,it is necessary to control the time for the first defecation. After repairing urinary fistula and perineal third-degree laceration, take a low-residue semi-liquid diet within 5 d. General control of the bowel movements within 5－7 d. After the patient has exhausted anus, take compound camphor tincture orally according to the doctor's instructions to inhibit bowel movements and control bowel movements. On the 5th day after the operation, liquid paraffin can be used for the patient to soften the stool and avoid difficulty in defecation.

● Urinary catheter care: Urinary catheters are generally needed after vulvar and vaginal operations. Care should be taken to keep the catheters unobstructed, and to observe and record the urine output, especially for patients undergoing urinary fistula repair, and pay attention to whether there is vaginal leakage. Before removing the urinary catheter, help the patient to train the bladder function. If there is difficulty in urination, take measures such as induction and hot compress to help the urination. If necessary, the catheter can be re-indwelled.

【健康教育】

①出院后 1 个月复查,了解术后康复情况及伤口愈合情况。②外阴部伤口常需间断拆线,回家后应保持外阴部清洁,注意休息,避免重体力劳动,预防便秘、久蹲等增加腹压的危险因素。③3 个月内禁止性生活。若发现会阴部异常出血或分泌物等情况,应及时就诊。

任务实施

妇科术前准备内容见表 13-1。

表 13-1　妇科术前准备

项目	内容
妇科手术方式、部位、麻醉方式	1. 腹腔镜手术;盆、腹腔;全身麻醉
	2. 宫腔镜手术;子宫;全身麻醉
	3. 子宫颈环扎术;子宫颈;腰麻
	4. 阴式手术;经阴道;全身麻醉
	5. 经腹手术;腹部;全身麻醉
术前功能锻炼	1. 术前护理人员应指导患者学会胸式呼吸,老年患者还应学习咳嗽和排痰,预防发生术后坠积性肺炎
	2. 疼痛:手术所致疼痛是一种急性疼痛,严重影响患者手术的恢复,增加术后并发症的发生。术前指导患者如何应对术后的疼痛,如何使用自控式镇痛泵,以减轻疼痛对患者的刺激,加快术后的恢复过程,减少或避免并发症的发生
	3. 翻身和起床:指导患者翻身、起床和活动的技巧,鼓励术后早期活动,以利术后康复。术后早期活动是避免下肢静脉血栓形成的有效方法
	4. 排泄:术前应指导患者在床上练习使用便器,以免术后发生排尿困难
饮食	手术前日中午不宜进食太多,宜选择清淡、易消化食物,如蒸鸡蛋羹,粥等;晚餐应以流质为主,如米汤,鱼汤;术前需禁食、禁饮 8 h,防止麻醉意外

续表 13-1

项目	内容
肠道准备	妇科一般手术患者肠道准备于术前 1 d 开始。手术前日清洁肠道,可口服磷酸钠盐口服溶液 90 mL 加温开水 750 mL 导泻,也可用 1% 肥皂水清洁灌肠,服药或灌肠后护士注意观察患者的反应。妇科恶性肿瘤患者,特别是卵巢癌患者,由于肿瘤组织有可能侵犯肠道,术中要剥离癌组织或切除病变部位的部分肠管,肠道准备从术前 3 d 开始。术前 3 d 进半流食,口服磷酸钠盐口服溶液 90 mL 加温开水 750 mL 导泻,术前 2 d 患者进流食,其他内容同术前 3 d。手术当日清晨清洁灌肠,至排泄物中无粪渣。对年老、体弱者清洁灌肠应按其承受能力而定,警惕腹泻导致脱水
其他	1. 皮肤准备:手术前日进行皮肤准备。腹部皮肤备皮范围是上自剑突下缘,下至两大腿上 1/3,左右到腋中线,剃去阴毛,脐部用碘伏棉签清洁后再用酒精棉签擦拭。整个备皮过程中护理人员动作要轻柔,切忌损伤患者表皮,以免微生物侵入而影响手术。备皮完成后用温水洗净、拭干
	2. 手术前日抽血做血型及交叉配血试验,遵医嘱行药物过敏试验
	3. 手术前日晚上及手术当日清晨测量患者生命体征,注意有无月经来潮、上呼吸道感染,如有上述情况应及时与医生取得联系
	4. 阴道准备:术前 1 d 为患者冲洗阴道 2 次,阴道流血及未婚者不做阴道冲洗。阴道冲洗时护士动作要轻柔,注意遮挡患者
	5. 术前晚如患者难入眠应遵医嘱给予镇静催眠药,可用地西泮 10 mg,肌内注射
	6. 膀胱准备:术前患者应排空膀胱,需要为患者导尿时应注意无菌操作,见尿后固定尿管
	7. 其他:术前要了解患者有无药物过敏史,遵医嘱做药物过敏试验。进入手术室前患者要摘下义齿、发卡及首饰等并妥善保管,遵医嘱给予术前药物,核对患者姓名、床号、手术带药及手术名称,将患者及病历交给手术室的手术人员
	8. 床单位准备:患者入手术室后,护士应进行手术患者床单位的准备,铺好麻醉床,床上备有床垫,备好血压表、听诊器、沙袋、弯盘、吸氧用物、引流瓶等,必要时准备胃肠减压器等

微课

课件

练习题及参考答案

（王珏辉）

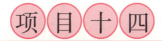

项目十四

女性生殖系统肿瘤患者的护理(Nursing of Patients with Female Reproductive System Tumor)

项目描述

　　女性生殖系统肿瘤包括良性肿瘤和恶性肿瘤,它们可以发生在生殖道内的任何部位,但主要发生在子宫和卵巢。子宫平滑肌瘤和卵巢囊肿是最常见的良性肿瘤,而子宫颈癌、子宫内膜癌和卵巢癌是3种最常见的恶性肿瘤,其中卵巢癌的死亡率最高。主要的治疗方式包括手术、化疗、放疗和免疫治疗。

　　Noplasm of the female genital tract is a kind of common disease that undermines women's health and even endangers women's lives. They may arise at any site within the genital tract, however predominantly occurring at uterus and ovary. They are divided into two categories: the benign and the malignant. Leiomyomas and ovarian cysts are the commonest benign tumors, while cervical cancer, endometrial cancer and ovarian cancer are the three commonest malignancies, of which ovarian cancer represents the highest mortality. The major therapeutic modalities include operation, chemotherapy, radiotherapy, and immunotherapy. In general, nursing interventions focus on preventive instruction, psychological counseling, and peri-therapeutic care.

任务一　　子宫颈癌(Cervical Cancer)

工作情景

　　患者,45岁,因性生活后阴道流血3个月前来就医。发病以来,无腹胀、腹痛,无消瘦、乏力及体重减轻,大小便及饮食正常。13岁月经初潮,(4~6)/(26~31)d,经量中等,无明显痛经,G_4P_1,人工流产3次,节育环避孕。既往体健,爱人及父母无特殊病史。妇科检查:子宫颈前唇见直径4.0 cm菜花状肿物,表面有脓血性分泌物,子宫颈质脆,触之易出血。子宫大小正常,双附件(-)。液基薄层细胞学(TCT)检查:子宫颈鳞状细胞癌。

　　请对该患者进行护理评估,并为患者提供护理措施。

任务内容

子宫颈癌是最常见的妇科恶性肿瘤,高发年龄为 50～55 岁。由于子宫颈癌筛查的普及,得以早期发现和治疗子宫颈癌和癌前病变,其发病率和死亡率明显下降。

任务目标

◆ 能叙述子宫颈癌的病因、病理及分类、转移途径、临床表现、护理措施。
◆ 能对子宫颈癌进行评估。

【概述】

1. 病因　引起子宫颈癌的确切病因不清,临床研究表明与下列因素相关。

(1)人乳头瘤病毒(HPV)感染　HPV 感染,尤其是高危型 HPV 感染与子宫颈鳞状上皮内病变(squamous intraepithelial lesion,SIL)和子宫颈癌发病密切相关。已在接近 90% 的 SIL 和 99% 的子宫颈癌组织中发现有高危型 HPV 感染,其中约 70% 与 HPV16 和 HPV18 型相关。接种 HPV 预防性疫苗可以实现子宫颈癌的一级预防。

(2)性行为及分娩次数　多个性伴侣、初次性生活<16 岁、早年分娩、多产与子宫颈癌发生有关。与有阴茎癌、前列腺癌或其伴侣曾患子宫颈癌的高危男子性接触的妇女,也易患子宫颈癌。

(3)其他　吸烟可增加感染 HPV 效应,屏障避孕法有一定的保护作用。

2. 病理及分类　子宫颈上皮是由位于子宫颈管内的柱状上皮和位于子宫颈阴道部的鳞状上皮组成,两者在子宫颈外口处形成鳞-柱交界部,鳞-柱交界部可随体内雌激素水平的变化内外移动。在原始鳞-柱交界部和生理性鳞-柱交界部之间形成的区域被称为转化区,是子宫颈癌的好发部位。转化区成熟的化生鳞状上皮对致癌物的刺激相对不敏感,但未成熟的化生鳞状上皮却代谢活跃,在 HPV 等的作用下,发生细胞异常增生、分化不良、排列紊乱、细胞核异常、有丝分裂增加,最后形成 SIL。

(1)子宫颈鳞状上皮内病变　SIL 是与子宫颈浸润癌密切相关的一组子宫颈病变,常发生于 25～35 岁妇女,分低级别鳞状上皮内病变(low-grade squamous intraepithelial lesion,LSIL)和高级别鳞状上皮内病变(high-grade squamous intraepithelial lesion,HSIL)。LSIL:细胞核极性轻度紊乱,有轻度异型性,核分裂象少,局限于上皮下 1/3,P16 染色阴性或在上皮内散在点状阳性(图 14-1)。HSIL:细胞核极性紊乱,核质比增加,核分裂象增多,异型细胞扩展到层上皮下 2/3 层甚至全层,P16 在上皮>2/3 层面内呈弥漫连续阳性(图 14-2)。SIL 反映了子宫颈癌发生发展中的连续过程,通过筛查发现 SIL,及时治疗高级别病变,是预防子宫颈浸润癌的有效措施。SIL 既往称为"子宫颈上皮内瘤变"(cervical intraepithelial neoplasia,CIN),分为 CIN Ⅰ 级、CIN Ⅱ 级和 CIN Ⅲ 级。LSIL 相当于 CIN Ⅰ 级,HSIL 包括 CIN Ⅲ 级和大部分 CIN Ⅱ 级。SIL 形成后继续发展,突破上皮下基底膜,浸润间质,形成子宫颈浸润癌(图 14-3)。

(2)子宫颈浸润癌

1)鳞状细胞癌:占 75%～80%。

巨检:肉眼观察无明显异常,或类似子宫颈炎,随着病变逐步发展,有以下 4 种类型(图 14-4)。①外生型:最常见。病灶向外生长,状如菜花,又称菜花型。组织脆,初起为息肉样或乳头状隆起,触之易出血。②内生型:癌灶向子宫颈深部组织浸润,使子宫颈扩张并侵犯子宫峡部。子宫颈肥大而硬,表面光滑或仅有柱状上皮异位,整个子宫颈段膨大如桶状。③溃疡型:上述两型癌灶继续发展,癌组织坏死脱落形成凹陷性溃疡或空洞样形如火山口。④颈管型:癌灶发生在子宫颈外口内,隐蔽在子宫颈管,侵入子宫颈及子宫峡部供血层及转移到盆壁的淋巴结,不同于内生型,后者是由特殊的浸润性生长扩散到子宫颈管。

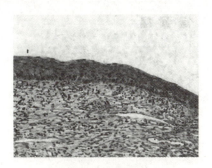

图 14-1　LSIL

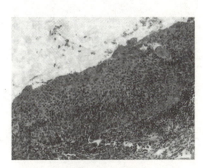

图 14-2　HSIL

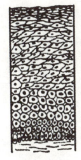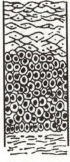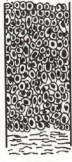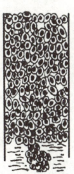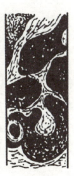

正常上皮　　上皮内病变　　原位癌　　微小浸润癌　　浸润癌

图 14-3　子宫颈正常上皮—上皮内病变—浸润癌

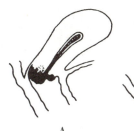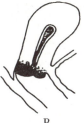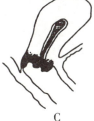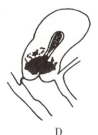

A　　　　B　　　　C　　　　D

A.外生型;B.内生型;C.溃疡型;D.颈管型。

图 14-4　子宫颈癌大体病理

镜检:①镜下早期浸润癌。原位癌基础上,在镜下发现癌细胞小团似泪滴状、锯齿状突破基底膜,或进而出现膨胀性间质浸润。②子宫颈浸润癌。根据细胞分化程度分3级:Ⅰ级,分化较好;Ⅱ级,中度分化;Ⅲ级,多为未分化的小细胞(相当于子宫颈上皮底层的未分化细胞)。

2)腺癌:近年来子宫颈腺癌的发生率有上升趋势,占 20%~25%。

3)其他:少见类型有腺鳞癌、腺样基底细胞癌、绒毛状管状腺癌、内膜样癌等上皮性癌,神经内分泌肿瘤,间叶性肿瘤等。

（3）临床分期　见表14-1。

表14-1　子宫颈癌临床分期

分期	解释
Ⅰ期	癌灶局限在宫颈（是否扩散至宫体不予考虑）
ⅠA期	仅在显微镜下可见浸润癌，最大浸润癌深度<5 mm
ⅠA1期	间质浸润深度<3 mm
ⅠA2期	间质浸润深度≥3 mm，<5 mm
ⅠB期	浸润癌浸润深度≥5 mm（超过ⅠA期），癌灶仍局限在子宫颈
ⅠB1期	间质浸润深度≥5 mm，病灶最大径线<2 cm
ⅠB2期	癌灶最大径线≥2 cm，<4 cm
ⅠB3期	癌灶最大径线≥4 cm
Ⅱ期	癌灶超越子宫，但未达阴道下1/3或未达骨盆壁
ⅡA期	侵犯上2/3阴道，无宫旁浸润
ⅡA1期	癌灶最大径线<4 cm
ⅡA2期	癌灶最大径线≥4 cm
ⅡB期	有宫旁浸润，未达盆壁
Ⅲ期	癌灶累及阴道下1/3和（或）扩展到骨盆壁和（或）引起肾盂积水或肾无功能和（或）累及盆腔和（或）主动脉旁淋巴结
ⅢA期	癌肿累及阴道下1/3，没有扩散到骨盆壁
ⅢB期	癌肿扩散到骨盆壁和（或）引起肾盂积水或肾无功能
ⅢC期	不论肿瘤大小和扩散程度，累及盆腔和（或）主动脉旁淋巴结
ⅢC1期	仅累及盆腔淋巴结
ⅢC2期	主动脉旁淋巴结转移
Ⅳ期	肿瘤侵犯膀胱黏膜或直肠黏膜（活检证实）和（或）超出真骨盆（泡状水肿不分为Ⅳ期）
ⅣA期	转移至邻近器官
ⅣB期	转移到远处器官

3.转移途径

（1）直接蔓延　最常见。癌组织直接侵犯相邻组织和器官，向下蔓延至阴道，向上经子宫颈管累及宫腔；也可向两侧蔓延至子宫主韧带、阴道旁组织甚至骨盆壁；向前、后蔓延侵犯膀胱、直肠等，可形成生殖道瘘。

（2）淋巴转移　癌组织通过病灶周围的淋巴管侵入局部淋巴结，向子宫旁或子宫颈旁、闭孔、髂内、髂外、髂总、骶前、腹股沟、腹主动脉旁淋巴结蔓延，晚期可出现锁骨上淋巴结转移。

（3）血行转移　极少见，发生在晚期。癌组织破坏小静脉后，随体循环转移到肺、肝或骨骼等处。

4.临床表现　早期子宫颈癌常无明显症状和体征。子宫颈管型患者因子宫颈外观正常易漏诊或误诊。随病变发展，可出现以下表现。

（1）阴道流血　常表现为接触性出血，即性生活或妇科检查后阴道流血。也可表现为不规则阴道流血，或经期延长、经量增多。老年患者常为绝经后不规则阴道流血。出血量根据病灶大小、侵及间质内血管情况而不同,若侵蚀大血管可引起大出血。一般外生型癌出血较早,量多;内生型癌出血较晚。

(2)阴道排液 多数患者有白色或血性、稀薄如水样或米汤状、有腥臭味的阴道排液。晚期患者因癌组织坏死伴感染,可有大量米汤样或脓性恶臭白带。

(3)疼痛 子宫颈癌晚期,根据癌灶累及范围出现不同的继发性症状,如尿频、尿急、便秘、下肢肿痛等。癌肿压迫或累及输尿管时,可引起输尿管梗阻、肾盂积水及尿毒症。晚期可有贫血、恶病质等全身衰竭症状。

5. 处理原则 根据患者的年龄、有无生育要求、临床分期、全身情况等综合分析确定治疗方案,原则是手术和放疗为主,化疗为辅的综合治疗。

(1)SIL 的处理

1)LSIL 约 60% 会自然消退,细胞学检查为 LSIL 及以下者可仅观察随访。在随访过程中病变发展或持续存在 2 年者宜进行治疗。细胞学为 HSIL,阴道镜检查充分者可采用冷冻和激光等消融治疗;若阴道镜检查不充分或不能排除 HSIL 或子宫颈管搔刮术(endocervical curettage,ECC)阳性者采用子宫颈锥切术。

2)HSIL 可发展为浸润癌,需要治疗。阴道镜检查充分者可行子宫颈锥切术或消融治疗;阴道镜检查不充分者宜采用子宫颈锥切术,包括子宫颈环形电切术(loop electrosurgical excision procedure,LEEP)和冷刀锥切术。经子宫颈锥切术确诊、年龄较大、无生育要求、合并有其他妇科良性疾病手术指征的 HSIL 也可行筋膜外子宫全切术。

(2)子宫颈浸润癌的处理

1)手术治疗:适用于ⅠA～ⅡA期无手术禁忌证的患者。根据病情选择不同手术方式,一般采用子宫根治术加盆腔淋巴结清扫术。优点为年轻患者可保留卵巢及阴道。

2)放疗:是子宫颈癌的主要治疗方法,适用于各期患者。放疗分为腔内及体外照射两种。外照射和腔内放疗的合理结合,可提高局部控制率。

3)全身治疗:包括全身化疗和靶向治疗、免疫治疗。化疗主要用于晚期、复发转移患者和根治性同期放化疗,也可用于手术前、后的辅助治疗。常用抗癌药物有顺铂、卡铂、紫杉醇、拓扑替康等,多采用静脉联合化疗,也可用动脉局部灌注化疗。靶向药物主要是贝伐珠单抗,常与化疗联合应用。免疫治疗如 PD-1/PD-L1 抑制剂等也已在临床试用中。

Etiology and Risk Factors

The exact etiology remains unknown. But there are numerous risk factors for cervical cancer: early onset of sexual activity, multiple sexual partners, high risk sexual partner, HPV infection, lower genital tract neoplasia, history of STDs (sexually transmitted diseases) cigarette smoking, HIV infection, AIDS and others form of immunosuppression, multiparity.

Pathology and Categories

The epithelium of the cervix consists of columnar epithelium located primarily in the endocervical canal and squamous epithelium found predominantly on the ectocervix. The squamocolumnar junction, which is located near the external cervical os, is the site of ongoing squamous metaplasia and is the site at most risk of neoplasia.

• Squamous intraepithelial lesion (SIL): SIL refers to anintraepithelial lesion of squamous epithelium that represents the clinical and morphological manifestation of a productive HPV infection. Female genital tract squamous intraepithelial lesions including the cervical, vaginal and vulvar squamous intraepithelial lesions, three or two of these lesions often co-exist at the same time.

SIL was traditionally called cervical intraepithelial neoplasia (CIN) or dysplasia, means disordered growth and development of the epithelial lining of the cervix. SIL is divided into two grades (low – grade squamous intraepithelial lesion, LSIL; high – grade squamous intraepithelial lesion, HSIL) according to the different pathogenesis, mature degree of cell differentiation and the risk of development to invasive cancer. A two tier system of low – and high – grade intraepithelial lesions is more biologically relevant and histologically more reproducible than the three – tier CIN I , CIN II and CIN III terminology used in the prior edition and is therefore recommended.

- Invasive cervical cancers: Progression from dysplasia to invasive cancer requires several years. Histologically, 75% –80% of invasive cervical cancers are defined as squamous cell in origin; the other 20% – 25% comprise various adenocarcinomas. Squamous cell carcinomas are divided into well – differentiated (grade I); moderately differentiated (grade II); and poor–differentiated (grade III).

Tumor Spread

Cancer of the cervix spreads by direct invasion; lymphatic metastasis; blood – borne metastasis. Squamous cell cancers spread by direct extension to the vaginal mucosa, the lower uterine segment, the parametrium, the pelvic wall, the bladder, and the bowel. Metastasis is usually confined to the pelvis, but distant metastases can occur through lymphatic spread and, rarely, via the circulatory system to the liver, the lungs, or bones.

Clinical Manifestations

Signs and symptoms of cervical cancer will vary with the size and extent of the primary lesion or metastatic sites. The very smallest cancers will produce no symptoms and will only be detected by Pap test.

- Symptoms: Vaginal bleeding, vaginal discharge, pain. The other clinical manifestations that develop as the disease progresses relate to the areas involved in the malignant process. These include pressure on the bowel, bladder, or both; bladder irritation; rectal discharge and manifestations of ureteral obstruction. Fistula formation may occur as the malignancy erodes through the walls of adjacent organs. Weakness, weight loss, and anemia are characteristic of the late disease, although acute blood loss and anemia may occur in an ulcerating stage I lesion.

- Signs: In early stage, there is no locally difference from the normal cervix. However, as the local disease progresses, physical signs appear. Infiltrative cancer produces enlargement, irregularity, and a firm consistency of the cervix and eventually of the adjacent parametria. An exophytic growth generally appears as a friable, bleeding, cauliflower–like lesion of the portio vaginalis. Ulceration may be the primary manifestation of invasive carcinoma, in the early stages the change often is superficial, so that it may resemble chronic cervicitis. With further progression of the disease, the ulcer becomes deeper and necrotic, with indurated edges and a friable, bleeding surface. The adjacent vaginal fornices may become involved next. Eventually, extensive parametrial involvement by the infiltrative process may produce a nodular thickening of the uterosacral and cardinal ligaments with resultant loss of mobility and fixation of the cervix.

Treatment

- Treatment plan for SIL: Current treatment of SIL is limited to local ablationsor excisional procedure. Selection of treatment modality depends on multiple factors including patient's age, parity, desire for future fertility, size and severity of lesion, contour of the cervix, prior treatment for SIL and coexistingmedical condition as immunocompromised status.

● Invasive cancer：Invasive cancer cervix spreads mainly by direct extension and lymphatic dissemination. Like in any other types of cancer，both primary lesions and potential sites of spread should be evaluated and treated. The therapeutic modalities achieving this goal include primary treatment with－surgery，radiotherapy，chemotherapy or chemo－radiation. Radiation therapy can be used in all stages of disease；surgery is limited to patients with stage Ⅰ to Ⅱ.

【护理评估】

1. 健康史　询问患者的一般情况,如年龄、职业、文化程度、饮食、家庭经济状况等,了解患者的月经史、婚育史、性生活史、既往史、家族史等,特别注意与子宫颈癌发病有关的高危因素。重视年轻女性的接触性阴道出血病史,年老患者的绝经后阴道不规则流血史或异常排液情况。

2. 身体状况　早期患者一般无自觉症状,多由普查中发现异常的子宫颈刮片报告。患者随病程进展出现典型的临床症状,表现为点滴样出血或因性交、阴道灌洗、妇科检查而引起接触性出血,出血量增多或出血时间延长可致贫血;恶臭的阴道排液使患者难以忍受;当恶性肿瘤穿透邻近器官壁时可形成瘘管;晚期患者则出现消瘦、贫血、发热等全身衰竭症状。早期子宫颈癌局部可无明显表现,子宫颈光滑或与慢性子宫颈炎无明显区别。随着疾病的进展,妇科检查可见外生型、内生型或溃疡型等子宫颈局部病变。癌组织侵及阴道壁可见阴道壁赘生物,向宫旁组织侵犯时,妇科检查可扪及两侧盆腔组织增厚,结节状,癌组织浸润达盆壁,可形成"冰冻"盆腔。

3. 心理－社会支持状况　早期子宫颈癌患者多在体检中发现,得知病情后会表现出震惊、怀疑、愤怒等复杂情绪。因出现接触性出血和大量阴道排液,使患者不能正常性生活,担心会影响夫妻关系,产生巨大的心理压力;随着诊断治疗的深入,还会出现悲观、厌世的表现;害怕手术,担心治疗费用。另外,患者家属得知情况后,会表现出恐惧、焦虑,无法处理与患者沟通交流等问题,从而采取隐瞒、回避等做法。

4. 辅助检查　根据病史和身体状况,尤其有接触性出血者,应首先想到子宫颈癌的可能,需做详细的全身检查及妇科三合诊检查,并采用以下辅助检查。

(1)子宫颈细胞学检查　是 SIL 及早期子宫颈癌筛查的基本方法,细胞学检查特异性高,但敏感性较低。可选用巴氏涂片法或液基薄层细胞学检查法。筛查应在性生活开始 3 年后开始,或 21 岁以后开始,并定期复查。子宫颈细胞学检查的报告形式主要为 TBS(the Bethesda system)分类系统,该系统较好地结合了细胞学、组织学与临床处理方案,推荐使用。

液基薄层细胞学检查

(2)HPV 检测　敏感性较高,特异性较低。目前,国内外已将高危型 HPV 检测作为常规的子宫颈癌筛查手段。

(3)阴道镜检查　筛查发现有异常,如细胞学 ASC－US(意义未明的不典型鳞状细胞)伴 HPV 检测阳性或细胞学 LSIL 及以上或 HPV 检测 16/18 型阳性者,建议行阴道镜检查。

(4)子宫颈活组织检查　是确诊子宫颈鳞状上皮内病变和子宫颈癌的可靠方法。任何肉眼可疑病灶,或阴道镜诊断为高级别病变者均应行单点或多点活检。若需要了解子宫颈管的病变情况,应行 ECC。

(5)子宫颈锥切术　对子宫颈活检为 HSIL 但不能除外浸润癌者或活检为可疑微小浸润癌需要测量肿瘤范围或除外进展期浸润癌者,需行子宫颈锥切术。

(6)其他检查　子宫颈癌确诊后,应进一步做胸部 X 射线检查、淋巴造影、膀胱镜检、直肠镜检等,以帮助确定临床分期。

通过筛查和对癌前病变及时有效的治疗可以预防大部分的宫颈癌。世界卫生组织推荐,30～65 岁的妇女应进行子宫颈癌及其癌前病变的筛查,有 HIV 感染、器官移植、长期应用皮质醇激素的高危妇女筛查的起始年龄应提前。青春期女孩不推荐 HPV 检测作为筛查方法。在 30~65 岁无高危因素的妇女中,若细胞学及 HPV 检测均为阴性,筛查间隔时间可为 5 年;若仅行子宫颈细胞学检查,则筛查间隔时间为 3 年。有高危因素的妇女则可根据具体情况增加筛查频次。妊娠期 SIL 仅作观察,产后复查后再处理。

【护理诊断】

1. 恐惧　与担心子宫颈癌危及生命有关。

2. 疼痛　与癌肿浸润或手术创伤有关。

3. 有感染的危险　与生殖道流血、机体抵抗力下降有关。

4. 排尿异常　与癌肿浸润、转移及手术损伤有关。

【护理措施】

1. 一般护理　注意饮食与营养。子宫颈癌术前流血较多、手术创伤大,有的患者会出现贫血,应鼓励进食富含高能量及营养素全面的食物,根据患者的身体状况、饮食习惯,协助患者及家属计划合理食谱,贫血严重者适当输血。协助患者维持个人卫生,保持会阴清洁,勤换内衣、内裤。指导卧床的患者进行床上肢体活动,预防并发症。

2. 病情观察　注意观察阴道出血量及阴道排液情况,注意腰骶部疼痛的性质及范围,还应注意双侧腹股沟有无扪及质软的包块(淋巴囊肿)。术后患者应观察伤口渗血及渗液情况,盆腔引流管是否通畅,引流液的量、颜色、性质等。

3. 对症护理

(1)阴道流血　便后及时冲洗并更换会阴垫,每天冲洗会阴 2 次。有活动性血者需消毒纱布填塞止血,要做好交接班,按时如数取出纱布。出现阴道大出血时,配合医生做好急救处理。

(2)恶病质　消瘦者加强营养,高热时物理降温,防止并发症。

(3)手术患者　术前需每日阴道冲洗 2 次,冲洗时动作应轻柔,以免损伤子宫颈癌组织引起阴道大出血。肠道按清洁灌肠准备。术前教会患者进行肛门、阴道肌肉的缩紧与舒张练习。术后协助患者膀胱功能康复,一般留置尿管 7~14 d,甚至 21 d。术后第 2 天开始做盆底肌肉的练习。在拔尿管的前 3 d 开始夹尿管,连续 3 d 每 2 h 放 1 次尿,锻炼膀胱功能,促进排尿功能的恢复。患者于拔管后 1~2 h 自行排尿 1 次;如不能自解应及时处理,必要时重新留置尿管。拔尿管后 4~6 h 测残余尿量 1 次,若超过 100 mL 则需继续留置尿管;少于 100 mL 者每日测 1 次,2~4 次均在 100 mL 以内者说明膀胱功能已恢复。保持负压引流管的通畅:子宫颈癌根治术的患者,由于创面大,渗出较多,以及清扫了盆腔淋巴结,使淋巴回流受阻,术后常在盆腔放置引流管,一般 48~72 h 拔除。

(4)放疗　按放疗常规护理方法进行护理。放疗的近期反应有放射性直肠炎和膀胱炎,但一般能自愈。

4. 化疗用药护理　按化疗常规护理方法进行护理。

5. 心理护理　协助患者接受各种诊治方案,评估患者目前的身心状况及接受诊治方案的反应,向患者介绍有关子宫颈癌的医学常识;介绍各种诊治过程、可能出现的不适及有效的应对措施。为患者提供安全、隐蔽的环境,鼓励患者提问,与护理对象共同讨论健康问题,解除其疑虑,缓解其不安情绪,使患者能以积极态度接受诊治。术后向患者讲解较长时间留置导尿管的重要性,待膀胱功能恢复后尽早拔出导尿管,消除插导尿管导致的不良心理反应。

It is imperative that nursing staff administer health care to women be familiar with screening techniques, diagnostic procedures, and risk factors for cervical cancer, especially its premalignant precursors. Women should be informed of premalignant precursors and abnormal conditions implicating cervical cancer, so early diagnosis and treatment for them can be obtained. In addition, every woman should be involved in the cancer-prevention net and often take part in screening program. Smoking cessation, late sexual activity and low parity are recommended to decrease the risk of cervical cancer. In addition, nurses may instruct women to limit the number of sexual partners and use condoms to limit the transmission of sexually transmitted diseases and human papillomavirus.

Papanicoloau test is suggested to be performed annually during routine physical examinations. Women in high-risk groups may be advised to have semiannual examinations. The American Cancer Society (ACS) advises all asymptomatic women older than 20 years and younger than 20 years who are sexually active to have a Pap test at least every 3 years after they have had two negative test results 1 year apart. The Pap test should be scheduled between the woman's menstrual periods so that the menstrual flow does not interfere with the test interpretation. The women should not douche, use vaginal medications, or have sexual intercourse for at least 24 h before the test.

Preparation for cervical biopsy and conization. The woman should be scheduled for the biopsy in the early proliferative phase of the menstrual cycle, when the cervix is least vascular. The chosen procedure should be explained to the woman. Because a biopsy evaluates potentially malignant cells, most women become anxiety and need time to discuss their feelings and fears. The use of relaxation techniques may facilitate the woman's comfort preparation for conization is similar to preparation for cervical biopsy.

Follow-up care for the woman undergoing cervical biopsy or conization. Instruct the woman to rest and avoid activity for the next 24 h. Tell her that some vaginal discharge (often blood-tinged) usually occurs after 3-5 d and that her next two or three menstrual periods may be prolonged, heavier than usual, and possibly preceded by a dark-brown premenstrual discharge. Bleeding can occur about 1 week after the procedures when the absorbable suture placed in the surgical bed reabsorbs. Any excessive bleeding should be reported to the physician immediately. Advise her to abstain from vaginal sexual activity, avoid tampons, and avoid douching for 2 weeks to achieve hemostasis, lessen trauma, and promote healing. Risks associated with conization also include infection, uterine perforation, cervical stenosis, preterm labor in future pregnancies. The patient should be informed of the risks. Meticulous perineal hygiene minimizes the risk of infection and makes the woman more comfortable. Showers or sponge baths should be taken after the procedure, avoid tub or sitz baths.

Usually, by the end of the first postoperative week, the woman begins expressing grief about her mutilated body. At first, she may deny changes by refusing to look at the wound or stoma sites. Later, she may become depressed or withdrawn or even angry or hostile. She may then move to reality testing by asking questions about her care, learning wound care, and becoming actively involved in self-care. The woman may have mood swings, and the nurse is alert when the woman becomes depressed so that interventions can be implemented to reorient the woman to other activities. The woman needs intense emotional support if she is to adapt to her altered body image and functions.

【健康教育】

1. 提供预防保健知识,做好子宫颈癌的预防　HPV 预防性疫苗接种(一级预防),通过阻断 HPV 感染预防子宫颈癌的发生;普及、规范子宫颈癌筛查,早期发现 SIL(二级预防);及时治疗高级别病变,阻断子宫颈浸润癌的发生(三级预防);开展预防子宫颈癌知识宣教,提高预防性疫苗注射率和筛查率,建立健康的生活方式。

2. 出院后康复指导 宫颈癌患者出院后 1 个月进行首次随访;治疗后 2 年内应每 3～6 个月复查 1 次;3～5 年内每 6 个月复查 1 次;第 6 年开始每年复查 1 次。随访内容包括妇科检查、阴道脱落细胞学检查、胸部 X 射线摄片、血常规及子宫颈鳞状细胞癌抗原(SC-CA)、超声、CT 或磁共振等。如有症状随时到医院检查。少数患者出院时导尿管未拔出,应教会其保留导尿管的护理,多饮水,保持外阴清洁,活动时勿使尿袋高于膀胱口,避免尿液倒流。继续进行盆底、膀胱功能锻炼,及时到医院拔导尿管、导残余尿。康复后应逐步增加活动强度,适当参加社交活动或恢复日常工作。

任务实施

子宫颈细胞学检查操作流程见表 14-2。

表 14-2　子宫颈细胞学检查操作流程

项目	内容	
操作前准备	1. 检查者准备:洗手,戴口罩	
	2. 环境准备:关闭门窗或屏风遮挡,保护患者隐私,室内温度适宜	
	3. 物品准备 (1)一般物品:一次性垫单、阴道扩张器、一次性手套、洗手液 (2)子宫颈涂片所需特殊物品:干燥棉球、长弯钳、特殊形状的刮板、毛刷、玻片(一侧为毛玻璃)、95% 乙醇、含检查介质的小瓶 注意:根据需要选择所用形状刮板	
操作步骤	患者取膀胱截石位,臀部紧邻检查床沿,头部稍高,双手臂自然放置在床两侧,腹部放松。检查者面向患者,站立在其两腿之间。如患者病情危重,不能搬动时也可在病床上检查,检查者站立在病床的右侧	
	1. 涂片法	(1)将一张干燥的玻片取出,标记好患者姓名
		(2)正确放置阴道扩张器,暴露子宫颈后,用干棉球轻轻擦拭子宫颈表面黏液样分泌物后进行涂片做细胞学检查。注意:擦拭力度要轻柔以免子宫颈脱落细胞丢失
		(3)用特制的小刮板的一头伸入子宫颈管,另一头贴附在子宫颈表面,以子宫颈外口为圆心沿一个方向轻轻旋转一周,将其沿一个方向涂在已准备好的玻片上
		(4)95% 乙醇固定标本,待巴氏染色后显微镜下观察细胞形态
	2. 液基薄层细胞学检查	(1)取一个装有细胞保存液体的小瓶,标记患者信息
		(2)正确放置阴道扩张器,暴露子宫颈时避免阴道扩张器触碰子宫颈,勿用干棉球等擦拭子宫颈表面
		(3)用专用的特制毛刷伸入子宫颈管约 1 cm,以子宫颈外口为中心,旋转 360°～720° 后取出并将毛刷头浸泡至保存液体中备检
		(4)如遇子宫颈肥大患者,应注意刷取子宫颈表面旋转毛刷不能刷到的区域,特别是鳞-柱上皮交界处。如有必要可使用刮板补充抹片
操作后	1. 撤去中单橡胶布及一次性垫单,协助患者整理衣裤及床单位	
	2. 整理用物,处理污物	
	3. 洗手,记录	

续表14-2

项目	内容
注意事项	1. 采集标本前24~48 h内应禁性生活、阴道检查、阴道灌洗及阴道上药
	2. 使用的阴道扩张器不得涂润滑剂
	3. 采集器等用品应保持干燥
	4. 阴道流血量非常多时，除特别需要应暂缓进行子宫颈涂片
	5. 阴道炎的急性期：应先治疗阴道炎后再行子宫颈涂片检查，否则不仅易发生感染，还会影响细胞学检查结果的准确性

任务二　子宫肌瘤（Uterine Myoma）

工作情景

患者，32岁，月经量多3年，有大血块，每次经期需用3~4包卫生巾（每包20片），常感头晕、乏力。查体：面色苍白，血压90/60 mmHg，既往体健。妇科检查：子宫前位，增大如妊娠8周大小，质硬，于子宫左前方可触及一直径4 cm的硬结，无压痛，双附件（-）。Hb 80 g/L。

①该患者需做哪些辅助检查？②护理时应注意哪些事项？

任务内容

子宫肌瘤是女性生殖系统最常见的良性肿瘤，主要由子宫平滑肌和结缔组织组成，多见于30~50岁的妇女。

任务目标

◆能叙述子宫肌瘤的分类、病因、病理及继发变性、临床表现及护理措施。

◆能对子宫肌瘤患者进行护理评估。

【概述】

1.病因　子宫肌瘤确切的病因尚不清楚，可能与女性雌激素水平过高或长期刺激有关。此外，研究还证实孕激素有促进肌瘤有丝分裂、刺激肌瘤生长的作用。细胞遗传学研究显示25%~50%的子宫肌瘤患者存在染色体异常。

2.病理

（1）巨检　肌瘤多为球形实质性的结节，单个或多发，大小不一，表面光滑，与周围肌组织有明显界限。外表有被压缩的肌纤维和结缔组织构成的假包膜。肌瘤表面色淡，质地较硬，切面呈灰白色漩涡状结构。

（2）镜检　可见梭形平滑肌细胞呈漩涡状或栅状排列，中间有不等量的纤维结缔组织，细胞大小均匀，核为杆状。

（3）肌瘤变性 当肌瘤生长过快时，由于其供血不足使肌瘤失去原有典型结构，称为肌瘤变性。最多见的是玻璃样变，又名透明变性。玻璃样变之后继发囊性变。红色样变为一种特殊类型的坏死，多见于妊娠期或产褥期。患者可突发剧烈腹痛，伴发热、白细胞升高等，检查肌瘤迅速增大、压痛等；肌瘤剖面呈暗红色，如半熟的牛肉，质软、腥臭，漩涡状结构消失。蒂细的浆膜下肌瘤及绝经后妇女的肌瘤可发生钙化。少数肌瘤会发生肉瘤变。

3.分类

（1）按肌瘤所在部位分类 分为子宫体肌瘤（90%）及子宫颈肌瘤（10%）。

（2）按肌瘤与子宫肌壁的关系分类 分为以下3种类型（图14-5）。

1）肌壁间肌瘤：瘤体位于子宫肌层内，周围被正常的子宫肌层包围，两者界限清楚，为最常见的类型，占60%～70%。

2）浆膜下肌瘤：肌瘤突向子宫表面向腹腔方向生长，表面由浆膜层覆盖，约占子宫肌瘤的20%。如肌瘤基底部形成蒂与子宫相连，称带蒂浆膜下肌瘤，易发生蒂部扭转，可并发急腹症。如肌瘤向阔韧带内生长，称为阔韧带肌瘤。

3）黏膜下肌瘤：肌瘤向子宫腔突出，表面由子宫黏膜覆盖，可改变宫腔的形状，但子宫外形可无明显变化，占子宫肌瘤的10%～15%。黏膜下肌瘤易形成蒂与子宫相连，称为带蒂的黏膜下肌瘤。当蒂细长时，肌瘤可脱出于子宫颈口或延伸阴道内达外阴口。

子宫肌瘤可单发，也可多发，几种类型的肌瘤可发生在同一子宫，称为多发性子宫肌瘤。

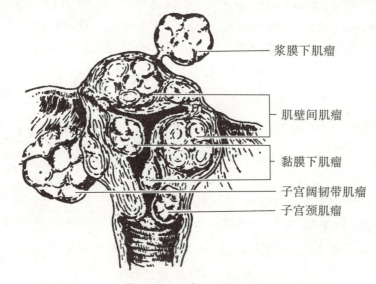

图14-5 子宫肌瘤的分类

4.临床表现 与肌瘤发生的部位、生长速度及肌瘤有无变性有关，而与肌瘤的大小、数目关系不大。一般浆膜下肌瘤或小型的肌壁间肌瘤多无症状，而黏膜下肌瘤症状出现较早。多数患者无明显的症状，仅妇科检查时发现。

（1）月经改变 多见于黏膜下肌瘤和大的肌壁间肌瘤。主要为月经量增多、经期延长、周期缩短及不规则阴道流血等，是肌瘤使子宫内膜面积增大、子宫收缩受影响或子宫内膜增生过多所致。如肌瘤发生坏死、溃疡、感染时，可有持续性或不规则阴道流血或脓血样排液。

（2）下腹包块 在肌瘤较小时常扪不到下腹部包块，当肌瘤增大超过3个月妊娠子宫大小时可在下腹部扪及。

（3）压迫症状　肌瘤长大后压迫膀胱时,可出现尿频、排尿困难或尿潴留;如压迫直肠,可出现里急后重、排便困难;压迫输尿管,可致肾盂积水。

（4）白带增多　肌壁间肌瘤使宫腔面积增大,内膜腺体分泌增多,导致白带增多,如黏膜下肌瘤脱出于阴道,表面易感染、坏死,可排出大量脓血性液体及腐肉样组织,伴臭味。

（5）继发性贫血　长期月经过多可出现全身乏力、面色苍白、气短、心悸等症状。

（6）其他　腰酸、腹痛及下腹坠胀,经期加重;当肌瘤发生蒂扭转时,患者可出现急性腹痛;肌瘤红色样变时,腹痛剧烈,并伴发热、白细胞升高等;当肌瘤压迫输卵管,或肌瘤使宫腔变形,妨碍受精、着床可造成不孕;子宫肌瘤使子宫内膜充血,胚胎供血不足,导致流产。

5. 处理原则　根据患者的年龄、生育要求、全身情况,以及肌瘤的部位、大小、数目、有无症状及症状的轻重等选择适当的治疗方案。

（1）保守治疗

1）随访观察:适用于子宫肌瘤小、无症状或症状较轻者,尤其是近绝经期妇女,因激素水平下降,肌瘤可自然萎缩。每3～6个月定期随访1次,如肌瘤增大或症状加重,应积极治疗。

2）药物治疗:适用于肌瘤小、症状轻、近绝经期或全身情况不能耐受手术者。一般采用:①促性腺激素释放激素类似物,如亮丙瑞林或戈舍瑞林,可抑制垂体、卵巢功能,降低雌激素水平,使肌瘤缩小或消失;②抗孕激素药物,如米非司酮,与孕激素竞争受体,拮抗孕激素作用。

（2）手术治疗　是目前子宫肌瘤的主要治疗方法,适用于肌瘤压迫症状严重,月经过多致继发贫血,药物治疗无效,有蒂肌瘤发生蒂扭转致急腹症,肌瘤致严重腹痛,引起不孕或反复流产及疑似恶变者等。年轻未生育、需保留子宫者,可经腹或经腹腔镜下切除肌瘤;突出子宫颈口或阴道内的黏膜下肌瘤经阴道或经宫腔镜切除。肌瘤较大、症状明显、药物治疗无效、不需保留生育功能或怀疑有恶变者,可行子宫次全切除术或子宫全切术。年龄50岁以下、卵巢外观正常者应保留卵巢。

（3）其他治疗　近年还有子宫动脉栓塞术（uterine artery embolization, UAE）、高能聚焦超声（high-intensity focused ultrasound, HIFU）、子宫内膜切除术（transcervical resection of endometrium, TCRE）等。

Etiology

The exact cause of leiomyomas is unknown. Steroid hormones, particularly estrogen, have long been recognized as promoting growth of myomas.

Pathophysiology

Leiomyomata are usually multiple, discrete and either spherical or irregularly lobulated. Their pseudocapsule usually clearly demarcates them from the surrounding myometrium. On gross examination in transverse section, myomas are buff colored, rounded, smooth and usually firm and lighter in color than the myometrium. On microscopy nonstriated muscle fibers are arranged in interlacing bundles of varying size running in different directions (whorled appearance). Individual cells are spindle shaped, have elongated nuclei and uniform in size. Varying amount of connective tissues is intermixed with the smooth muscles bundles.

Classification

Leiomyomas in the uterine body are much more frequent than in the cervix, only about 10% may appear in the cervix. Leiomyomas may be classified according to their location.

- Interstitial or intramural leiomyomas: Intramural lesions are found in the uterine wall, surrounded by myometrium. They are the most common category, representing 60%–70% of leiomyomas.

- Subserous leiomyomas: Subserous lesions represent 20% of leiomyomas. They are found on the outer surface（under the serosa）of the uterus. These tend to become pedunculated, to wander, and to be large. If a leiomyoma arises from the lateral wall of the uterus it may grow outwards between the layers of the broad ligament. This tumor is usually referred to as an intraligamentary leiomyoma. Rarely, a pedunculated leiomyoma twists on its pedicle and breaks off, when it attaches to other tissues, particularly the omentum, it is called parasitic leiomyoma.

● Submucous leiomyomas：Submucous lesions represent 10% – 15% of leiomyomas. They occur directly under the endometrium, involving the endometrial cavity. Leiomyomas may develop pedicles and protrude fully into the uterine cavity. Occasionally they may even pass through the cervical canal while still attached with the corpus by a long stalk. When this occurs, leiomyomas are subject to torsion, necrosis or infection.

Clinical Manifestations

Most uterine leiomyomas produce no any symptoms, which may be found incidentally during physical examination, during laparotomy or at autopsy. Symptoms directly attributable to leiomyomas depend mainly upon their number, size, and site and upon the presence and nature of secondary changes in the tumors.

● Abnormal uterine bleeding：The most common symptom associated with leiomyoma is abnormal uterine bleeding. The typical change is the heavier flow and the prolongation of the periods. It is most caused by intramural myomas and submucous myomas, which enlarge the surface area of endometrium and meanwhile hinder the uterine constraction. Menstrual irregularity or intermenstrual bleeding is commonly thought to be associated with submucous or peduculated myomas on the basis of either ulceration or necrosis. However, the incidence of submucous myomas is too low to explain the incidence of these conditions. Some studies demonstrate alterations in vasculature in the areas of leiomyomas that may alter normal hemostatic mechanisms. Prolonged bleeding may cause progressive anemia and debility.

● Vaginal discharge：Submucous leiomyomas enlarge the surface area of endometrium and thus the glands of the endometrium increase, secreting more fluids, so vaginal discharge increase. When infection of a pedunculated submucous myomas occurs it is always accompanied by vaginal discharge. As the infected tissues are necrotic and sloughing the discharge is purulent and frequently blood-stained.

● Abdominal swelling：Sometimes, the only complaint is of gradual enlargement of the abdomen. This symptom will obviously result from a leiomyomas of considerable size, most frequently of the subserous variety.

● Pain：Pain is not common with uncomplicated uterine myomas but may occur intermittently in cases of submucous myomas. The pain may be caused by powerful and painful uterine contractions endeavoring to expel the tumor from the wall or cavity of the uterus and generally become heavier when menstruation is present. Acute pain may result from torsion of a pedunculated leiomyoma or infarction and red or sarcomatous degeneration.

● Pressure effects：Pressure from large tumors may affect the other pelvic organs, especially bladder and rectum. Gradual pressure upon the bladder causes urinary incontinence, frequency, dysuria, and even retention of urine. Posterior myomas may lead to dyschezia, constipation or, in extreme case, obstruction.

● Infertility and spontaneous abortion：Leiomyomas are an infrequent primary cause of infertility and have been reported as a sole cause in only a small percentage of infertile patients. A large interstitial or subserous tumor may obstruct the fallopian tube, a submucous tumor may distort the uterine cavity, unsatisfactory embedding of a fertilized ovum and early spontaneous abortion may result.

Treatment

The choice of treatment depends upon the severity of symptoms, the age and general condition of the patient, the types of tumor present, or the presence of secondary changes and the type.

- Conservative management.

Expectant or observational management：Expectant or observational management is appropriate for the majority of women who have small, asymptomatic leiomyomas, especially those who are close to menopause. However, the patients should be examined at 3 – 6 months intervals to determine that rapid growth is not taking place.

Medical management：For women whose leiomyomas produce slighter symptoms, or whose poor performance status allow no surgery, GnRH agonistmay be chosen to try. The side effects of GnRH agonists are those associated with hypoestrogenism/menopause, most of which will disappear 3 – 6 months after cessation of GnRH agonist therapy. However, prolonged use of GnRH agonists has been definitely associated with significant bone loss over several months. Therefore, the use of these agents for more than 6 months has not been recommended.

- Surgical management：A pedunculated submucous leiomyoma which protrudes into the uterine cavity can be removed through the cervix, provided that the cervical canal can be dilated sufficiently to gain access to the tumor. The choice of operation in all other types of leiomyomas lies between myomectomy and hysterectomy. Where it is desirable to retain the uterus, particularly when pregnancy is desired, myomectomy or enucleation of the tumors is ideal. However, long – term problem associated with performing a myomectomy is recurrence of myomas necessitating subsequent surgery. In the older patient and where pregnancy is not desired, hysterectomy is the best method of treatment. Pre – operative treatment, especially of anemia, is most important. This may, in a few cases, necessitate curettage to stop uterine hemorrhage and thus allow time to give iron therapy or a blood transfusion, usually of packed cells.

【护理评估】

1. 健康史　了解患者月经史、生育情况、流产史及有无长期服用雌激素等用药史；询问家族史，家族中有无子宫肌瘤发病史。

2. 身体状况

（1）症状　详细评估患者的月经情况，包括何时月经发生改变，与以往比较经量和经期的变化情况；对长期经量增多的患者还要评估有无嗜睡、乏力、心悸等症状的发生及发生时间。同时还需评估白带有无改变或有无异味，有无接触性阴道流血和阴道不规则流血或血样脓性排液等现象发生。对腹部触及包块的肌瘤患者主要评估有无下腹坠胀、排尿异常或便秘等现象发生。当浆膜下肌瘤患者出现急性腹痛、恶心等急腹症表现时，应评估有无肌瘤蒂扭转发生。对妊娠和产褥期肌瘤患者出现症状，应首先评估有无肌瘤红色样变的发生。

（2）体征　肌瘤较大者可在下腹扪及质硬、不规则、结节状突起。妇科检查：子宫呈不规则或均匀性增大，质硬，表面可扪及数个结节状的突起。浆膜下肌瘤的子宫表面有球状物，可活动。黏膜下肌瘤的子宫多为均匀性增大，当肌瘤脱出于子宫颈口或阴道口时，可见有红色、表面光滑的实质性肿物，如伴有感染，表面可见溃疡，排液有臭味。

3. 辅助检查　B型超声为常用的辅助检查方法，可帮助了解肌瘤的大小、个数及部位等。也可用腹腔镜、宫腔镜、子宫输卵管碘油造影等协助诊断。

4.心理-社会支持状况　由于大多数患者无明显临床症状,是体检偶然发现,缺少思想准备。一部分患者在得知诊断时表现出惊讶、恐惧心理,会去多家医院看病重复检查,或是坚决要求住院手术切除;另一部分患者因为子宫肌瘤是良性肿瘤而表现出轻视的态度,不能按期随诊观察,配合医生治疗。有月经改变、阴道不规则流血的患者,由于影响起居和性生活,可表现出焦虑、烦躁、失眠等社会心理现象。

【护理诊断】

1.营养失调:低于机体需要量　与月经量过多,长期失血有关。

2.焦虑　与担心病情恶变及手术后遗症有关。

3.有感染的危险　与月经量增多,机体抵抗力下降有关。

4.舒适度改变　与肿瘤压迫症状及月经改变有关。

【护理措施】

1.一般护理　注意休息,加强营养,贫血者应予以高蛋白、含铁丰富的食物,减少活动量。禁止吃含有雌激素类的药品、食品或补品。

2.病情观察　对出血多的患者,严密观察患者面色、生命体征,评估并记录出血量。黏膜下肌瘤脱出者,注意观察阴道分泌物的性质、量、颜色。浆膜下肌瘤者应注意观察患者有无腹痛,腹痛部位、程度及性质,若出现剧烈腹痛,应考虑肌瘤蒂扭转,并立即通知医生,做好急诊手术准备。

3.对症护理

(1)阴道出血　保持外阴清洁与干燥,防止感染。加强营养,纠正贫血。

(2)压迫症状　压迫膀胱出现尿潴留者,应给予导尿,压迫直肠出现便秘者可行灌肠。遵医嘱做好术前准备。经阴道行黏膜下肌瘤摘除术的患者按阴道手术患者护理。子宫全切或肌瘤切除的患者,术后按妇科腹部手术患者护理。

(3)剧烈腹痛　应联系医生及时处理,必要时做好经腹急症手术的准备。

(4)白带增多　黏膜下肌瘤脱出于阴道口者,每日用消毒液行外阴冲洗,并做好外阴皮肤准备,协助医生行蒂部留置止血钳24～48 h,摘除黏膜下肌瘤。

4.用药护理　按医嘱给予止血药和子宫收缩剂止血,对贫血严重者遵医嘱输血、补液,维持正常血压并纠正贫血状态。对应用激素治疗的患者,讲明药物作用原理、剂量、用药方法、可能出现的不良反应及应对措施,告之服药过程中不能擅自停服、漏服或用药过多,以免出现撤药性出血或男性化。

5.心理护理　建立良好的护患关系,给患者及家属讲解疾病的有关知识,使患者和家属确信子宫肌瘤为良性肿瘤。对症状重需手术者,让患者及家属了解手术的必要性,纠正错误认识,共同配合治疗与护理,增强康复的信心。

Nursing Interventions

• Nursing for the women receiving conservative management: For women who don't need to receive any treatment, follow-up every 3-6 months should be informed by the nurse. For women receiving medical treatment, the nurse should make sure that they understand the effects of the medication, the way to administer the medicine, and the possible side effects of the medicine. Generally, the side effects are minor and self-limited and abate when drug is discontinued. GnRH agonist should not be used for longer than 6 months.

• Preoperative care: Frequently, a woman undergoing gynecologic surgery needs assistance in understanding her problem and the surgery being performed to correct it. She needs to understand her option and the difference between a myomectomy and a hysterectomy. Advantages and disadvantages of myomectomy versus hysterectomy should be discussed with the patient. She needs information as to what to expect postoperatively and how to care for herself. If a woman is going to have a hysterectomy, she needs to understand that her reproductive capacity will be lost. If a woman is having her ovaries removed as well, a surgical menopause should be discussed with her. It is important to remember, however, that some women are relieved at the loss of the risk of unwanted pregnancy and the disappearance of severe manifestations.

●Postoperative care: After a pedunculated submucous myoma is removed transvaginally, a hemostatic forceps should be kept on the vestige of the pedicle for 24–48 h immediately after the surgical procedure to prevent bleeding. After the hemostatic forceps is removed, the nurse should observe the vaginal bleeding and frequently change pads for the patient. Postoperative nursing care of the woman having an abdominal hysterectomy or myomectomy is similar to that of any woman having abdominal surgery. For the patients who have undergone abdominal myomectomy, the nurse should closely assess vaginal bleeding and vital signs specifically because the surgical procedure tends to interfere uterine contraction. Specific interventions for a vaginal hysterectomy include assessment of vaginal bleeding, foley catheter care, perineal care.

【健康教育】

①嘱手术患者 1 个月后到门诊复查,了解术后康复的情况,并给予自我保健指导。术后 3 个月内禁止性生活和重体力劳动。告知子宫肌瘤切除术的患者,术后应避孕 2 年以上才能考虑妊娠。让保守治疗者明确随访的时间、目的及联系方式,按时接受随访指导,以便根据病情需要修正治疗方案。②鼓励患者多参加社会活动,保持心情开朗、情绪乐观。对生育期女性做好月经相关知识宣传,增强女性自我保护意识,积极接受定期的妇科普查工作。③建立女性正确使用美容保健品的健康理念。

任务三　子宫内膜癌(Endometrial Carcinoma)

工作情景

张女士,55 岁,停经 2 年,不规则阴道流血 1 周,量少。妇科检查:子宫略大,子宫颈、阴道无明显异常。怀疑子宫内膜病变。

①确定诊断的辅助检查有哪些? ②目前患者主要存在哪些护理问题? ③该疾病应如何处理及护理?

任务内容

子宫内膜癌是发生于子宫内膜的一组上皮性恶性肿瘤,以来源于子宫内膜腺体的腺癌最常见。子宫内膜癌为女性生殖道三大恶性肿瘤之一,占女性全身恶性肿瘤 7%,占女性生殖道恶性肿瘤 20%～30%,平均发病年龄为 60 岁,其中 75% 发生于 50 岁以上妇女。近年子宫内膜癌发病率在世界范围内呈上升趋势。

任务目标

◆ 能叙述子宫内膜癌病因、临床表现、常见护理诊断、护理措施。
◆ 能对子宫内膜癌进行护理评估。

【概述】

1. 病因 病因不十分清楚,目前认为子宫内膜癌有两种发病类型。

(1)雌激素依赖型 其发生可能与长期雌激素作用而无孕激素拮抗,致使子宫内膜过度增生,继而癌变。这种类型多见,均为子宫内膜样腺癌,预后好。该类型患者较年轻,常伴有肥胖、高血压、糖尿病、不孕或绝经延迟。

(2)非雌激素依赖型 发病与雌激素无明显关系,多见老年体瘦妇女,肿瘤恶性程度高,分化差,预后不良。

2. 病理

(1)巨检 不同组织学类型内膜癌的肉眼观无明显区别。大体可分为弥散型和局灶型。弥散型:子宫内膜大部或全部为癌组织侵犯,并突向宫腔,常伴有出血、坏死,较少有肌层浸润。晚期癌灶可侵及深肌层或子宫颈,若阻塞子宫颈管可引起宫腔积脓。局灶型:多见于宫腔底部或宫角部,癌灶小,呈息肉或菜花状,易浸润肌层。

(2)镜检及病理类型 包括内膜样腺癌(占80%~90%)、腺癌伴鳞状上皮分化、透明细胞癌和浆液性乳头状腺癌。

3. 转移途径 多数子宫内膜癌生长缓慢,局限于内膜或在宫腔内时间较长,部分特殊病理类型(浆液性腺癌、鳞腺癌)和低分化腺癌可发展很快,短期内出现转移。其主要转移途径为直接蔓延、淋巴转移,晚期可有血行转移。

(1)直接蔓延 癌灶初期在子宫内膜蔓延生长,向上可沿子宫角波及输卵管,向下可累及子宫颈管及阴道。若癌瘤向肌壁浸润,可穿透子宫肌层,累及子宫浆膜层,种植于盆腹膜、直肠子宫陷凹及大网膜。

(2)淋巴转移 为子宫内膜癌的主要转移途径。

(3)血行转移 晚期经血行转移至全身各器官,常见部位为肺、肝、骨等。

4. 临床分期 采用国际妇产科联盟(FIGO,2014年)修订的手术病理分期(表14-3)。

表14-3 子宫内膜癌手术病理分期(FIGO,2014年)

分期	标准
Ⅰ期	肿瘤局限于子宫体
ⅠA期	肿瘤浸润深度<1/2肌层
ⅠB期	肿瘤浸润深度≥1/2肌层
Ⅱ期	肿瘤侵犯子宫颈间质,但无宫体外蔓延
Ⅲ期	肿瘤局部和(或)区域扩散
ⅢA期	肿瘤累及浆膜层和(或)附件
ⅢB期	阴道和(或)宫旁受累

续表 14-3

分期	标准
ⅢC 期	盆腔淋巴结和(或)腹主动脉旁淋巴结转移
ⅢC1 期	盆腔淋巴结阴性
ⅢC2 期	腹主动脉旁淋巴结阳性伴或不伴盆腔淋巴结阳性
Ⅳ 期	肿瘤侵及膀胱和(或)直肠黏膜,和(或)远处转移
ⅣA 期	肿瘤侵及膀胱和(或)直肠黏膜
ⅣB 期	远处转移,包括腹腔内和(或)腹股沟淋巴结转移

5.临床表现

(1)症状　约90%的患者出现阴道流血或阴道排液症状,在诊断时无症状者不足5%。

1)阴道流血:主要表现为绝经后阴道流血,量一般不多。尚未绝经者可表现为月经增多、经期延长或月经紊乱。

2)阴道排液:多为血性液体或浆液性分泌物,合并感染则有脓血性排液,恶臭。因阴道排液异常就诊者约占25%。

3)下腹疼痛及其他:若肿瘤累及子宫颈内口,可引起宫腔积脓,出现下腹痛及痉挛样疼痛。晚期浸润周围组织或压迫神经可引起下腹及腰骶部疼痛。晚期可出现贫血、消瘦及恶病质等相应症状。

(2)体征　早期患者妇科检查可无异常发现。晚期可有子宫明显增大,合并宫腔积脓时可有明显压痛,子宫颈管内偶有癌组织脱出,触之易出血。癌灶浸润周围组织时,子宫固定或在宫旁扪及不规则结节状物。

6.处理原则　根据患者年龄、全身情况、肿瘤累及范围和组织学类型制订适宜的治疗方案。早期以手术为主,术后根据高危因素选择辅助治疗。晚期采用手术、放疗及药物等综合治疗。

(1)手术治疗　手术治疗是首选治疗方法,手术目的是进行病理分期,Ⅰ期行筋膜外全子宫及双附件切除术;Ⅱ期行改良广泛全子宫和双附件切除术、盆腔淋巴结切除及腹主动脉旁淋巴结取样术。

(2)放疗　放疗是治疗子宫内膜癌的有效方法之一,分为腔内照射及体外照射。适用于已有转移、可疑淋巴结转移或复发的患者。

(3)化疗　化疗是晚期或复发子宫内膜癌综合治疗措施之一。也可用于有术后复发高危因素患者的治疗,以减少盆腔外远处转移。

(4)孕激素治疗　主要用于晚期或复发癌患者,也适用于极早期需要保留生育功能的年轻患者。孕激素以高效、大剂量、长期应用为宜,至少用12周以上才可评价疗效。常用药物:口服醋酸甲羟孕酮200～400 mg/d;乙酸孕酮500 mg,每周2次肌内注射。

Etiology

Classically, endometrial cancer affects the obese, nulliparous, infertile, hypertensive and diabetic women, but it can occur in absence of all these factors.

Pathology

Endometrial carcinoma may start as a discrete focal lesion as in a polyp, or it may also be diffuse in several different areas. In some situations it may involve the entire lining of the endometrial surface. Almost all endometrial carcinomas are primarily adenocarcinomas. Endometrioid adenocarcinomas are the most common carcinomas found in the endometrium, representing 80%–90% of all carcinomas.

Patterns of Spread

Most endometrial carcinomas grow slowly and are limited in uterus for a relatively long time, except some rare types. Endometrial carcinoma can spread by three routes: direct extension of tumor to adjacent sites, lymphatic dissemination, and hematogenous dissemination.

Clinical Manifestations

Endometrial carcinoma most commonly occurs in women in the sixth and seventh decades of life. About 90% of women with endometrial carcinoma have abnormal uterine bleeding, most common presentation is postmenopausal bleeding, 10% of patients may present with vaginal discharge. Occasionally patients with cervical stenosis may have a pyometra or hematometra. In more advanced disease, women may experience pelvic pressure or discomfort indicative of uterine enlargement or extra-uterine disease spread. Less than 5% of women diagnosed with endometrial cancer are asymptomatic and detected as the results of abnormal Pap smear, on pelvic sonography or CT scan for an unrelated reason.

Treatment

● Surgical therapy: The first step in the management of most endometrial cancer is surgery, which should be performed as early as possible. The extent of surgery is due to the stage of the disease. The cornerstone of treatment for endometrial carcinorma is total abdominal hysterectomy and bilateral salpingo-oophorectomy, and this operation should be performed in all cases whenever feasible. Now primary surgery followed by individualized radiation therapy has become the most widely accepted treatment for early-stage endometrial cancers.

● Irradiation therapy: For patients who are not able to undergo or tolerate a surgical procedure, radiation, including external bean and intracavitary implant, is an alternative to surgery. It should be noted, however, that radiation alone has a poorer overall survival rate as compared with surgery.

● Hormone therapy: Progestins are currently recommended as initial treatment for stage Ⅰ and stage Ⅱ cancers with positive hormone receptors and for stage Ⅳ cancer when palliative treatment may be needed. If an objective response is obtained, the long-term, high-dose progestin therapy is worth trying because of their low toxicity.

【护理评估】

1. 健康史　评估患者年龄、月经史和婚育史；有无肥胖、高血压、糖尿病、不孕或绝经延迟等高危因素存在；有无长期服用雌激素或子宫内膜癌家族史。

2. 身体状况　评估患者阴道流液的特点，特别是绝经后阴道流血及尚未绝经者月经异常的情况。评估患者阴道流血的性质和量，有无下腹及腰骶部疼痛，有无食欲减退、消瘦等。盆腔检查评估有无子宫增大、变软、子宫固定等，有无癌组织自子宫颈口脱出，是否可于子宫旁扪及结节状不规则肿块。

3. 辅助检查

（1）B 型超声检查　经阴道 B 型超声检查可了解子宫大小、宫腔形状、宫腔内有无赘生物及子宫内膜厚度、肌层有无浸润及深度，为进一步检查提供参考。

（2）诊断性刮宫　是最有价值的诊断方法。如果临床怀疑有子宫颈转移或鉴别子宫内膜癌和子宫颈癌，应行分段诊刮。组织学检查是确诊子宫内膜癌的主要依据。

（3）宫腔镜检查　可直视观察子宫颈及子宫颈管内有无癌灶，其大小及部位，且可活检取材，对局灶子宫内膜癌的确诊更为准确。

4.心理状况　子宫内膜癌多发生于绝经后妇女,由于此年龄段妇女处于生理特殊时期,常有孤独无助感,在诊疗过程中面对各种检查表现出紧张不安和恐惧心理。

【护理诊断】

1.恐惧　与确诊子宫内膜癌,担心手术及预后有关。

2.舒适度减弱　与阴道排液及癌肿浸润周围组织导致疼痛有关。

【护理措施】

1.治疗配合

(1)手术治疗的护理　按照妇科腹部手术的要求,做好术前准备和术后护理。尤其注意术后阴道残端愈合情况,严密观察阴道流血量、颜色、性状等,若有出血或感染应及时通知医生处理,并做好记录。

(2)放疗的护理　患者按放疗常规护理。接受盆腔内放疗者,为避免放射性损伤,事先灌肠并留置导尿管,以保持直肠及膀胱空虚。腔内照射期间,在保证患者卧床同时,在床上适当进行肢体活动,以免因长期卧床出现并发症。取出放射源后,鼓励患者渐进性下床活动。

(3)药物治疗的护理　化疗者,按化疗护理常规护理;孕激素用药时间长、用药量大,鼓励患者应具备足够的信心配合治疗,告知患者长期使用孕激素可有水钠潴留、水肿或药物性肝炎等不良反应,但停药后可恢复,不必担心。

2.一般护理　提供安静舒适的病房环境,嘱患者充分休息,合理饮食,增强疾病抵抗能力。阴道流血及排液多时,嘱患者取半卧位,保持外阴清洁,勤换会阴垫,每天擦洗会阴2次。

3.心理护理　积极做好沟通工作,介绍疾病的相关知识,让患者及家属能正确认识疾病,增强治疗信心。关心体贴患者,尽量陪伴,缓解患者恐惧心理。

Nursing of Patients Receiving Radiotherapy

If intracavitary radiation therapy is selected, a radiologist places an applicator within the woman's uterus through the vagina while she is anesthetized. After the correct position of the applicator is confirmed by X-ray, the radiologist places a radioactive isotope in the applicator, which remains for 1–3 d. Before the implant, the nurse instructs the patient on postprocedure activities, such as deep breathing and leg exercises. While the implant is in place, the woman is strictly isolated, usually in a private room. The nurse informs the patient that she is restricted to bed rest on her back with the head of the bed flat or slightly elevated (more than 20°). Movement in bed is restricted to prevent dislodgment of the radioactive source. The nurse inserts a Foley catheter into the bladder to prevent dislodgment of the implant, which can be caused by a full bladder or attempts to void. The nurse carefully assesses the skin for breakdown over the bony pressure points during the patient's activity restriction period. The patient is usually placed on a low-residue diet (to prevent bowel movements that might dislodge the implant), and fluid intake is encouraged (to prevent stasis of urine and possible infection).

After intracavitary radiation implant, the teaching plan includes the following information. Side effects should be reported to the physician, such as vaginal bleeding, rectal bleeding, foul-smelling discharge, abdominal pain or distention, hematuria. The high dose of radiation causes sterility, and vaginal shrinkage can occur. Vaginal dilators can be used with water-soluble lubricants for 10 min/d until sexual activity resumes. Vaginal douching may decrease inflammation. A normal diet may be resumed.

Radiation precautions are practiced while the implant is in place. The nurse organizes care so that minimal time is spent at the bedside. Care is given as far away from the radioactive source as possible.

Nurses who are pregnant or attempting to become pregnant are usually not assigned to these patients. Visitors are restricted to brief visits, and pregnant women and children younger than 18 years old should not be allowed to visit.

Specific instructions for the woman having external radiation for endometrial cancer include watching for signs of skin breakdown, especially in the perineal area, no sunbathing, and no bathing over the markings outlining the treatment site. The woman also needs to know that cystitis and diarrhea are common complications, as are nutritional problems that result from alteration in taste and anorexia. Corresponding supportive care should be given to the patients with these complications.

Nursing of Patients Receiving Hormone Therapy

For the patient receiving hormone therapy, the nurse should underline the significance of strict medication and explain any medication prescribed in terms of dosage, schedule of administration, therapeutic effects, and possible side effects. Progestin therapy may give rise to retention of water and sodium, edema, drug hepatitis, which, however, can disappear gradually after cessation of medication. Some symptoms similar to climacteric syndrome, such as hot flashes, osteoporosis and irritable mood, are associated with the long-term use of Tamoxifen. Some patients also have nausea and vomiting, mild vaginal bleeding, even amenorrhea. When the side effects are severe, the physician should be informed and management should be performed correspondingly in time. Other nursing interventions include encourage low-salt diet; monitor weight; caution if hypertension or cardiac disease is present so patient comply with follow-up care needed.

【健康教育】

①普及防癌知识,已婚女性每年接受1次防癌检查。②积极治疗高血压、糖尿病等高危因素,绝经后阴道流血者应及时就诊。③严格掌握雌激素应用指征,指导患者正确用药及自我监护。④加强对林奇综合征妇女的监测,建议在30~35岁后每年进行1次妇科检查、经阴道超声检查和内膜活检,甚至建议在完成生育后可预防性切除子宫和双侧附件。⑤指导患者定期随访:子宫内膜癌术后2~3年内每3个月随访1次;3年后每6个月1次;5年后每年1次。随访内容包括详细询问病史、妇科检查、阴道细胞学涂片、血清CA125检测等。

任务实施

分段诊断性刮宫操作流程见表14-4。

表14-4　分段诊断性刮宫操作流程

项目	内容
操作前准备	1. 医务人员准备:穿工作服,戴口罩、帽子,洗手
	2. 核对患者床号、姓名
	3. 自我介绍
	4. 取得患者知情同意并签字,测量生命体征,评估术前无禁忌证
	5. 嘱患者排尿并清洗外阴
	6. 用物准备:诊刮包、络合碘、无菌棉签、臀下巾、棉球、纱布,手套等。检查包装是否完好,是否在有效期内
	7. 评估环境,保护患者隐私

续表 14-4

项目	内容
操作步骤	1. 垫好臀下巾,协助患者取膀胱截石位
	2. 打开诊刮包,检查灭菌指示卡
	3. 将此次操作需要的棉球及纱布取出,络合碘倒入相应容器中,包布无渗湿
	4. 正确戴手套
	5. 常规消毒外阴,顺序正确(小阴唇→大阴唇→阴阜→大腿内侧 1/3→会阴及肛周)
	6. 消毒方向:从内到外,从上到下
	7. 消毒次数 3 次,不留空隙
	8. 铺孔巾
	9. 正确选择阴道扩张器
	10. 消毒阴道
	11. 双合诊了解子宫及附件情况
	12. 用阴道扩张器暴露子宫颈,固定阴道扩张器
	13. 子宫颈钳夹持子宫颈前唇
	14. 消毒子宫颈管 2 次
	15. 纱布垫于阴道后穹隆处,用小刮匙刮子宫颈管一周,收集标本
	16. 探宫,探针弯曲方向正确,报告深度
	17. 用扩宫棒依次扩张子宫颈管至 6 号
	18. 用小刮匙刮宫腔(注意两侧宫角及宫底),收集标本
操作步骤	19. 再次探宫,探针弯曲方向正确,注意深度有无改变
	20. 检查无活动性出血,再次消毒
	21. 检查阴道内无异物残留后取下子宫颈钳、阴道扩张器
	22. 分瓶收集子宫颈和宫腔标本组织,10% 甲醛溶液固定,标记姓名、内容送检
	23. 脱手套,撤臀下巾
	24. 协助患者复位,复原衣物、被褥
	25. 交代术后注意事项:禁性生活、盆浴 2 周,追踪病理结果
	26. 做好操作记录
注意事项	1. 手套未碰触非无菌区
	2. 器械未碰触非手术区
	3. 操作熟练,操作过程中注意询问患者感受

任务四　卵巢肿瘤(Ovarian Tumor)

工作情景

患者,36岁,已婚,G_2P_1,平时月经规律。今晨无意中发现左侧下腹部有一肿块,约鸡蛋大小,按压无痛感,光滑,活动度好。遂来院检查。

①该患者最有可能发生什么情况?②为了帮助明确诊断,指导该患者进行必要的检查。③检查过后,该患者内心恐惧,此时护士应该如何进行护理?

任务内容

卵巢肿瘤是妇科常见的肿瘤,可发生于任何年龄。卵巢恶性肿瘤是女性生殖器常见的三大恶性肿瘤之一,由于卵巢位于盆腔深部,早期病变不易被发现,晚期缺乏有效治疗手段,因此卵巢恶性肿瘤死亡率居妇科恶性肿瘤之首,已成为当今严重威胁妇女生命和健康的主要肿瘤。

任务目标

◆ 能叙述卵巢肿瘤的分类及病理、临床表现、并发症、护理措施。
◆ 能对卵巢肿瘤进行评估。

【概述】

1.病因　卵巢肿瘤确切病因尚不清楚,可能与生育史、高胆固醇饮食、内分泌因素、持续排卵及家族遗传等有关。

2.分类及主要卵巢肿瘤病理特点　卵巢肿瘤组织学类型繁多,是全身各脏器原发肿瘤类型最多的器官。分类方法很多,最常用的是世界卫生组织(WHO)的卵巢肿瘤组织学分类(2014年),主要组织学类型为上皮性肿瘤、生殖细胞肿瘤、性索间质肿瘤及转移性肿瘤。

(1)卵巢上皮性肿瘤　常见,占原发性肿瘤的50%~70%,占卵巢恶性肿瘤的85%~90%,多见于中老年妇女。可分为浆液性、黏液性、子宫内膜样、透明细胞、移行细胞和浆黏液性肿瘤5类,各类别依据生物学行为进一步分类,即良性肿瘤、交界性肿瘤(不典型增生肿瘤)和癌。

1)浆液性肿瘤

• 浆液性囊腺瘤:约占卵巢良性肿瘤的25%。单侧居多,大小不等,呈球形,表面光滑,多为单房,囊内充满淡黄色清亮液体。镜下见囊壁为纤维结缔组织,内衬单层柱状上皮。

• 交界性浆液性囊腺瘤:多为双侧,中等大小。镜下见乳头分支纤细而密,无间质浸润。

• 浆液性囊腺瘤:占卵巢上皮性癌75%。多为双侧,体积较大,囊实性,腔内充满乳头状物。镜下囊壁上皮增生明显,复层排列,癌细胞异型明显,并向间质浸润。

2)黏液性肿瘤

• 黏液性囊腺瘤:占卵巢良性肿瘤的20%。多为单侧,体积较大,呈圆形或卵圆形,表皮光滑,切面常为多房,囊内充满胶冻样黏液。镜下囊壁为纤维结缔组织,内衬单层柱状上皮。

• 交界性黏液性囊腺瘤:一般较大,多为单侧,表面光滑。常为多房,镜下见细胞轻度异型性,细胞核大,无间质浸润。

● 黏液性囊腺癌:占卵巢上皮癌20%,单侧居多,瘤体较大,囊液混浊或呈血性。镜下见腺体密集,细胞异型明显,并有间质浸润。

(2)卵巢生殖细胞肿瘤　是来源于生殖细胞的肿瘤,占原发性肿瘤的20%～40%,可分为畸胎瘤、无性细胞瘤、卵黄囊瘤、胚胎性癌、非妊娠性绒癌、混合型生殖细胞肿瘤等,多发生于儿童及年轻妇女。

1)畸胎瘤:由多胚层组织构成,偶见只含有一个胚层成分。分为成熟畸胎瘤和未成熟畸胎瘤两类,肿瘤的良恶性及恶性程度取决于组织的分化程度。

● 成熟畸胎瘤:又称皮样囊肿,属于良性肿瘤,可发生于任何年龄,以20～40岁多见。多为单侧,中等大小,呈圆形或卵圆形。切面多为单房,腔内充满油脂和毛发,有时可见牙齿和骨质。恶变率2%～4%,多见于绝经后妇女。

● 未成熟畸胎瘤:属于恶性肿瘤,多见于青少年,肿瘤多为实性,由分化程度不同的未成熟胚胎组织构成,主要为原始神经组织。

2)无性细胞瘤:中度恶性,好发于青春期及生育期女性,中等大小,实性,触之如橡皮样,表面光滑,切面呈淡棕色。对放疗敏感。

3)卵黄囊瘤:又称内胚窦瘤,较罕见,常见于儿童及年轻妇女。多为单侧,肿瘤较大,呈圆形或卵圆形。镜下见疏松网状和内皮窦样结构。瘤细胞能产生甲胎蛋白(AFP),故患者血清AFP升高是诊断及监测病情的重要标志物。该肿瘤恶性程度高,预后差。

(3)卵巢性索间质肿瘤　来源于原始性腺中的性索间质组织。此类肿瘤能分泌性激素,又称功能性卵巢肿瘤。其中颗粒细胞瘤与卵泡膜细胞瘤能分泌雌激素,支持细胞-间质细胞瘤又称为睾丸母细胞瘤,具有男性化作用。

1)颗粒细胞瘤:低度恶性肿瘤,可发生于任何年龄,肿瘤能分泌雌激素。青春期前患者可出现性早熟,生育年龄患者出现月经紊乱,绝经后患者可出现不规则阴道流血,常合并子宫内膜增生,甚至癌变。镜下见颗粒细胞环绕成小圆形囊腔,呈菊花样排列。预后较好,5年生存率达80%。

2)卵泡膜细胞瘤:常与颗粒细胞瘤同时存在。切面为实性、灰白色。镜下见瘤细胞呈梭形,细胞交错排列呈漩涡状。恶性较少见,预后比卵巢上皮性癌好。

3)纤维瘤:常见于中年妇女,中等大小,表面光滑或呈结节状。镜下可见梭形瘤细胞排列呈编织状。若纤维瘤伴有胸腔积液或腹腔积液,称为梅格斯综合征(Meigs syndrome),一旦手术切除后,腹腔积液、胸腔积液自行消失。

(4)转移性肿瘤　体内任何部位如乳腺、胃、肠、生殖道、泌尿道等的原发性癌,均可能转移到卵巢。库肯勃瘤是一种特殊的转移性腺癌,原发部位在胃肠道,肿瘤为双侧,中等大小,保持卵巢原状或呈肾形。一般与周围器官无粘连,切面实性、胶质状。镜下见典型的能产生黏液的印戒细胞。

3.恶性肿瘤的转移途径　主要通过直接蔓延、腹腔种植及淋巴转移。其转移特点是盆、腹腔内广泛转移灶,以上皮性癌表现最为典型。晚期可通过血行转移至肺、胸膜及肝实质。

4.恶性肿瘤分期　目前多采用国际妇产科联盟(FIGO)的手术病理分期(表14-5)。

表14-5　原发性卵巢恶性肿瘤的手术-病理分期(FIGO,2014年)

分期	标准
Ⅰ期	肿瘤局限于卵巢
ⅠA期	肿瘤局限于一侧卵巢,包膜完整,卵巢表明无肿瘤;腹水或腹腔积液中未见癌细胞

续表 14-5

分期	标准
Ⅰ B 期	肿瘤局限于双侧卵巢,包膜完整,卵巢表明无肿瘤;腹水或腹腔积液中未见癌细胞
Ⅰ C 期	肿瘤局限于单侧或双侧卵巢并伴有如下任何一项:
Ⅰ C1 期	手术导致肿瘤破裂
Ⅰ C2 期	手术前包膜已破裂或卵巢表面有肿瘤
Ⅰ C3 期	腹水或腹腔冲洗发现癌细胞
Ⅱ 期	肿瘤累及单侧或双侧卵巢并伴有盆腔内扩散(在骨盆入口平面以下)
Ⅱ A 期	肿瘤蔓延或种植到子宫和/或卵巢
Ⅱ B 期	肿瘤蔓延到其他盆腔内组织
Ⅲ 期	肿瘤累及单侧或双侧卵巢,伴有细胞学或组织学证实的盆腔外腹膜转移或证实存在腹膜后淋巴结转移
Ⅲ A1 期	仅有腹膜后淋巴结转移(细胞学或组织学证实)
Ⅲ A1(i) 期	淋巴结转移最大直径≤10 mm
Ⅲ A1(ii) 期	淋巴结转移最大直径>10 mm
Ⅲ A2 期	显微镜下盆腔外腹膜受累,伴或不伴腹膜后淋巴结转移
Ⅲ B 期	肉眼盆腔外腹膜转移,病灶最大直径≤2 cm,伴或不伴腹膜后淋巴结转移
Ⅲ C 期	肉眼盆腔外腹膜转移,病灶最大直径>2 cm,伴或不伴腹膜后淋巴结转移(包括肿瘤蔓延至肝包膜和脾,但未转移到脏器实质)
Ⅳ 期	超出腹腔外的远处转移
Ⅳ A 期	胸腔积液细胞学阳性
Ⅳ B 期	腹腔外器官实质转移(包括肝实质转移和腹股沟淋巴结和腹腔外淋巴结转移)

5.并发症

(1)蒂扭转　为常见的妇科急腹症。约10%卵巢肿瘤可发生蒂扭转,好发于瘤蒂较长、中等大小、活动良好、重心偏向一侧的肿瘤,如成熟畸胎瘤。常发生在体位突然改变或妊娠期、产褥期子宫大小、位置发生改变时(图14-6)。扭转的蒂由骨盆漏斗韧带、卵巢固有韧带和输卵管组成。典型症状为患者突发一侧下腹部剧痛,伴恶心、呕吐甚至休克。妇科检查可触及张力较大、压痛明显的肿物,并有肌紧张。确诊后立即手术切除。

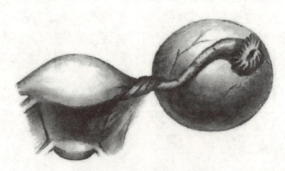

图 14-6　卵巢肿瘤蒂扭转

（2）肿瘤破裂　包括自发性破裂和外伤性破裂。症状的轻重主要取决于破裂口大小及流入腹腔囊液的量和性质。轻者无症状，严重者囊液流入腹腔，产生剧烈疼痛和腹膜刺激症状。疑有肿瘤破裂，应立即剖腹探查，切除肿瘤并彻底清洗腹腔。

（3）感染　较少见，多继发于蒂扭转或破裂后，或邻近器官感染（如阑尾脓肿）扩散。患者可有发热、腹膜刺激征及白细胞升高等。控制感染后行肿瘤切除术。

（4）恶变　若肿瘤生长迅速尤其是双侧性的，应考虑有恶变的可能，应尽快手术。

6.临床表现

（1）症状

1）卵巢良性肿瘤：肿瘤较小时一般多无症状，常在妇科检查时偶然发现。肿瘤增大时，可感觉腹胀或腹部扪及肿块。肿瘤继续增大占据盆、腹腔时，可出现尿频、便秘、气短、心悸等压迫症状。

2）卵巢恶性肿瘤：早期常无症状，晚期主要症状为腹胀、腹部肿块、腹腔积液及消化道症状。肿瘤向周围组织浸润或压迫时，可引起腰骶部或下肢部疼痛；压迫盆腔静脉可出现下肢水肿；功能性肿瘤可出现不规则阴道流血或绝经后出血；部分患者可有消瘦、贫血等恶病质表现。

（2）体征

1）卵巢良性肿瘤：检查见腹部膨隆，包块活动度好，叩诊实音，无移动性浊音。盆腔检查可在子宫一侧或双侧触及圆形或类圆形肿块，多为囊性，活动良好，表面光滑，与子宫无粘连。

2）卵巢恶性肿瘤：肿块多为双侧，三合诊检查在直肠子宫陷凹处可触及质硬结节或肿块，表面凹凸不平，实性或囊实性，与子宫分界不清，活动差，常伴有腹腔积液。有时可在腹股沟、腋下或锁骨上触及肿大的淋巴结。

7.处理原则　卵巢肿瘤一经发现，首选手术治疗。根据患者年龄、生育要求、肿瘤性质及对侧卵巢情况决定手术范围。

（1）良性肿瘤　年轻患者单侧肿瘤可行患侧卵巢肿瘤剥除或卵巢切除术；双侧肿瘤应行肿瘤剥除术。绝经后妇女宜行全子宫及双侧附件切除术。术中需判断肿瘤良恶性，必要时做冰冻切片组织学检查，明确肿瘤的性质以确定手术范围。

（2）交界性肿瘤　主要采用手术治疗。对年轻希望保留生育功能的Ⅰ期患者，可保留子宫和对侧卵巢。

（3）恶性肿瘤　以手术治疗为主，辅以化疗、放疗。晚期卵巢上皮性癌行肿瘤细胞减灭术，手术目的为尽可能切除所有原发灶和转移灶，使残余的肿瘤病灶达到最小，必要时可切除部分肠管、膀胱、脾脏等脏器。常用的化疗药物有顺铂、卡铂、紫杉醇、环磷酰胺等。

Etiology and Risk Factors

- Family history：Family history of breast or ovarian cancer is the most important risk factor. 5% – 10% of patients have an inherited genetic predisposition.

- Incessant ovulation：For other 90% –95% , most risk factors are related to a pattern of uninterrupted ovulatory cycles during the reproductive years.

- Diet：Diet high in saturated animal fats seem to confer an increased risk by unknown mechanism.

- Tubal ligation and hysterectomy：Have been associated with a substantial reduction in the risk of developing ovarian cancer.

- Genetic risk：Approximately 90% of ovarian cancer are sporadic in which familial or hereditary patterns account for 5% –10% of all malignancies.

Common Categories

- Epithelial neoplasm：Epithelial neoplasm accounts for more than 60% of all ovarian neoplasm and for more than 90% of malignant ovarian tumor.

- Germ cell neoplasm: Germ cell tumors are derived from the primordial germ cells of the ovary. Although 20% –25% of all benign and malignant ovarian neoplasm are of germ cell origin, out of which only about 3% of these tumors are malignant.

- Sex cord stromal tumors of the ovary: They account for 5% – 8% of all ovarian malignancies. This group is derived from sex cords and the ovarian stroma or mesenchyme. The tumors usually are composed of various combination of elements, including the female cells (i. e., granulosa and thecacells), and male cells (Sertoli and Leydig cells).

- Neoplasm metastatic to the ovary: Cancer metastasizing to the ovary accounts for 5% –6% of all ovarian malignancies. Most common sites are female genital tract, breast or the gastrointestinal tract.

Patterns of Spread

Ovarian cancers spread primarily by direct extension, by exfoliation of cells into the peritoneal cavity, by lymphatic dissemination, and by hematogenous spread. The most common and earliest mode of dissemination of ovarian epithelial cancer is by exfoliation of cells that implant along the surfaces of the peritoneal cavity.

Clinical Manifestations

Most tumors produce few or only mild, no specific symptoms. The most common symptoms include abdominal distension, abdominal pain or discomfort, lower abdominal pressure sensation, and urinary or gastrointestinal symptoms. If the tumor is hormonally active, symptoms of hormonal imbalance, such as vaginal bleeding and sexual precocity related to estrogen production, may be present. Acute pain may occur with adnexal torsion, cyst rupture, or bleeding into a cyst. Pelvic findings in patients with benign and malignant tumors differ. Masses that are unilateral, cystic, mobile, and smooth are most likely to be benign, whereas those that are bilateral, solid, fixed, irregular, and associated with ascites, culdesac nodules, and a rapid rate of growth are more likely to be malignant. Most often, the diagnosis of malignancies is made after abdominal dissemination has taken place, leading to impaired bowel function, decreased appetite, nausea, vomiting, changing bowel habits, and signs of peritoneal carcinomatosis, i. e., weight loss, abdominal distention, and ascites. Pain can also be caused by rapid enlargement of the ovarian tumor, as well as leakage of fluid into the peritoneal cavity and bleeding. This is more commonly seen in fast–growing tumors such as germ–cell malignancies. Often patients are initially referred for gastrointestinal evaluation, which is usually negative. Ultimately, ascites develops and the diagnosis of ovarian cancer is obvious. Decreased performance status and weakness are often present at this stage.

Treatment

- Benign tumor: Treatment of ovarian tumors that are suspected to be functional is expectant. Generally an interval of no more than 2 months is allowed, the tumor regresses if it is really functional. If the tumor does not regress or if it increases in size, it must be presumed to be neoplastic and must be removed surgically because of the risk of malignancy and other serious complications. Suspected ovarian torsion needs immediate transabdominal surgery. The type and extent of the operation to be performed depends on the type of tumor and the age of the patient. In a patient before menopause it is generally correct to remove the affected ovary for an ovarian tumor. In peri–menopausal or postmenopausal patients the uterus and the other ovary are recommended to be removed. In young women, even with bilateral tumors, ovarian cystectomy is chosen so as to conserve normal healthy ovarian tissue.

● Malignant tumor.

Surgery：In general，surgery is the cornerstone of therapy for malignant ovarian tumors. For early stage malignancies，the extent of the operation performed depends on the type of tumors，the surgical staging，the degree of differentiation，and the age of the patient. For advanced stage malignancies，cytoreductive surgery should be undertaken to remove as much of tumor and its metastases as possible. The operation to remove the primary tumor as well as the associated metastatic disease is also referred to as de-bulking surgery.

Chemotherapy：Because most ovarian malignancies are relatively sensitive to chemotherapy，chemotherapy is considered an important method to treat ovarian malignancies. Even when wide metastases or recurrence occur，chemotherapy may play an important role in controlling tumor-growth and relieving symptoms，resulting in better quality of life.

Radiotherapy：Different categories of ovarian malignancies are differently sensitive to radiation. Dysgerminomas are very sensitive to radiation therapy and may be curative by radiotherapy even for gross metastatic disease. Granulosa cell tumor and epithelial cancer are also partly sensitive to radiation.

【护理评估】

1.健康史　评估患者有无发病的高危因素，如卵巢癌家族史，高胆固醇饮食，有无乳腺癌、胃癌等其他恶性肿瘤史。了解患者的月经史和生育史。

2.身体评估

(1)症状　仔细评估患者有无腹痛、发热、腹水、下肢水肿、消瘦、贫血等症状。

(2)体征　检查评估患者腹部包块的大小、性质、和周围组织是否有粘连等。在腹股沟、腋下或锁骨上是否扪及肿大的淋巴结。

3.辅助检查

(1)B型超声检查　B型超声检查可了解肿块的大小、部位、形态、囊性或实性、囊内有无乳头。临床诊断符合率>90%，但是不易测出直径<1 cm 的实性肿瘤。

(2)肿瘤标志物

1)血清 CA125：80%卵巢上皮性癌患者血清 CA125 水平升高，90%以上患者 CA125 水平与病程进展相关，故可用于病情监测及疗效评估。

2)血清甲胎蛋白：甲胎蛋白对卵黄囊瘤有特异性诊断价值。

3)血清 hCG：血清 hCG 水平对非妊娠性卵巢绒癌诊断具有特异性。

4)性激素：颗粒细胞瘤、卵泡膜细胞瘤可产生较高水平雌激素。浆液性囊腺瘤、黏液性囊腺瘤或勃勒纳瘤有时也可分泌一定量的雌激素。

5)血清 HE4：HE4 是继 CA125 后被高度认可的卵巢上皮性肿瘤标志物。可与 CA125 联合应用判断盆腔肿块的良恶性。

(3)细胞学检查　抽取腹腔积液或腹腔冲洗液和胸腔积液，行细胞学检查。

(4)腹腔镜检查　腹腔镜检查可以直接观察肿块外观和盆腔、腹腔及横膈等部位，可在可疑部位进行多点活检，抽取腹腔积液进行细胞学检查。

4.心理-社会支持状况　卵巢肿瘤可以是良性，也可以是恶性的，检查期间患者容易焦虑、恐惧，一旦被确诊为恶性肿瘤，患者常出现悲观、绝望等心理反应。患者会因为切除卵巢影响其生育功能及出现卵巢功能衰退症状而焦虑。

【护理诊断】

1.恐惧　与卵巢肿瘤诊断有关。

2.舒适度减弱　与肿瘤压迫、腹腔积液、术后伤口疼痛等有关。

3.营养失调:低于机体需要量　与肿瘤晚期恶病质和化疗不良反应等有关。

4.自我形象紊乱　与子宫和卵巢切除、雌激素分泌不足和化疗脱发等有关。

【护理措施】

1.一般护理　加强营养,给予高蛋白、高维生素及易消化的饮食。对进食不足或全身状况极差者应给予支持治疗,必要时静脉补充营养,如输血、白蛋白、氨基酸等。避免高胆固醇饮食。创造安静的休养环境,排除不必要的刺激,使患者得到充分的休息。肿瘤过大或腹部过度膨隆的患者,应给予半卧位。

2.病情观察　注意观察患者腹痛的特点,如发生蒂扭转、破裂等,则可发生急性剧烈腹痛;恶性肿瘤浸润周围组织或压迫神经,可产生腰痛、下腹痛。重视盆腔肿块生长速度、质地,观察是否有气短、心悸、尿频、便秘等压迫症状出现及明显消瘦、贫血、水肿、衰竭等恶病质的表现。

3.心理护理　护士应该关心体贴患者,建立良好的护患关系,为患者提供安静、舒适、整洁环境,避免各种不良刺激。耐心向患者及家属介绍疾病特点及治疗方法,及时解答患者和家属提出的问题,帮助患者以积极心态配合各种治疗。鼓励患者坚持治疗,定期检查,以乐观心态融入正常生活、工作中。

4.手术患者的护理　按照腹部手术护理内容做好术前及术后护理,包括与病理科联系行快速切片组织学检查及应对必要时扩大手术范围的准备。对于巨大卵巢肿瘤患者,应备沙袋,术后腹部放置沙袋压迫,以防腹压骤然下降引起休克。

5.放腹水时的护理　对于需放腹水患者,备好腹腔穿刺用物,并协助医生完成操作。放腹水过程中,严密观察患者反应、生命体征变化及腹水性状,并记录。1次可放腹水3 000 mL左右,不宜放过多,速度宜慢。放腹水后腹部用腹带包扎,以免腹压骤降发生虚脱。

6.腹腔化疗患者的护理　注意术后留在腹腔的化疗管是否脱落。及时更换敷料,保持敷料干燥。腹腔化疗前抽腹水,将化疗药物稀释后注入腹腔,注入后指导患者更换体位,使药物尽量接触腹腔每个部位。严密观察药物对机体的毒性反应,如发现有骨髓、肝、肾、心、肺及神经系统的不良反应,应及时报告医生。

Nursing Interventions

● Psychological support:The woman who is faced with the diagnosis of advanced ovarian cancer may be concerned about dying. She needs to be encouraged to ventilate her feelings about her diagnosis. Realistic assurance, as well as accurate information about treatments, can be provided. Often, providing the woman with information about ovarian cancer and its treatment decreases her fears. Providing continuity of care, with at least one regular caregiver, may be helpful. The nurse encourages the patient to use her support system, including family members, friends, and a spiritual leader. A visit from another woman who has survived a similar disease may decrease fears. If there is recurrence, the woman may deny symptoms at first or express feelings of anger and grief. The family is often fearful of the outcome. The nurse needs to provide encouragement and support during this difficult time and help the family and the woman work through their grief and prepare for death.

● Chemotherapy nursing:For the woman receiving chemotherapy, nursing care is similar to that of the patient with choriocarcinoma. For the woman with intraperitoneal therapy, caution should be instructed that if there is a great deal of watery fluid coming out from the rectum during the instillation of the chemotherapeutic agents, the woman must report it immediately to the medical staff because the needle possibly penetrated the intestine and thus the chemotherapeutic agents entered the intestinal cavity. At that time, the installation should be stopped immediately and close observation should be given to the woman to find whether an acute abdominal pain and high temperature occur. After instillation, the woman is asked to turn frequently to facilitate the distribution of the chemotherapeutic agents throughout the peritoneal cavity (e. g., turning to the right, to the left, head down, feet down, prone, and supine).

【健康教育】

①指导患者术后 2 个月内注意休息，逐步增加运动量，避免重体力劳动。②根据术后恢复情况指导性生活，子宫全切者一般术后 3 个月内禁止性生活，以免发生感染。③大力宣传防癌知识，饮食中应增加蛋白质、维生素 A，减少胆固醇食物，预防感染。高危妇女口服避孕药有利于预防卵巢癌的发生。④开展普查普治凡 30 岁以上妇女每年进行 1 次妇科检查，高危人群不论年龄大小，最好每半年接受 1 次检查，以排除卵巢肿瘤。⑤及早手术切除实质性或囊实性，或直径>8 cm 的囊性附件包块。⑥卵巢恶性肿瘤易复发，应长期监测和随访。术后第 1 年，每 3 个月随访 1 次；术后第 2 年每 4~6 个月 1 次；第 5 年后每年随访 1 次。

任务实施

卵巢良恶性肿瘤的鉴别见表 14-6。

表 14-6　卵巢良恶性肿瘤的鉴别

疾病	病史	体征	一般情况	超声
卵巢良性肿瘤	病程长，逐渐增大	多为单侧，活动；囊性，表面光滑；常无腹腔积液	良好	为液性暗区，可有间隔光带，边缘清晰
卵巢恶性肿瘤	病程短，迅速增大	多为双侧，固定；实性或囊实性，表面不平，结节状；常有腹腔积液，多为血性，可查到癌细胞	恶病质	液性暗区内有杂乱光团、光点，或囊实性，肿块边界不清

微课　　　　　　　课件　　　　　　练习题及参考答案

（任　美）

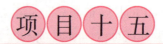

项目十五

妊娠滋养细胞疾病患者的护理（Nursing of Patients with Gestational Trophoblastic Disease）

项目描述

　　妊娠滋养细胞疾病是一组来源于胎盘绒毛滋养细胞的疾病。根据组织学特点可将其分为葡萄胎、侵蚀性葡萄胎和绒毛膜癌（简称绒癌）。虽然侵蚀性葡萄胎在组织学分类中属于交界性或不确定行为肿瘤，但其临床表现、诊断及处理原则与绒癌有相似性，临床上仍将其与绒癌一起合称为妊娠滋养细胞肿瘤。病变局限于子宫者称为无转移性滋养细胞肿瘤，病变出现在子宫以外部位者称为转移性滋养细胞肿瘤。

　　Gestational trophoblastic disease (GTD) refers to the spectrum of proliferative abnormalities of the placental trophoblast. It includes the hydatidiform mole, invasive mole, choriocarcinoma and placental site trophoblastic tumor (PSTT), which is a rare tumor has the potential to metastasize and cause death. The benign hydatidiform mole can develop into invasive hydatidiform or choriocarcinoma. Choriocarcinoma can also be derived directly from hydatidiform mole, term pregnancy, abortion or ectopic pregnancy. Trophoblastic tissue normally shares certain characteristics with malignancies, such as the ability to divide rapidly, to invade locally, and occasionally to metastasize to distant sites such as the lung, yet these activities usually cease at the end of pregnancy, and the trophoblast disappears. However, in GTD, abnormal growth and development continue beyond the end of pregnancy.

任务一　　葡萄胎（Hydatidiform Mole）

工作情景

　　结婚3年的小王终于盼来了怀孕的喜讯，心里充满了幸福感。可她刚刚怀孕10周却出现了阴道流血，急忙在丈夫的陪同下到医院就诊。医生对她进行妇科检查后又让小王化验尿 hCG 和做 B 型超声检查，然后告诉她患了葡萄胎，需立即住院治疗。小王夫妇感到十分震惊，这是怎么回事？

任务内容 //

　　葡萄胎是一种良性滋养细胞病变,主要为妊娠后胎盘绒毛滋养细胞增生,间质水肿变性,形成大小不一的水泡,水泡间借蒂相连成串,形如葡萄,故称葡萄胎,又称水泡状胎块。

任务目标 //

　　◆能叙述葡萄胎的病因、病理、临床表现、护理措施。
　　◆能对葡萄胎患者进行评估。

【概要】

　　1.病因　葡萄胎可见于任何年龄的生育期妇女,年龄<20岁及>35岁妊娠妇女的发病率明显增高,可能与该年龄阶段易发生异常受精有关。另外,营养因素、感染、孕卵异常、细胞遗传异常等可能与发病有关。

　　2.病理　葡萄胎分完全性葡萄胎和部分性葡萄胎两类,多数为完全性葡萄胎。葡萄胎病变大多局限于子宫腔内,不侵入肌层,也不发生远处转移。完全性葡萄胎大体检查见水泡状物充满宫腔,形如葡萄(图15-1),直径数毫米至数厘米不等,其间混有血块及蜕膜碎片,无胎儿及其附属物;镜下检查为滋养细胞不同程度的增生,绒毛间质水肿呈水泡样,间质内胎源性血管消失。部分性葡萄胎仅部分绒毛变为水泡,常合并胚胎或胎儿组织,胎儿多发育畸形或已死亡;镜下见部分绒毛水肿,轮廓不规则,滋养细胞增生程度轻,间质内可见胎源性血管。

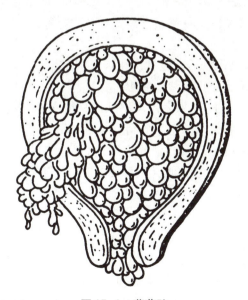

图15-1　葡萄胎

　　3.临床表现　由于诊断技术的迅速发展,越来越多的患者在未出现症状或仅有少量阴道流血时已能明确诊断并治疗,所以症状典型的葡萄胎患者已少见。典型症状如下。

　　(1)停经后阴道流血　最常见的症状,多在停经后8～12周开始出现不规则阴道流血,量多少不定,若母体血管破裂可造成大出血导致休克,有时可在阴道出血中发现水泡。若出血时间长又未及时治疗,可继发贫血和感染。

(2)子宫异常增大、变软　约半数以上患者的子宫大于正常妊娠停经月份子宫,质地极软;约1/3患者的子宫大小与正常妊娠停经月份子宫相符;极少数患者子宫小于正常妊娠停经月份子宫,其原因可能与水泡退行性变有关。

(3)卵巢黄素化囊肿　由于绒毛滋养细胞过度增生,产生大量的人绒毛膜促性腺激素(hCG)刺激卵巢内膜细胞,产生过度黄素化反应,形成卵巢黄素化囊肿(图15-2)。囊肿常为双侧,囊壁薄,表面光滑,一般无症状,偶可发生扭转。黄素化囊肿在葡萄胎清除后2~4个月可自行消退。

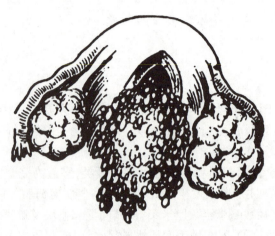

图15-2　卵巢黄素化囊肿

(4)妊娠呕吐及妊娠期高血压疾病征象　妊娠呕吐出现时间早且严重,持续时间长。妊娠期高血压疾病多发生于子宫异常增大和hCG异常升高者。可在妊娠早期出现高血压、蛋白尿和水肿,容易发展为子痫前期。

(5)腹痛　为葡萄胎增长迅速致子宫过度快速扩张所致,多为阵发性下腹痛,常发生于阴道流血之前。若黄素化囊肿扭转或破裂可出现急性腹痛。

(6)甲状腺功能亢进征象　约7%患者出现甲状腺功能亢进,表现为心动过速、皮肤潮热和震颤,三碘甲腺原氨酸(T_3)、甲状腺素(T_4)水平升高。

4.处理原则　葡萄胎一经确诊应及时清除宫腔内容物。对具有高危因素和随访有困难的患者,可考虑预防性化疗。对于有高危因素且无生育要求者可行子宫全切术,保留双侧附件。卵巢黄素化囊肿在葡萄胎清宫后会自行消退,一般不需处理。

Etiology

Hydatidiform mole may occur in any women during childbearing years. The etiology of hydatidiform mole is still unclear. The genetics of molar pregnancy has been extensively studied. Chromosomal banding techniques have provided useful information regarding the development of these tumors. Recurrent spontaneous abortion, lower socioeconomic status, poor nutrition, women younger than 20 years or older than 35 years, race and ethic origin are also the risk factors for hydatidiform mole.

Pathology

Hydatidiform molar pregnancies may be complete or partial and differentiated on the basis of histologic and cytogenetic features. In classic gross appearance of a well-developed complete hydatidiform mole, one finds the uterus enlarged and distended by thousands of watery, pale, smooth grapelike clusters of translucent villi with no trance of the embryo. In partial hydatidiform mole, only a very limited number of villi are affected. In such cases a small cluster of hydatidiform villi is found at some point in an otherwise normal placenta.

Clinical Manifestations

* Irregular vaginal bleeding: The most classic presentation is vaginal bleeding. Abnormal bleeding is present in over 90% of patients with molar pregnancies. The pathologic changes begin early, but they rarely produce symptoms until vaginal bleeding appears after 2−4 months of amenorrhea (average 12 weeks). The bleeding varies in character, as well as in the amount of blood lost. When intermittent spotting occurs, the bloody discharge is usually blackish in color, grading off to a brown, red or pink, depending on the amount loss. Bleeding may be profuse and red. Occasionally, the vaginal bleeding mixed with hydatidiform mole can be found and the passage of vesicular tissue becomes the first evidence. The associated symptoms often mimic an incomplete or threatened abortion. The prolonged bleeding without appropriate treatment will lead to anemia and subsequent infection.

* Excessive uterine size: Disproportionate uterine size is the most common sign of molar gestation. Approximately more than half of these patients have excessive uterine size for gestational date because the endometrial cavity may be expanded by chorionic tissue and retained. Excessive uterine size is generally associated with markedly elevated hCG levels. However, one fourth of the uterus is smaller than expected. Sequelae appear to be more common among those with an enlarged uterus. The rapidly expanded uterus often leads to the lower abdominal pain before vaginal bleeding. It is usually endurable and not very serious.

* Theca lutein ovarian cysts (ovary luteinizing cyst): Multiple theca cysts causing enlargement of one or both ovaries occur in some women with molar pregnancies, which is associated with a higher frequency of future sequelae as compared to those without ovarian enlargement. The development of these theca lutein cysts is believed to be secondary to the lutenizing hormone−like effect of excessive hCG stimulation on the ovary, commonly without clinical manifestation. In about half the cases, both ovaries are enlarged and may be a source of acute abdominal pain. Involution of the cysts proceeds over several weeks, usually paralleling the declining of hCG level.

* Hyperemesis gravidarum and hypertensive disorders: Nausea and vomiting are common complaints to be reported to occur in 14% − 32% of patients with hydatidiform mole. As is true in normal pregnancy, frequently excessive but at times difficult to distinguish from similar complaints. And hyperemesis gravidarum has been reported, 10% of patients with molar pregnancies have nausea and vomiting severe enough to require hospitalization. And if not correct in time, it can cause electrolyte, metabolic, and nutritional imbalances. Preeclampsia occurs in 1/4 patients. Signs of hypertensive disorder complicating pregnancy as increased blood pressure, edema, proteinuria occur before 28 gestational weeks in hydatidiform mole. But eclamptic convulsions rarely occur. The hypertensive disorder complicating pregnancy develops almost exclusively in patients with markedly elevated hCG values and excessive uterine enlargement.

* Hyperthyroidism: Mild clinical hyperthyroidism manifested by tachycardia, tremor is seen in 7% of patients with molar pregnancies. The manifestations disappear following evacuation of the mole. An occasional patient may require brief antithyroid therapy.

Principle of Management

The uterus should be emptied promptly once the diagnosis of a hydatidiform mole has been made beyond the shadow of a doubt. But to those with serious complication as pregnancy-induced hypertension syndrome, electrolyte imbalance, severe anemia, the complications should be treated first and then hydatidiform mole. The treatment of hydatidiform mole includes evacuation, treatment of complication, the prevention of malignant sequelae and follow-up after evacuation.

【护理评估】

1.健康史 询问患者的月经史、生育史,有无滋养细胞疾病史;本次妊娠早孕反应发生的时间和程度,有无阴道流血,流血的量和时间,是否有水泡状物排出。

2.身体评估 患者往往有停经后阴道流血症状,询问阴道流血的时间、出血量、是否在血中发现水泡,有无继发贫血和感染的表现。多数患者子宫大于正常妊娠停经月份子宫,质软,扪不到胎体。患者因子宫过度快速扩张可有腹部不适或阵发性隐痛,发生黄素化囊肿扭转或破裂可出现急性腹痛。少数患者可有高血压、蛋白尿和水肿等妊娠期高血压疾病征象。

3.心理-社会状况 患者及家属会担心清宫手术是否安全,是否需要进一步治疗,对今后生育有无影响,加之对妊娠滋养细胞疾病知识的缺乏和预后的不确定性等,均增加了患者的焦虑和恐惧情绪。

4.辅助检查

(1)hCG 测定 患者血清及尿中的 hCG 均增高且持续不降或超出正常妊娠水平。

(2)B 型超声检查 是诊断葡萄胎的重要检查方法。超声可见增大的子宫腔内充满不均质密集状或短条状回声,呈"落雪状",若水泡较大则呈"蜂窝状",无妊娠囊或胎心搏动。

【护理诊断】

1.功能障碍性悲哀 与妊娠的愿望得不到满足及对将来妊娠担心有关。

2.有感染的危险 与长期阴道流血、贫血造成机体抵抗力下降有关。

3.知识缺乏 缺乏葡萄胎的治疗及术后随访知识。

【护理措施】

1.心理护理 热情接待患者,详细评估患者对疾病的心理承受能力,鼓励患者表达对疾病的感受及对治疗手段的认识,确定其主要心理问题。讲解关于葡萄胎的性质、治疗、预后等疾病知识,说明尽快行清宫术的必要性。告知清宫术后应坚持随访,治愈 2 年后可正常生育,使患者消除悲哀心理,增强信心,以坦然的心态接受清宫术和术后随访。

2.严密监测病情,预防感染 观察腹痛及阴道流血情况,记录出血量,对流血多者注意血压、脉搏、呼吸等生命体征。保持外阴清洁,勤换消毒会阴垫,清宫术时,严格执行无菌技术操作和消毒隔离制度,有感染者应予隔离。

3.做好清宫术护理 告知患者清宫术的重要性,取得患者的理解和配合。清宫应由有经验的妇科医师操作。停经大于16 周的葡萄胎清宫术应在超声引导下进行。一般选用吸刮术,其具有手术时间短、出血少、不易发生子宫穿孔等优点。清宫前备血、缩宫素、抢救药品及物品,并建立静脉通路,以防治术中大出血休克。术中充分扩张子宫颈管,选用大号吸管吸引,开始吸宫后加缩宫素10 U于液体中静脉滴注。子宫颈管未扩张者不能用缩宫素,以防将水泡挤入血管,导致肺栓塞。通常 1 次刮宫即可刮净葡萄胎组织。若有持续子宫出血或超声提示有妊娠物残留,需要第二次刮宫。每次刮出物选取靠近宫壁的组织送病理检查。

Nursing Interventions

● Psychological counseling: Women need to discuss their concerns about the presence of hydatidiform mole and the potential for malignancy. The nurse provides emotional support and tries to create an atmosphere that encourages the woman to ask questions or express her fears and concerns. Significant others are included in discussions when possible. She needs information as to what to expect postoperatively and how to care for herself. If a woman is going to have a hysterectomy, she needs to understand that her reproductive capacity will be lost. It is particularly important for the woman to know that sexual intercourse will be perfectly normal following a hysterectomy. Answer honestly any questions the woman has and encourage her to express her feelings and concerns.

● Nursing for women before evacuation: The nurse helps the doctor obtain a complete history and physical examination to rule out the classic symptoms and signs that would lead to a diagnosis of severe anemia, dehydration, preeclampsia and/or hyperthyroidism. The patient should be stabilized hemodynamically and known the significance of appropriate laboratory and radiologic examination. Helps the patients do pre-evacuation hCG, a complete blood count, electrolytes, renal function, liver function tests, thyroid function test, pelvic ultrasound and chest X-ray. And evaluates these outcomes carefully and patiently.

● Nursing for women receiving evacuation: Hydatidiform mole is a benign trophoblastic disease. In general, it has a good prognosis. It is imperative that nursing staff be familiar with the diagnostic methods and risk factors for hydatidiform mole. When the diagnosis is confirmed, the uterus should be evacuated. Tell the patient the process of evacuation, the times of evacuation related to the uterus size. Assess the vaginal bleeding during and after evacuation.

【健康教育】

(1)加强随访。向患者和家属讲解坚持正规治疗和随访葡萄胎的重要性,以便尽早发现滋养细胞肿瘤并及时处理,懂得定期监测 hCG 的重要性。①意义:葡萄胎排空后,有 10% ~25% 患者可发生恶变,通过随访可及早发现滋养细胞肿瘤,以及早治疗,提高治愈率。②随访内容:监测血、尿 hCG,同时应注意有无异常阴道流血,有无咳嗽、咯血等转移症状,妇科检查及 B 型超声观察子宫复旧、黄素囊肿消退情况,必要时行胸部 X 射线检查。③随访时间:定期监测 hCG,葡萄胎清宫术后每周 1 次,直至连续 3 次监测为阴性,随后仍每个月监测 1 次,共 6 个月,然后每 2 个月监测 1 次,共 6 个月,自第一次阴性后共随访 1 年。④避孕指导:避孕时间为 6 个月,可选择避孕套和口服避孕药,一般不选宫内节育器,以免混淆子宫出血的原因。

(2)随访困难且有葡萄胎恶变的高危因素(年龄大于 40 岁,hCG>100 000 U/L,子宫明显大于相应孕周子宫,卵巢黄素囊肿直径大于 6 cm,反复葡萄胎)的患者可行预防性化疗。

(3)告知患者进食高蛋白、高维生素、易消化食物,适当活动,保证充足睡眠,以增强机体抵抗力。注意保持外阴清洁,清宫术后禁止性生活和盆浴 1 个月,以预防感染。

任务实施

出院指导是整体护理的重要组成部分,也是患者出院后继续接受护理的前提和保证。做好出院指导,保证了整体护理的连续性、系统性及完整性,能调动患者主观能动性,从而做好自我调护,避免疾病复发和并发症的发生。葡萄胎清宫术后的出院指导见表 15-1。

表 15-1　葡萄胎清宫术后的出院指导

项目	内容
出院指导方法	1. 语言教育指导：语言教育是最直接、最简洁、效果最好的方法之一。在出院前 1~2 d，根据患者的具体情况，针对不同人群的共性问题进行教育。指导患者认识影响疾病恢复的因素。教会患者有关疾病的护理知识，重点突出，形象生动。语言宜通俗易懂，反复强调重点。对内向性格者，语言适度，对患者提出的问题耐心解释；对外向性格者多讲道理。对忽视自己疾病者，重点讲明疾病的危害性及预防的重要性
	2. 书面教育指导：根据葡萄胎清宫术后患者病情观察、健康教育及随访内容、生活护理方面的注意事项，印制宣传单，要通俗易懂，患者易于理解接受
出院指导内容	1. 心理护理指导：告诉患者葡萄胎发生、发展过程，同时让患者了解葡萄胎的治疗过程，如清宫、随访等，以解除顾虑，减轻不良心理反应。告知患者虽然此次妊娠不成功，但经治疗后能恢复正常，还可以再次妊娠，增加患者战胜疾病的信心，使其能积极配合治疗
	2. 病情观察指导：患者出院后应密切观察阴道流血量、质、色及有无葡萄状内容物，有无腹痛。还应注意体温的变化，并按时服药，以预防和治疗感染。保持外阴清洁。如出现腹痛、阴道流血多或流出物有异常等情况应及时到医院治疗
	3. 生活指导 (1) 饮食指导：指导患者禁烟酒，忌食辛辣刺激食物，应进食高蛋白、高维生素、易消化的食物。并鼓励患者合理饮食，多吃水果、蔬菜，保证足够的营养 (2) 保证充足的睡眠：指导患者保证充足的睡眠，避免过度劳累。阴道流血较多或身体虚弱者，应绝对卧床休息 (3) 健康指导：患者出院后应保持外阴的清洁，并勤换内裤，预防感染。清宫术后 1 个月内禁止性生活和盆浴，严格避孕 6 个月。避免使用宫内节育器，可以采用阴茎套和口服避孕药
	4. 随访指导：定期监测 hCG，葡萄胎清宫术后每周监测 1 次，直至连续 3 次监测为阴性，随后仍每个月监测 1 次，共 6 个月，然后每 2 个月监测 1 次，共 6 个月，自第一次阴性后共随访 1 年。随访期间坚持避孕，并注意观察自身症状，如出现不规则阴道出血、咳嗽、咯血等症状应及时就诊。定期做妇科检查、盆腔 B 型超声及胸片等。复诊时要带上病历资料，做好复诊记录，以便医生更好地了解疾病的康复情况

任务二　妊娠滋养细胞肿瘤(Gestational Trophoblastic Tumor)

工作情景

　　王女士，28 岁，葡萄胎清宫术后 6 个月，现停经 2 个月，阴道不规则流血 10 d，咳嗽、痰中带有血丝 1 周，经抗感染治疗不见好转。检查子宫增大、变软，尿 β-hCG 阳性，B 型超声显示子宫腔未见胚囊，肺部 X 射线检查有棉球状阴影。

　　①该患者最可能的诊断是什么？②针对该患者的护理要点有哪些？

任务内容

妊娠滋养细胞肿瘤是滋养细胞的恶性病变,临床常见妊娠滋养细胞肿瘤有侵蚀性葡萄胎和绒毛膜癌。侵蚀性葡萄胎恶性程度较低,预后较好。绒毛膜癌恶性程度极高,发生转移早而广泛,在化疗药物问世以前,其死亡率高达90%以上,但随着诊断技术及化疗的发展,预后已得到极大的改善。

任务目标

◆ 能叙述妊娠滋养细胞肿瘤的病理、临床表现、护理措施。
◆ 能对妊娠滋养细胞肿瘤患者进行评估。

【概要】

妊娠滋养细胞肿瘤60%继发于葡萄胎,30%继发于流产,10%继发于足月妊娠或异位妊娠。侵蚀性葡萄胎仅继发于葡萄胎清宫术后,绒毛膜癌可继发于流产、足月妊娠、异位妊娠、葡萄胎清宫术后。

1. 病理　妊娠滋养细胞肿瘤多原发于子宫,肿瘤常位于子宫肌层,在子宫肌层或转移灶中见到绒毛结构为侵蚀性葡萄胎,见成片滋养细胞而无绒毛结构者为绒毛膜癌。

2. 临床表现

(1)无转移妊娠滋养细胞肿瘤　多继发于葡萄胎后,仅少数继发于流产或足月产后。

1)不规则阴道流血:葡萄胎清宫术后或流产、足月产后出现不规则阴道流血,量多少不定,或月经恢复数月后又出现阴道流血。

2)子宫复旧不良或不均匀增大:葡萄胎清宫术后4~6周子宫未恢复正常大小,质软,也可因子宫肌层内病灶部位或大小影响表现为子宫不均匀增大。

3)卵巢黄素化囊肿:由于hCG持续升高或降至正常后又升高,在葡萄胎清宫术后、流产、足月产后,卵巢黄素化囊肿持续存在。

4)腹痛:肿瘤组织穿破子宫浆膜层,可引起大出血和宫腔积血导致急性腹痛。卵巢黄素化囊肿发生蒂扭转或破裂也可出现急性腹痛。

5)假孕症状:因hCG及雌激素、孕激素的作用,患者可有乳房增大,乳头及乳晕着色,外阴、阴道、子宫颈质地变软、着色。

(2)转移性妊娠滋养细胞肿瘤　多数为绒毛膜癌,症状和体征视转移部位而异。最常见的转移部位是肺部,其次依次为阴道、盆腔、肝、脑等。各转移部位的共同特点是局部出血。

1)肺转移:常见症状为咳嗽、血痰、反复咯血、胸痛及呼吸困难,常急性发作。

2)阴道转移:转移灶常位于阴道前壁,局部表现紫蓝色结节,破溃后可大出血。

3)肝转移:为不良预后因素之一,多同时伴有肺转移。病灶较小时可无症状,也可表现右上腹部或肝区疼痛、黄疸等,若病灶穿破肝包膜可出现腹腔内出血,导致死亡。

4)脑转移:预后凶险,为主要死亡原因。按病情进展分3期。①瘤栓期:表现为一过性脑缺血症状,如短暂失语、失明、突然跌倒等。②脑瘤期:表现为头痛、喷射性呕吐、偏瘫、抽搐、昏迷。③脑疝期:表现为颅内压明显升高,脑疝形成,压迫呼吸中枢而死亡。

3.处理原则　以化疗为主,手术和放疗为辅。

Ingestational trophoblastic tumor 60% is preceded by hydatidiform mole, 30% is preceded by spontaneous abortions, 10% by normal pregnancy and ectopic pregnancy. Invasive mole is reported in 5% – 20% of patients who have had primary molar pregnancy and most within 6 months after evacuation. Choriocarcinoma is preceded by hydatidiform mole, spontaneous abortions, normal pregnancy and ectopic pre-gnancy.

妊娠滋养细胞肿瘤的化疗

Pathology

Grossly, invasive mole, a benign tumor arising from a hydatidiform mole can invade myometrium or blood vessels, and infrequently is deported to distant sites, most commonly to the lung and vagina. Choriocarcinoma occurs most at uterus. It is an interesting and not too uncommon observation to find metastases from choriocarcinoma without any gross or microscopic evidence of disease in either the endometrium or myometrium. The difference between an invasive mole and choriocarcinoma is the preservation of the villous pattern in invasive molar disease, which may be sparse in number.

Clinical Manifestations

● Manifestations of original sites.

Vaginal bleedind: Because the tumor choriocarcinoma invades blood vessels and the vaginal nodule has a tendency to necrosis, the predominant symptom is vaginal bleeding. After delivery, abortion, especially evacuation of the hydatidiform mole, vaginal bleeding appears, differing in the volume. Amenorrhea may occur because of the effect of hCG. When the primary hydatidiform mole disappears while the secondary metastasis develops, there is no vaginal bleeding.

Abdominal pain: If the tumor tissues perforate uterine, abdomen pain and intraperitoneal hemorrhage manifest.

Pelvis masses: It is possible for a choriocarcinoma to be hidden in the wall of the uterus without involving the endometrium. The only suggestion other than the rising the titer of HCG will be the size of the uterus, which either fails to involute or increases in dimension. If the primary site disappears, the enlargement of uterus will not be detected. Because of the luteining cyst, parametrium metastasis, pelvis masses be tangible in gynecological examination.

● Manifestations of metastases: Choriocarcinoma metastasize mainly through blood vessels. The most common metastatic sites are lung (80%), vagina (30%), brain (10%), liver (10%) in turns. The symptoms and signs vary greatly according to the metastatic sites.

Pulmonary metastases: Pulmonary metastases are relatively common in women with high – risk gestational trophablastic tumors. Metastasis to the lung is extremely frequent with choriocarcinoma. The first indication of trouble is often the appearance of a persistent cough, hemoptysis or simply shortness of breath. Atelectasis occurs when bronchi obstructed. If metastasis is adjacent to pleura, chest pain and hemothorax manifest. The X–ray film will confirm the presence of a solitary nodule or wide–spread metastases in the lung fields.

Vaginal metastases: Vaginal metastasis or extension may occur in nearly 50% of cases, the vaginal lesion presenting as a dark, reddish or bluish raised nodule which may resemble an angioma or an old hematoma. Indeed, excision of such a nodule, with subsequent microscopic examination, may be the first clue to existence of choriocarcinoma. Because the tumor has a tendency to necrosis, vaginal metastasis will produce a heavy bleeding.

Cerebral metastases：Brain metastases are present in 10% –15% of patients with metastatic GTD. The most common clinical symptoms at presentation are headaches, paresis, vomiting, and seizures. Most patients with CNS lesions have concomitant metastatic disease in the lungs.

Hepatic metastases：Metastasis to liver is frequently accompanied by metastasis to lung and vagina. The presence of hepatic metastases at diagnosis portends a poor prognosis for women with gestational trophoblastic tumors. Hepatic bleeding is a potentially fatal complication that can occur during treatment.

Principle of Management

Chemotherapy is the main method and the operation is the assistant, especially to invasive trophobalstic mole. Surgery is still important in controlling complication as hemorrhage or infection. Radiation is rarely used, and is usually reserved as part of combination treatment for patients with brain or liver metastasis. Chemotherapy drugs can be administered as single – agent or combined according to the condition of the patient.

【护理评估】

1. 健康史　询问患者既往史,包括妊娠滋养细胞疾病史、用药史及药物过敏史。既往曾患葡萄胎者,应了解其清宫术的时间、水泡大小及吸出组织的量,是否做过预防性化疗,治疗后阴道流血的量、时间,子宫复旧情况。收集血、尿 hCG 随访资料及肺部 X 射线检查结果。

2. 身体评估　大多数患者有阴道不规则出血,量多少因人而异。当滋养细胞穿破子宫浆膜层时则有腹腔内出血及腹痛;若发生转移,要评估转移灶症状,不同部位的转移病灶可出现相应的临床表现。

3. 心理-社会状况　由于不规则阴道流血和转移灶症状,担心疾病的预后和化疗不良反应,以及多次化疗带来的经济负担,患者和家属不能接受现实,感到恐惧和悲哀,失去治疗信心。子宫切除者担心女性特征改变或不能生育而绝望,迫切希望得到家人的关心和理解。

4. 辅助检查

(1)血、尿 hCG 测定　血清 hCG 水平升高是葡萄胎后诊断妊娠滋养细胞肿瘤的主要依据。患者常于葡萄胎排空后 9 周以上,或流产、足月产、异位妊娠后 4 周以上,血、尿 hCG 持续高水平或一度下降后又升高,排除妊娠物残留或再次妊娠,结合临床表现,诊断为妊娠滋养细胞肿瘤。

(2)超声检查　子宫正常大小或不均匀增大,肌层内可见高回声团或回声不均区域,边界清楚,无包膜。

(3)胸部 X 射线摄片　肺转移的典型 X 射线表现为棉球状或团块状阴影。

(4)组织病理学检查　在子宫肌层或子宫外转移灶中见到绒毛或退化的绒毛阴影,诊断为侵蚀性葡萄胎;若仅见到大量滋养细胞出血、坏死,绒毛结构消失,则诊断为绒毛膜癌。

【护理诊断】

1. 恐惧　与担心疾病预后不良及化疗不良反应有关。
2. 潜在并发症　如肺转移、阴道转移、脑转移。
3. 活动无耐力　与转移灶症状及化疗不良反应有关。

【护理措施】

1. 心理护理　评估患者及家属对疾病的心理反应,鼓励其说出心里痛苦,介绍有关的化疗药物及护理措施。告知患者妊娠滋养细胞肿瘤目前通过化疗治愈率达 90%,减轻其心理压力和恐惧感,树立战胜疾病的信心,配合治疗。

2.严密观察病情 观察患者有无阴道流血、腹痛及转移灶症状。记录出血量,对于出血多者应密切观察患者的血压、脉搏、呼吸,并配合医生做好抢救工作,及时做好手术准备。发现有转移灶症状者立即通知医生并配合处理。

3.对有转移灶者的护理

(1)阴道转移 ①尽量卧床休息,禁止不必要的阴道检查,配血备用,备好各种抢救物品。②若发生破溃大出血,立即通知医生并配合抢救,用纱垫或长纱布条填塞阴道压迫止血,并输血、输液防治休克,填塞的纱布条须于24~48 h内取出。保持外阴清洁,预防感染。

(2)肺转移 ①卧床休息,有呼吸困难者采取半卧位并吸氧,按医嘱给予镇静剂。②若出现大咯血,立即让患者取头低患侧卧位并保持呼吸道通畅,轻拍背部,排出积血。

(3)脑转移 ①尽量卧床休息,起床时应有人陪伴,以防因瘤栓期的一过性脑缺血而突然跌倒。②观察颅内压增高症状,记录出入水量,严格控制补液总量和速度,以防颅内压增高。③遵医嘱给予止血剂、脱水剂、吸氧等,并采取必要的措施预防抽搐及昏迷状态下的坠地损伤、咬伤及吸入性肺炎等。④做好腰椎穿刺及脑脊液 hCG 测定等项目的检查配合。

4.治疗护理 对接受化疗的患者按化疗的护理常规护理,对手术治疗的患者按妇科手术护理常规护理。

Nursing Intervention

● Psychological counseling:Women need to discuss their concerns about the presence of cancer and the potential for metastases,their fear of chemotherapy and its side reaction. The nurse provides emotional support and tries to create an atmosphere that encourages the woman to ask questions or express her fears and concerns. If it is possible, significant others should be included in discussions, since the ideas of significant others especially her partner can effect the patient's feelings greatly.

● Preventive instruction:The nurse may have responsibility for instructing women with abnormal vaginal bleeding, persistent cough or hemoptysis to do early investigation for the possibility of choriocarcinoma,as well to the patients after term delivery,abortion or ectopic pregnancy. In addition,the nurse should make sure that women be well informed of diagnostic methods about choriocarcinoma. Since there is ideal examination of choriocarcinoma by β-hCG and other image methods,the early detection of early choriocarcinoma is practical. And special attention should be given to high-risk persons for early diagnosis.

【健康教育】

①鼓励患者进食高蛋白、高维生素、易消化的食物,以增强机体抵抗力。保持外阴清洁,预防感染,节制性生活。出现转移灶症状时,应卧床休息,病情缓解后再适当活动。②出院后严密随访,第1次随访在出院后3个月,然后每6个月1次至3年,此后每年1次至5年,随访内容同葡萄胎。随访期间严格落实避孕措施,一般于化疗停止≥12个月后方可妊娠。

任务实施

葡萄胎、侵蚀性葡萄胎、绒毛膜癌的鉴别见表15-2。

表 15-2 葡萄胎、侵蚀性葡萄胎、绒毛膜癌的鉴别

疾病	先行妊娠	潜伏期	绒毛	滋养细胞增生	浸润深度	组织坏死	转移	肝、脑转移	hCG
葡萄胎	无	无	有	轻→重	蜕膜层	无	无	无	+
侵蚀性葡萄胎	葡萄胎	多在6个月以内	有	轻→重,成团	肌层	有	有	少	+
绒毛膜癌	各种妊娠	常超过12个月	无	重,成团	肌层	有	有	较易	+

任务三　化疗患者的护理(Nursing of Patients Receiving Chemotherapy)

任务内容

化学药物治疗(简称化疗)是采用化学药物在分子水平上纠正和阻断各种致癌因素所致的细胞异常增殖、杀死肿瘤细胞、抑制肿瘤细胞生长繁殖和促进肿瘤细胞分化的一种治疗方式。通过化疗许多恶性肿瘤患者的症状得到缓解,有的甚至达到基本根治。妊娠滋养细胞肿瘤是所有肿瘤中对化疗最敏感的肿瘤,是迄今预后最好的恶性肿瘤,总治愈率达 90%。

任务目标

◆ 能叙述常用化疗药物种类,化疗患者临床表现、常见护理诊断、护理措施。
◆ 能对化疗患者进行评估。

【概要】

1. 常用化疗药物种类　①烷化剂;②抗代谢药;③抗肿瘤抗生素;④植物碱类抗肿瘤药;⑤铂类化合物。

2. 化疗患者常见临床表现

(1)造血功能障碍　造血功能障碍是最常见的化疗不良反应,主要表现为外周血白细胞和血小板计数减少,严重时也可引起贫血。由于严重的骨髓抑制,患者常继发感染及出血倾向,不仅造成继续化疗的困难,甚至可危及生命。骨髓抑制现象在停药后多可自然恢复。

(2)消化道反应　最常见的消化道反应是恶心、呕吐,多在用药后 2~3 d 开始,5~6 d 后达高峰,停药后逐步好转,一般不影响继续治疗。呕吐严重者可出现电解质紊乱现象,患者可有腹胀、乏力、精神淡漠及痉挛等。此外,还可出现消化道溃疡,以口腔溃疡为明显,多数在用药后 7~8 d 出现,一般于停药后能自然消失。

(3)肝功能损害　其主要表现为用药后血转氨酶值升高,偶可见黄疸。一般在停药后一定时期内恢复,但未恢复时不能继续化疗。

(4)肾功能损害　某些药物(如环磷酰胺)对肾脏有一定的毒性,表现为尿频、尿急、尿痛,严重者可现出血性膀胱炎。

（5）神经系统损害 长春新碱对神经系统有毒性作用，表现为指、趾端麻木，复视等。氟尿嘧啶大剂量用药可使患者发生小脑共济失调。

（6）脱发和皮疹 脱发最常见于应用放线菌素 D 时，1 个疗程头发可全部脱落，但停药后均可再生。皮疹最常见于应用甲氨蝶呤后，严重者可引起剥脱性皮炎。

3. 心理反应 患者（尤其是有化疗经历的患者）常对化疗反应产生恐惧，对疾病预后及化疗效果产生怀疑。因长期多次化疗加重经济负担而焦虑，表现出对支持及帮助的渴望。

4. 辅助检查

（1）血常规 在化疗前检测白细胞计数，为用药提供依据。如用药前白细胞计数$<4.0×10^9$/L，不能用药。用药过程中白细胞计数$<3.0×10^9$/L，应停药。

（2）尿常规、肝肾功能 了解化疗药物对肝肾的毒性反应，化疗前如有异常，应暂缓化疗。化疗期间，如出现明显的肝肾功能损害，应停药。

Side Effects of Chemotherapy

• Bone marrow suppression：The bone marrow is the tissue inside some bones that produces white blood cells（WBCs），red blood cells（RBCs），and blood latelets. Damage to the blood cell–producing tissues of the bone marrow is called bone marrow suppression，and is one of the most common side effects of chemotherapy.

• Digestive system：Nausea and vomiting are two of the most common and most dreaded side effects of chemotherapy. How often the patients feel these side effects and how severe they may be depend on the drugs. The nurse explains to the patients that nausea and vomiting usually start a few hours after treatment and last a short time. Chemotherapy drugs can cause sores in the mouth and throat and can make them dry and irritated or cause them to bleed. During chemotherapy factors as drugs，poor diet，bed rest，depression，length of treatment，etc. ，lead to constipation or diarrhea.

• Kidneys and bladder affections：Some chemotherapy drugs can irritate the patient's bladder or cause temporary or permanent kidney damage. They may cause pain or burning when urinate，frequent urination，reddish or bloody urine（some chemotherapy will change the color of urine），fever.

• Nerves and muscles affections：Certain drugs can produce peripheral neuropathy，a condition that causes tingling and burning sensations or weakness or numbness in the patient's hands and feet. In addition to affecting the nerves，certain chemotherapy drugs can also affect the muscles and make them weak，tired，or sore.

• Heart damage：Certain chemotherapy drugs can damage the heart. With heart damage caused by chemotherapy，the patient may feel these symptoms：puffiness or swelling in the hands and feet；shortness of breath；dizziness；erratic heartbeats；dry cough.

• Skin problems and hair loss：The patient may have minor skin problems during treatment，including redness，itching，peeling，dryness，and acne. Chemotherapy affects the rapidly growing cells of hair follicles. The hair may become brittle and break off at the surface of the scalp，or it may simply fall out from the hair follicle.

【护理诊断】

1. 营养失调：低于机体需要量 与化疗所致的消化道反应有关。

2. 有感染的危险 与化疗引起的骨髓抑制有关。

3. 自我形象紊乱 与化疗所致的脱发有关。

4. 有口腔黏膜损伤的危险　与化疗所致口腔溃疡有关。

5. 焦虑　与担心化疗不良反应及化疗效果有关。

【护理措施】

1. 生活护理　①提供安静、舒适的休息环境,病室每日通风,病室及患者用物定期消毒,防止交叉感染。②指导患者合理进食,注意休息,保证充足的睡眠。③化疗期间,根据患者实际情况,指导其适当活动并逐渐增加活动量。

2. 改善营养状况　①与患者及家属一起制订合理营养方案。鼓励患者进食高蛋白、高热量、高维生素、易消化的食物。②尽可能照顾患者的饮食习惯,提供适合患者口味的饭菜,以增加食欲。嘱患者少量多餐,以保障能量及营养物质的摄入。③必要时遵医嘱静脉补充能量及所需营养物质。

3. 预防感染　①保持环境清洁、空气清新,病房每天通风、消毒;②加强营养,提高机体抵抗力;③保持床单清洁、平整,防止擦伤皮肤,勤洗澡,保持皮肤清洁;④限制探陪人员,嘱患者少去公共场所,以防感染;⑤监测体温、血常规变化,对全血细胞减少或白细胞减少的患者遵医嘱少量多次输新鲜血或成分输血,并进行保护性隔离;⑥遵医嘱应用抗生素。

4. 用药护理

(1)准确计算药量,保证疗效　①准确测量体重,在每个疗程的用药前及半疗程时各测1次体重,以便计算和调整药量。方法:清晨、空腹、排空大小便后测体重,并减去衣着的重量。②按医嘱剂量准确输入,在配药、输液、拔针过程中,严防药液浪费,以保证疗效。

(2)执行"三查七对",正确给药　①认真执行"三查七对"制度,特别核对化疗方案和用药顺序;②药物现配现用,一般常温放置不超过1 h;③避光药物(如放线菌素D、顺铂等)应用避光输液管及避光套,严格按医嘱控制给药速度,按计算剂量保证药物全部输入。

(3)注意保护静脉,处理药液外渗　①注意保护静脉血管,从远端开始有计划穿刺,并尽可能减少穿刺次数;②用药前先注入少量0.9%氯化钠注射液,确认穿刺无误再滴入化疗药物,发现药物外渗立即停止滴入,局部冷敷并用0.9%氯化钠注射液或1%普鲁卡因局部封闭,以减轻疼痛,防止局部组织坏死。

5. 药物不良反应的观察与护理

(1)消化道反应的护理　①合理安排用药时间,创造良好的进餐环境。②提供清淡、易消化、可口的饮食,遵医嘱给镇静止吐剂。对呕吐严重不能进食者,静脉补充营养物质。③口腔黏膜有溃疡者,应保持口腔清洁,进食前后用消毒液漱口,使用软毛牙刷刷牙,避免进食刺激性食物,必要时遵医嘱全身或局部用药。

(2)造血功能障碍的护理　按医嘱定期查血常规,对于白细胞计数$<3.0×10^9$/L者,应与医生联系考虑停药,并给予升白细胞药物。如白细胞计数$<1.0×10^9$/L,要采取保护性隔离措施,减少探视,净化空气,应用抗生素,输新鲜血或白细胞。当血小板减少到$50×10^9$/L时,应立即停药。

(3)肝肾损害的护理　定期检查肝肾功能,严密监护其功能受损时的症状及体征,以及时报告医生,采取相应措施。

6. 提供心理支持　经常巡视病房,解决患者生活需要,耐心解答患者的提问,建立良好的护患关系。向患者介绍所用药物及可能出现的不良反应、可采取的应对措施,并积极给予相应的帮助。解释脱发的原因,说明停药后头发能再生;指导患者不要用力梳理头发,为患者提供卫生帽或建议其戴假发,帮助患者修饰形象,维护自尊。

Nursing Care Before Chemotherapy

Estimate the empty abdomen weight before chemotherapy. Help the patient to do liver and renal function, blood regular test. Choose the appropriate chemotherapy schedule and calculate the exact dosage according to the weight and illness.

Nursing Care During Chemotherapy

Prepare the medication as what is prescribed, and use it instantly after preparation in case its invalidation open to air. Since many chemotherapy drugs are considered hazardous, the nurses who give chemotherapy will take precautions to avoid direct contact with the drugs while giving them to the patient. Those who are pregnant or attempting to become pregnant should pay more attention. Choose the blood vessels from the veinlet. Try to improve one's puncture skill to avoid the medication leakage. Pay attention to the drop speed and the concentration to alleviate the side effect. During the chemotherapy, observe the patients' reaction, explain any medication prescribed in terms of dosage, schedule of administration, therapeutic effects, possible side effects and the countercheck. Prepare rescue if it is necessary. Measure β-hCG titer weekly, surveillance the blood.

Nursing of Side Effects of Chemotherapy

• Bone marrow suppression: While the patient is getting chemotherapy, her blood will be regularly sampled, sometimes daily when necessary, so the numbers of these cells can be counted by a complete blood count (CBC). When WBC counts are very low, The nurse can give antibiotics to the patient as prescribed to prevent infections. Because of the risk of infections, additional chemotherapy doses may be delayed when a very low white blood cell count exists. In some situations, doctors may prescribe growth factors to keep the WBC from falling too low so that chemotherapy can be given on schedule.

• Digestive system: The best way to handle anticipatory nausea is through effective antiemetics to prevent vomiting and with relaxation techniques. It's important for nurse to take possible steps to help patients prevent mouth sore. Brush teeth and gums after every meal. Use an extra soft toothbrush and a gentle touch. Mouth, throat, and esophagus sores are temporary and usually develop 5–14 d after receiving chemotherapy. They will heal completely once chemotherapy is finished.

• Kidneys and bladder affections: Encourage the patient to drink plenty of fluids to prevent such problems. Water, juice, soup, soft drinks, broth, etc., are all considered fluids.

• Nerves and muscles affections: The nurse tells the patient to report any nerve or muscle symptoms immediately. Caution and common sense can help the patient deal with nerve and muscle problems. When the patient's fingers become numb, for example, be very careful when handling objects that are sharp, hot, or otherwise dangerous. If the patient's sense of balance is affected, move carefully and use handrails on stairs.

• Heart damage: During the treatments, heart function will be checked to ensure that no changes have occurred. Tests such as an electrocardiogram (ECG) should be performed. If problems develop, the chemotherapy drug will be stopped to prevent further permanent damage.

【健康教育】

①食物应尽量做到多样化，多吃高蛋白、高维生素、低脂肪、易消化的食物。为防止化疗引起的全血细胞下降，宜多食含铁食物，如动物肝脏、蛋黄、瘦肉等；同时可配合药膳，如党参、黄芪、当归、红枣、花生等。②告诉患者饮食前后漱口，常洗澡，更换内衣，保持皮肤清洁。③注意休息，保证充足睡眠以减少消耗。

任务实施

化疗药物应急处理流程见图15-3。

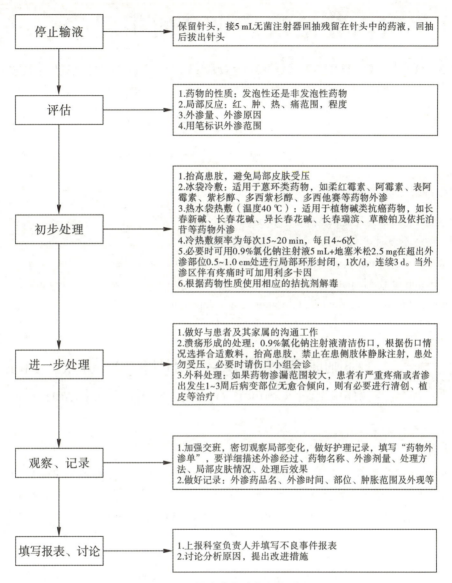

图 15-3　化疗药物应急处理流程

课件

练习题及参考答案

（张艳亭）

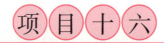

项目十六

女性生殖内分泌疾病患者的护理（Nursing of Patients with Female Reproductive Endocrine Disorders）

项目描述

　　女性生殖内分泌疾病是妇科常见病,通常由下丘脑-垂体-卵巢轴功能异常或靶器官效应异常所致,部分还涉及遗传因素、女性生殖器发育异常等。

　　Reproductive endocrine disorders is a common gynecological disease. It is usually caused by abnormal function of the hypothalamic-pituitary-ovarian axis or abnormal target organ effect, and also involves genetic factors, abnormal female genital development, etc.

任务一　排卵障碍性异常子宫出血（Abnormal Uterine Bleeding Caused by Ovulatory Dysfunction）

工作情景

　　女童,14 岁,自 12 岁初潮后月经一直不规律,月经周期 25～45 d,经期 7～15 d,量中,无痛经,未进行任何治疗。患者此次行经已有 20 余日,经量时多时少,昨日经量突然增多,故到医院就诊。体格检查:体温 36.5 ℃,脉搏 78 次/min,呼吸 18 次/min,血压 100/80 mmHg。盆腔检查:子宫前位,大小正常,活动度好,无压痛,附件未发现异常。实验室检查:红细胞计数 3.5×10^{12}/L,血红蛋白 105 g/L。既往无特殊病史。

　　①该患儿可能患有何种疾病? 如何治疗? ②护士应如何对患儿进行健康指导?

任务内容

　　正常月经的周期为 21～35 d,经期持续 2～8 d,平均失血量为 20～60 mL。凡不符合上述标准的均属异常子宫出血。引起异常子宫出血的病因很多,可由全身或生殖器官器质性病变所致,也可由生殖内分泌轴功能紊乱所致。临床上最常见的是排卵障碍性异常子宫出血,包括无排卵性和排卵性两类。

任务目标

◆ 能叙述排卵障碍性异常子宫出血的病因、分类、临床表现及处理原则。

◆ 能根据排卵障碍性异常子宫出血的临床表现选择恰当的辅助检查,从而判断其出血的类型。

◆ 能对排卵障碍性异常子宫出血患者进行整体护理。

【概述】

1. 病因

(1)无排卵性异常子宫出血　好发于青春期和绝经过渡期,但也可发生于生育期。

1)青春期:青春期下丘脑-垂体-卵巢轴激素间的反馈调节尚未成熟,大脑中枢对雌激素的正反馈作用存在缺陷,FSH 持续低水平,无 LH 高峰(排卵必须),导致无排卵。

2)绝经过渡期:因卵巢功能下降,卵泡数量极少,卵巢内剩余卵泡对垂体促性腺激素的反应低下,卵泡发育受阻而不能排卵。

3)生育期:有时因内、外环境刺激,如劳累、应激、流产、手术和疾病等引起短暂的无排卵,也可因肥胖、多囊卵巢综合征、高催乳素血症等引起持续无排卵。

各种因素造成的无排卵,均导致子宫内膜受单一的雌激素刺激,无孕激素拮抗而到达或超过雌激素的内膜出血阈值,发生雌激素突破性出血或撤退性出血。

(2)黄体功能异常

1)黄体功能不足:病因复杂,引起黄体功能不足的原因包括卵泡发育不良、LH 排卵高峰分泌不足、LH 排卵峰后低脉冲缺陷。

2)子宫内膜不规则脱落:由于下丘脑-垂体-卵巢轴调节功能紊乱或溶黄体机制失常,黄体萎缩不全,内膜持续受孕激素影响,以致不能如期完整脱落。

2. 临床表现

(1)无排卵性异常子宫出血　最常见的症状是子宫不规则出血,特点为月经周期紊乱,经期长短和经量多少不一,出血量少者仅为点滴出血,出血量多时间长者可能继发贫血,大量出血可导致休克。出血期间一般无腹痛或其他不适。

(2)黄体功能异常

1)黄体功能不足:月经周期缩短,表现为月经频发(周期<21 d)。有时月经周期虽在正常范围内,但卵泡期延长、黄体期缩短(<11 d),以致患者不易受孕或在妊娠早期流产。

2)子宫内膜不规则脱落:月经周期正常,经期延长,可达 9~10 d。

3. 治疗原则

(1)无排卵性异常子宫出血　出血期止血并纠正贫血,血止后调整周期预防复发和子宫内膜增生,有生育要求者促排卵治疗。青春期少女以止血、调整月经周期为主;生育期妇女以止血、调整月经周期和促排卵为主;绝经过渡期妇女则以止血、调整月经周期、减少经量、防止子宫内膜癌变为主。

(2)黄体功能异常

1)黄体功能不足:针对发生原因,调整性腺轴功能,促使卵泡发育和排卵,以利于正常黄体的形成。

2)子宫内膜不规则脱落:促进黄体功能,使黄体及时萎缩,内膜按时完整脱落。

Etiology

● Anovulatory abnormal uterine bleeding（AUB）：Abnormal uterine bleeding with anovulation is most common in the perimenopausal and adolescent woman.

For adolescent, immaturity of the hypothalamic-pituitary-ovarian axis（HPOA）, especially the defect to estrogen positive feedback is a common cause of AUB. Absence of LH peak results in anovulation.

For perimenopausal women, the number and quality of remaining ovarian follicles decrease. Perimenopausal women have lower follicular-phase estrogen levels in lieu to do negative feedback on pituitary. As a woman approaches menopause, at some point the peak estrogen level achieved is not of a magnitude sufficient to initiate an LH surge, and ovulation therefore does not occur.

In patients with anovulatory AUB there is continuous estrogen production without corpus luteum formation and progesterone production. The steady state of estrogen stimulation leads to a continuously proliferating endometrium, which may outgrow its blood supply or lose nutrients with varying degree of necrosis.

● Ovulatory AUB：For the patients with luteal phase defect, the FSH may be sufficient in quantity to develop an ovarian follicle and initiate ovulation, but the corpus luteum does not develop normally or does not function properly.

For the irregular shedding of endometrium patients, ovulation occurs in the menstrual cycle. Because of the dysfunction of HPOA, the corpus luteum develops well but the desquamation period prolonged.

Clinical Manifestation

● Anovulatory abnormal uterine bleeding：The clinical manifestations are different. The most common symptom is irregular uterine bleeding. In contrast to the bleeding that follows estrogen or progesterone withdrawal, the bleeding that results from chronic unopposed estrogen is not a universal event throughout the uterine cavity. Women with chronic anovulatory will present with a spectrum of menstrual irregularities. Some women remain amenorrheic, some present with heavy active bleeding after several months of amenorrhea, and some complain of light bleeding or spotting that occur at irregular intervals and can last for weeks at a time. No abdomen pain and other discomfort during bleeding. Anemia is often secondary to long-term or heavy bleeding. On bimanual examination, the uterus is in normal size and flexible when uterine bleeding occurs.

● Ovulatory abnormal uterine bleeding：For the patients with luteal phase defect, the menstrual cycle is short and the episodes of bleeding occur more frequently. The menstruation is in a normal range, and the luteal phase shortens while the follicular phase prolongs. It is difficult for them to be pregnant and abortion often occurs in early pregnancy. For the patients with irregular shedding of endometrium, the menstruation interval is normal while bleeding period prolongs to 9-10 d with heavy bleeding.

Management

● Anovulatory AUB：The management is different according to the age of the patient. The management of AUB in adolescent group is to control the hemorrhage, regulates menstruation cycle, the same time to treat the complication and to improve the holistic status of the patient. For the maternity period women is to control the hemorrhage, regulates menstruation cycle, to promote ovulate. For the perimenopausal women, the principle is to decrease hemorrhage and to regulate the menstruation cycle and to prevent endometrial cancer.

● Vulatory AUB：Promote the function of corpora lutea.

【护理评估】

1. 健康史　询问患者年龄、月经史、婚育史、避孕措施、既往史,了解患者发病前有无精神紧张、情绪打击、过度劳累及环境改变等诱发因素,了解发病时间、阴道流血情况、诊治经过等。

2. 身心状况　观察患者的精神和营养状态,有无肥胖、贫血貌、出血点、紫癜、黄疸和其他病态。进行全身体格检查,了解淋巴结、甲状腺、乳房发育情况。妇科检查常无异常发现。随着病程延长并发感染或止血效果不佳引起大量出血,患者易产生焦虑和恐惧;绝经过渡期者因担心疾病性质而焦虑不安。黄体功能不足常可引起不孕、妊娠早期流产,患者常感焦虑。

3. 辅助检查

(1) 基础体温测定(BBT)　是诊断无排卵性异常子宫出血最常用的手段,无排卵性异常子宫出血者基础体温呈单相型(图16-1)。黄体功能不全者基础体温呈双相型,但高温相上升缓慢,上升幅度偏低,高温相持续时间≤11 d(图16-2)。子宫内膜不规则脱落者基础体温呈双相型,但高温相下降缓慢(图16-3)。

(2) 刮宫或子宫内膜活组织检查　以明确子宫内膜病理诊断,而刮宫兼有诊断和止血双重作用。适用于年龄>35 岁、药物治疗无效或存在子宫内膜癌高危因素的异常子宫出血患者。为确定有无排卵或黄体功能,应在月经来潮前1~2 d或月经来潮6 h内刮宫;为尽快减少大量出血、除外器质性疾病,可随时刮宫;为确定是否子宫内膜不规则脱落,需在月经来潮第5~7天刮宫。

(3) 宫腔镜检查　可直接观察到子宫颈管、子宫内膜的生理和病理情况,直视下活检的诊断准确率显著高于盲取。

(4) 子宫颈黏液结晶检查　根据羊齿植物叶状结晶的出现与否判断有无排卵,月经前仍可见羊齿植物叶状结晶表示无排卵。目前已较少应用。

(5) 激素测定　测定雌激素、孕激素、雄激素、FSH、LH 等,了解有无排卵及卵巢功能。

(6) 其他　全血细胞计数、凝血功能检查确定有无贫血及血小板减少,排除凝血和出血障碍性疾病;尿妊娠试验或血 hCG 检测,除外妊娠相关疾病;超声检查了解子宫内膜厚度,明确有无宫腔占位性病变及其他生殖道器质性病变等。

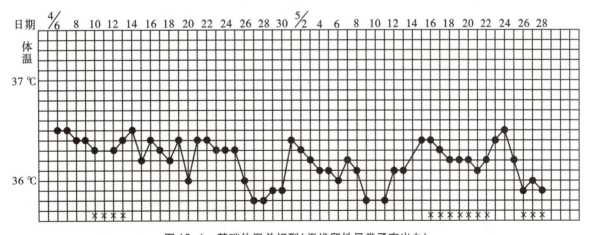

图 16-1　基础体温单相型(无排卵性异常子宫出血)

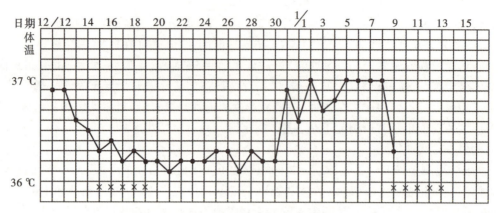

图 16-2　基础体温双相型(黄体功能不足)

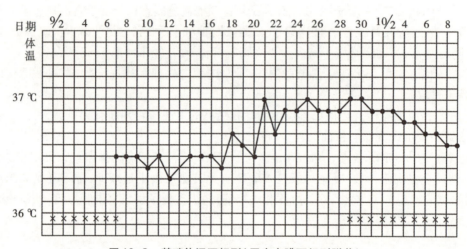

图 16-3　基础体温双相型(子宫内膜不规则脱落)

【护理诊断】

1. 疲乏　与子宫异常出血导致的贫血有关。

2. 焦虑　与反复阴道流血,担心预后有关。

3. 有感染的危险　与子宫不规则出血、出血量多导致贫血,机体抵抗力下降有关。

【护理措施】

1. 无排卵性异常子宫出血

(1)止血

1)性激素为首选药物:①孕激素,适用于流血不多、无贫血的患者。孕激素可使雌激素作用下持续增生的子宫内膜转化为分泌期,并有对抗雌激素作用,停药后出现撤药性出血,此种内膜脱落较彻底,故又称"药物性刮宫"。常用甲羟孕酮、甲地孕酮、炔诺酮等。②雌激素,可使子宫内膜增生,修复创面而止血,又称"子宫内膜修复法",适用于急性大量出血的患者。常用己烯雌酚或妊马雌酮,血止后逐渐减量,当血红蛋白达到 90 g/L 时需加用孕激素。③复方短效口服避孕药,适用于长期而严重的无排卵性出血。目前应用的是第三代短效口服避孕药,如复方屈螺酮片、去氧孕烯炔雌醇片、复方孕二烯酮片或复方醋酸环丙孕酮片。④孕激素内膜萎缩法。高效合成孕激素可使内膜萎缩,达到止血目的,此法不适用于青春期患者。

2)刮宫术:此为绝经过渡期和病程长的生育期患者的首选方法,能迅速止血,并将刮出的内膜送病理,还可明确诊断。

3)辅助治疗:①一般止血药,氨甲环酸、酚磺乙胺和维生素 K 等;②雄激素(丙酸睾酮),拮抗雌激素作用,减少盆腔充血和增加子宫血管张力,从而减少出血,适用于绝经过渡期异常子宫出血。

(2)调整月经周期 应用性激素止血后,必须调整月经周期。调整月经周期是治疗的根本,也是巩固疗效、避免复发的关键。

1)孕激素:使用范围相对广泛,适用于体内有一定雌激素水平的各年龄段的患者。可于撤退性出血第 15 天起,口服地屈孕酮 10 ~ 20 mg/d,用药 10 d;或微粒化孕酮 200 ~ 300 mg/d,用药 10 d;或甲羟孕酮 4 ~ 12 mg/d,每日分 2 ~ 3 次口服,连用 10 ~ 14 d。酌情应用 3 ~ 6 个周期。

2)口服避孕药:可很好地控制周期,尤其适用于有避孕需求的患者。一般在撤退性出血后,周期性使用口服避孕药 3 个周期,病情反复者酌情延至 6 个周期。生育期、有长期避孕需求、无避孕药禁忌证者可长期应用。

3)雌激素、孕激素序贯法:如孕激素治疗后不出现撤退性出血,考虑是否为内源性雌激素水平不足,可用雌孕激素序贯法,常用于青春期患者。

4)左炔诺孕酮宫内缓释系统:宫腔内局部释放左炔诺孕酮,抑制子宫内膜生长。适用于生育期或围绝经期、无生育需求的患者。

(3)促排卵 用于生育期、有生育需求者,尤其是不孕患者。常用促排卵药有氯米芬、人绒毛膜促性腺激素(hCG)、尿促性素(hMG)。

(4)手术治疗 手术治疗适用于药物治疗无效、无生育要求的患者,尤其是不易随访的年龄较大者。主要有子宫内膜切除术和子宫切除术。

2.有排卵性异常子宫出血 黄体功能不足患者促进卵泡发育、补充黄体功能;子宫内膜不规则脱落患者,调节下丘脑-垂体-卵巢轴的功能,促使黄体及时萎缩,内膜如期完整脱离。

(1)黄体功能不足 首选氯米芬促进卵泡发育,绒促性素促进和维持黄体功能,或选用天然孕酮补充黄体功能。

(2)子宫内膜不规则脱落 自下次月经前 10 ~ 14 d 开始,每日口服甲羟孕酮 10 mg,有生育要求者每日肌内注射黄体酮。也可用绒促性素促进黄体功能。

3.遵医嘱使用性激素 ①按时、按量正确服用性激素,保持药物在血中的稳定水平,不得随意停服和漏服。②药物减量必须按医嘱规定在血止后才能开始,每 3 d 减量 1 次,每次减量不得超过原剂量的 1/3,直至维持量。③维持量使用时间,通常结合停药后发生撤退性出血的时间与患者上次行经时间综合考虑。④告知患者在治疗期间如出现不规则阴道流血应及时就诊。

4.大出血患者的护理 观察并记录患者的生命体征,嘱患者保留出血期间使用的会阴垫及内裤,以便更准确地估计出血量。出血量较多者,督促其卧床休息,避免过度疲劳和剧烈活动。贫血严重者,遵医嘱做好配血、输血、止血等措施,以维持患者正常血容量。需要接受手术治疗的患者,按手术常规护理。

5.预防感染 严密观察与感染有关的征象,如体温、子宫体压痛等,监测白细胞计数和分类,同时做好会阴部护理,保持局部清洁。如有感染征象,应及时与医生联系并遵医嘱进行抗生素治疗。

6.心理护理 鼓励患者表达内心感受,耐心倾听患者的诉说。耐心向患者解释病情及提供相关信息,帮助其解除思想顾虑,摆脱焦虑。

Anovulatory AUB

- Control hemorrhage: To the acute heavy bleeding, hormone treatment should take effects within 6 h, control of hemorrhage within 24 – 48 h. If uterine bleeding continues beyond 96 h after hormone therapy, organic diseases should be taken into account. Progesterone (medical curettage), estrogen, oral contraceptives and progestogen endometrial atrophy method.

- Regulate the menstrual cycles: When the uterine hemorrhage has been corrected the next step is to ensure the restoration or the establishment of a normal regular cyclic menstrual pattern. This can be managed in two ways—either by employing substitution therapy until such time as the patient spontaneously ovulates and resumes a normal cycle, or attempting to induce ovulation if spontaneous recovery is too long delayed or seems unlikely to occur, especially to the adolescent, reproductive woman and the infertility.

- Stimulate the ovulation: Clomiphene, human chorionic gonadotropin, gonadotropin releasing hormone agonist are usually used.

- Surgical treatment: It is suitable for patients with ineffective drug treatment and no fertility requirements, especially for older patients who are not easy to follow-up. There are mainly endometrial removal and hysterectomy.

Ovulatory AUB

- Progesterone: In women with ovulatory AUB the progesterone receive from 10 to 14 d before next menstruation. Medroxyprogesterone in a dose of 10 mg daily for 10 d each month is a successful therapeutic regimen that produces regular withdrawal bleeding in patients with adequate amounts of endogenous estrogen to cause endometrial growth.

- hCG: hCG acts on the promotion of luteal function.

任务二　闭经（Amenorrhea）

工作情景

王某,女,18 岁,因近半年无月经来潮而就诊。月经史:12 岁初潮,周期 30 ~ 32 d,经期 5 ~ 6 d,无痛经。既往史:无特殊。半年前离家异地求学后,一直没有行经。体格检查和盆腔检查未见异常。

①该患者发生闭经的可能原因是什么? 有哪些治疗方法? ②护士要如何对患者进行健康教育?

任务内容

闭经为常见的妇科症状,表现为无月经或月经停止。根据既往有无月经来潮,分为原发性闭经和继发性闭经两类。原发性闭经指年龄超过 14 岁,第二性征未发育;或年龄超过 16 岁,第二性征已发育,月经还未来潮。继发性闭经指正常月经建立后月经停止 6 个月,或按自身原有月经周期计算停止 3 个周期以上者。原发性闭经较少见,多为遗传因素或先天性发育缺陷引起。继发性闭经发生率明显高于原发性闭经。

任务目标

◆ 能叙述闭经的概念、原因及分类。

◆ 能通过恰当的辅助检查判断闭经的部位。

【概述】

1. 病因

（1）原发性闭经　较少见，多为遗传原因或先天性发育缺陷引起。约30%患者伴有生殖道异常。根据第二性征的发育情况，分为第二性征存在和第二性征缺乏两类。

（2）继发性闭经　病因复杂，根据控制正常月经周期的5个主要环节，以下丘脑性闭经最常见，其次为垂体、卵巢、子宫性及其他内分泌功能异常引起的闭经。

1）下丘脑性闭经：指中枢神经系统及下丘脑各种功能和器质性疾病引起的闭经。常见原因有精神应激、体重下降和神经性厌食、运动性闭经、药物性闭经和颅咽管瘤等。

2）垂体性闭经：腺垂体器质性病变或功能失调，均可影响促性腺激素分泌，继而影响卵巢功能引起闭经。常见原因有希恩综合征（sheehan syndrome）、垂体肿瘤等。

3）卵巢性闭经：卵巢分泌的性激素水平低下，子宫内膜不发生周期性变化。如卵巢功能早衰、卵巢功能性肿瘤、多囊卵巢综合征等。

4）子宫性闭经：包括感染、创伤导致宫腔粘连引起的闭经。如阿谢曼（Asherman）综合征（子宫性闭经最常见原因）、手术切除子宫或放疗。

5）其他：甲状腺、肾上腺、胰腺等功能紊乱也可引起闭经。

2. 处理原则　明确病变环节及病因后，针对病因给予治疗。改善全身健康情况，进行心理治疗，给予相应激素治疗，达到治疗目的。

Etiology and Classification

A complex hormonal interaction must take place in order for normal menstruation to occur. If any of the components （hypothalamus, pituitary, ovary, outflow tract, and feedback mechanism） or the cyclic endometrium responding to steroid hormone are nonfunctional, dysfunctional menstruation even amenorrhea can occur.

● Primary amenorrhea: Primary amenorrhea is relatively uncommon. Approximately 30% of patients with primary amenorrhea have an associated genetic abnormality.

● Secondary amenorrhea: Normal female reproductive function requires intimate interaction between the hypothalamus, pituitary, ovaries, and uterus. In addition, the integrity of adrenal and thyroid gland function is essential for reproductive homeostasis. Failure of menses to appear in a woman who previously has had regular periods is called secondary amenorrhea. The incidence is 10 times to primary amenorrhea. According to the 4 sites of menstruation modulation, the hypothalamic amenorrhea （55%） is the most common one to encounter in clinic, the pituitary （20%）, ovarian （20%）, and the uterine amenorrhea （5%） in turns.

Management

● Primary amenorrhea: Absence of the uterus and ovarian dysgenesis caused by chromosomal abnormalities cannot be altered, but in some patients morale can be improved by the use of intermittent estrogen therapy. This will cause breast enlargement, and monthly withdrawal bleeding if the uterus is present by sexual hormone therapy.

- Secondary amenorrhea: The possible causes of secondary amenorrhea are many and varied. It may be due to systemic or psychic unrest. The primary source for the difficulty may rest in the ovary, thyroid, adrenal or central nervous system. The kind of treatment and the prognosis expected from it depend on the cause. Treatment includes correction of the underlying causes, such as the administration of female hormones or thyroid hormone (if the client is hypothyroid), and the improvement of the patient health status.

- Hormone therapy: According to the hormone changes, different schedules should be selected.

【护理评估】

1. 健康史　详细询问月经史，了解发病前有无导致闭经的诱因，如精神因素、环境改变、体重变化、有无剧烈运动及各种疾病、用药情况等。已婚妇女需询问生育史及产后并发症史。原发性闭经应询问第二性征发育情况，了解生长发育史，有无先天缺陷或其他疾病及家族史。

2. 身心状况　注意观察患者精神状态、营养、全身发育状况，测量身高、体重、智力情况、躯干和四肢的比例，检查五官生长特征及第二性征发育情况，有无多毛、溢乳等。妇科检查应注意内、外生殖器发育，有无先天缺陷、畸形等。长时间闭经患者会产生很大压力，患者会担心闭经对自己的健康、性生活和生育能力的影响。病程过长及反复治疗效果不佳时心理压力会加重，情绪低落，对治疗和护理丧失信心，这反过来又会加重闭经。

3. 辅助检查　生育期妇女闭经首先需排除妊娠。

(1) 子宫功能的检查

1) 影像学检查：盆腔超声检查、子宫输卵管造影，了解有无宫腔病变。

2) 宫腔镜检查：能精确诊断宫腔粘连。

3) 药物撤退性试验。①孕激素试验：用黄体酮 20 mg，每日肌内注射 1 次，连续 5 d；或口服甲羟孕酮，每日 10 mg，连续 5 d。停用后 3~7 d 出现撤药性出血为阳性，说明子宫内膜已受一定水平的雌激素影响；若无撤药性出血为阴性，应进一步做雌-孕激素序贯试验。②雌-孕激素序贯试验：每晚睡前服妊马雌酮 1.25 mg，连续 20 d，最后 10 d 每日加服醋酸甲羟孕酮 10 mg，若停药 3~7 d 有撤药性出血为阳性，提示子宫内膜功能正常，可排除子宫性闭经；若无撤药性出血则为阴性，重复试验后若仍无出血，提示子宫内膜有缺陷或被破坏，可诊断为子宫性闭经。

(2) 卵巢功能检查　包括基础体温测定、子宫颈黏液结晶检查、阴道脱落细胞检查、性激素测定、B 型超声监测等以了解卵巢排卵及分泌雌激素、孕激素的功能。

(3) 垂体功能检查　雌激素试验阳性时，提示病变不在子宫，为确定病变是在卵巢、垂体或下丘脑，需做血催乳素(PRL)、FSH、LH 放射免疫测定。当 FSH、LH 均低时做垂体兴奋试验，又称促性腺激素释放激素(GnRH)刺激试验，了解垂体对促黄体素释放激素(LHRH)的反应性。注射 LHRH 后 LH 升高，说明垂体功能正常，病变在下丘脑。如 LH 值仍无升高或升高不显著，提示病变在垂体。

(4) 其他　疑有垂体肿瘤时应做蝶鞍摄片、CT 或 MRI 检查，疑有多囊卵巢综合征、肾上腺皮质肿瘤等应行 B 型超声检查。

【护理诊断】

1. 长期低自尊　与长期闭经，治疗效果不明显，月经不能正常来潮而出现自我否定等有关。

2. 焦虑　与担心疾病对健康、性生活、生育的影响有关。

【护理措施】

1. 治疗配合　鼓励患者积极遵医嘱治疗。手术治疗者,做好术前准备和术后护理。性激素治疗者,指导患者按时按量用药,说明性激素的作用、不良反应、具体用法等,嘱患者不得随意停用或漏服。

2. 心理护理　建立良好的护患关系,鼓励患者说出内心感受,倾听患者诉说。及时向患者提供诊疗信息,帮助纠正一些错误观念,消除顾虑。鼓励患者多与他人交往,保持心情舒畅,正确对待疾病。

Nursing Interventions

- Amenorrhea prevention: In many cases, teenage girls can help to prevent primary amenorrhea by following a sensible exercise program and by maintaining a normal weight for their height and age. Primary amenorrhea caused by anatomic abnormalities of the reproductive tract usually cannot be prevented. To prevent secondary amenorrhea that is related to diet, over-exercise or stress, the nurse advises the patient to take the following steps: Eat a low-fat diet that meets the recommended daily nutritional needs; Exercise moderately, but not excessively, to maintain an ideal body weight and muscle tone; Find healthy outlets for emotional stress and daily conflicts; Balance work, recreation and rest; Avoid excessive alcohol consumption and cigarette smoking.

- Help the patient do diagnostic examination: The nurse helps doctors to acquire the thorough history of the patient. Since the causes of amenorrhea are complex, the nurse should explain the significance of the diagnostic examination and helps them to complete the examinations.

- Psychological support: It is important that the nurse provides the psychological support for the patient. If amenorrhea is caused by stress or psychological factors, the nurse instructs the patient's significant ones to take part in the support group and provider psychological supports for the patient.

【健康教育】

①告诉患者性激素治疗是有效的治疗方法,服用性激素可以使月经按期来潮,促进子宫发育,维持第二性征,并能有效缓解阴道干涩、性欲低下、潮热出汗等低雌激素症状,维持女性健康。若使用不当,会引起子宫异常出血等不良反应,嘱其严格遵医嘱服用并定期复查。②指导患者保持心情舒畅,避免忧愁思虑。适当锻炼,合理饮食,保持标准体重。对营养不良者需增加营养,而肥胖者常并发内分泌失调,应低脂肪、低碳水化合物饮食,注意补充维生素和矿物质。

任务实施

闭经部位的诊断流程见图16-4。

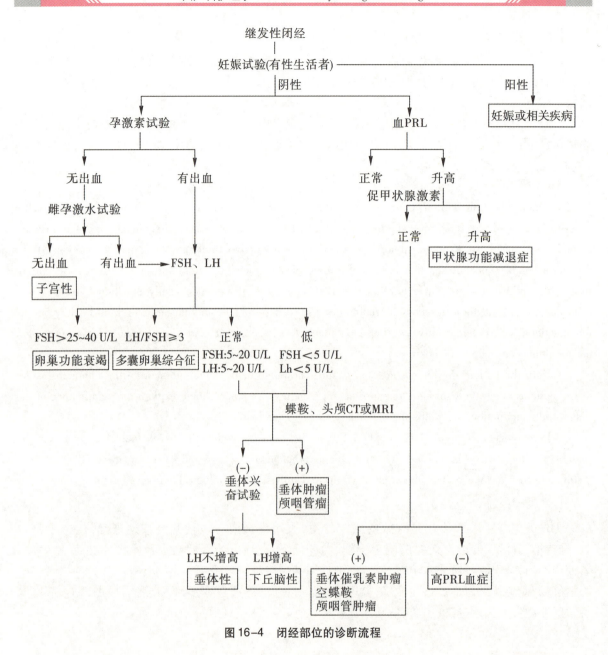

图16-4　闭经部位的诊断流程

任务三　痛经（Dysmenorrhea）

工作情景

李某,女,15岁,学生。因月经期下腹疼痛2年来就诊。自述月经12岁初潮,30 d左右1次,经期5~6 d,量中等。开始行经时下腹疼痛轻,近一年行经时下腹疼痛渐进性加重,行经当日胀痛明显,痛而拒按,持续1~2 d。经色暗红,有小血块,随经血增多,血块流出疼痛减轻。

①该患者可能出现了什么问题? 如何治疗? ②护士应如何对患者进行健康指导?

任务内容

痛经为常见的妇科症状之一,指行经前后或月经期出现下腹部疼痛、坠胀,伴有腰酸或其他不适。症状严重者影响生活和工作。痛经分为原发性和继发性两类,原发性痛经指生殖器无器质性病变的痛经,占痛经90%以上;继发性痛经指由盆腔器质性疾病引起的痛经。本节仅叙述原发性痛经。

任务目标

- ◆ 能叙述痛经的分类及原因。
- ◆ 能指导痛经患者掌握缓解疼痛的方法。

【概述】

1. 病因　原发性痛经的发生主要与月经来潮时子宫内膜前列腺素(prostaglandin,PG)含量增高有关。研究表明,痛经患者子宫内膜和月经血中$PGF_{2\alpha}$和PGE_2含量均较正常妇女明显升高,$PGF_{2\alpha}$含量升高是造成痛经的主要原因。

2. 临床表现　下腹疼痛是痛经的主要症状。原发性痛经在青春期多见,常在初潮后1~2年内发病。疼痛多自月经来潮后开始,最早出现在经前12 h,以行经第1天疼痛最剧烈,持续2~3 d后缓解。疼痛常呈痉挛性,通常位于下腹部耻骨上,可放射至腰骶部和大腿内侧,可伴有恶心、呕吐、腹泻、头晕、乏力等症状,严重时面色发白、出冷汗。妇科检查无异常发现。

3. 治疗原则　以对症治疗为主,避免精神刺激和过度疲劳。

Etiology

Dysmenorrhea is related to the strong uterine contractions. During strong contractions, the uterus may contract too strongly or too frequently, causing the blood supply to the uterus to be temporarily cut off and pain occurs. The cause of primary dysmenorrehea is of the increased endometrial prostaglandin production. These compounds especially $PGF_{2\alpha}$ and PGE_2 are found in higher concentration in secretory endometrium than in proliferative endometrium.

Clinical Manifestation

Primary dysmenorrhea is common at the adolescents, 1−2 years after menarche. The low abdomen pain of primary dysmenorrhea usually begins a few hours before or just after the onset of a menstrual period and may last up to 2−3 d. The onset and severity of primary dysmenorrhea mimics the menstrual flow itself, beginning within a few hours of the onset of flow and reaching maximal severity during the heaviest portion of the period. The pain is similar to labor, with suprapubic cramping, and may be companied by lumbosacral backache, pain radiating down the anterior thigh. Sometimes, dysmenorrhea accompanies with nausea, vomiting, diarrhea, fatigue, and rarely syncopal episodes. The pain of dysmenorrhea is colicky in nature and is improved with abdominal massage, movement of the body. The abdomen examination is normal. Occasionally, the normal uterine position changes, from anteversion and anteflexion to excessive anteversion and anteflexion.

Management

Symptomatic treatment is mainly used, mental stimulation and excessive fatigue should be avoided.

【护理评估】

1. 健康史　了解患者的年龄、月经史与婚育史，询问有无精神紧张等诱发痛经的相关因素，疼痛与月经的关系。

2. 身心状况　评估下腹痛严重程度及伴随症状，注意与其他原因造成的下腹部疼痛症状相鉴别。妇科检查无阳性体征。因反复疼痛影响生活质量，患者常常会感到焦虑。

3. 辅助检查　为排除继发性痛经和其他原因造成的疼痛，可做盆腔超声检查、腹腔镜、宫腔镜检查、子宫输卵管造影，以排除器质性病变。

【护理诊断】

1. 急性疼痛　与经期子宫收缩，子宫缺血缺氧有关。

2. 焦虑　与反复痛经造成的精神紧张有关。

【护理措施】

1. 心理护理　说明月经时的轻度不适是生理反应，消除紧张和顾虑可缓解疼痛。

2. 对症护理　腹部局部热敷和进食热饮料可缓解疼痛。疼痛不能忍受时指导患者遵医嘱使用镇痛、镇静、解痉的药物，如前列腺素合成酶抑制剂布洛芬，月经来潮即开始服用，连服 2~3 d，该类药物治疗有效率可达 80%；有避孕要求的痛经妇女还可以选择口服避孕药，通过抑制排卵减少月经血前列腺素含量，疗效达 90% 以上。

Psychological treatment is important. When the pain is intolerable, analgesics, or other drugs can be used. Prostaglandin synthase inhibitors are effective for the treatment of primary dysmenorrhea in about 80% of women. For the patients with primary dysmenorrhea who has no contraindications to oral contraceptive agents or who desires contraception, the oral contraceptives are the agent of choice. When the pharmacology is administered, the nurse explains the medication effect, dosage, frequency, side effects to the patients, and supervises the client during medication. The nurse discusses diagnosis, explains any scheduled procedures or surgeries with patient including their impact on child-bearing. The patient should be told that menstrual pain responds well to non-narcotic.

【健康教育】

注意经期清洁卫生，经期禁止性生活和盆浴。保证足够的休息和睡眠，保证营养的摄入，进行规律而适度的锻炼，戒烟。

任务四　绝经综合征(Menopause Syndrome)

工作情景

张女士,49 岁,潮热、出汗加重半年。1 年前无明显诱因出现月经周期延长为 60~85 d,继而出现颈部、颜面部发热,随后出汗的症状,每日 3~5 次,未经治疗。近半年来症状较前有所加重,每日可达 20 余次,今来就诊。月经史:13 岁初潮,周期 30~35 d,经期 5~6 d,量中,无痛经。既往无高血压、糖尿病等病史。妇科检查:外阴已婚已产型,子宫颈光滑,子宫前位,大小如常,质地软,活动度好,无压痛,双侧附件无异常。实验室检查:FSH 32 U/L,E$_2$ 15 ng/L。

①患者可能患有何种疾病？②发生该疾病的主要原因是什么？

任务内容

绝经指卵巢功能停止所致永久性无月经状态。绝经综合征指妇女绝经前后出现性激素波动或减少所致的一系列躯体及精神心理症状。绝经分为自然绝经和人工绝经。自然绝经指卵巢内卵泡生理性耗竭所致的绝经，人工绝经指两侧卵巢经手术切除或放射线照射等所致的绝经。人工绝经者更易发生绝经综合征。

任务目标

◆能叙述绝经综合征的原因及临床表现。
◆能指导患者使用激素替代治疗缓解近期症状，预防远期症状。

【概述】

1.病因　卵巢功能衰退是引起绝经期综合征的主要原因。绝经前后最明显的变化是卵巢功能衰退，随后表现为下丘脑-垂体功能退化，正常的下丘脑-垂体-卵巢轴之间的平衡失调，影响了自主神经中枢及其支配下的各脏器功能，从而出现一系列自主神经功能失调的症状。此外，还与患者体内神经递质含量异常、个体神经类型、健康状态、社会环境，以及职业、文化水平等有关，神经类型不稳定、精神压抑或受过较强烈精神刺激的女性易发生绝经综合征，而体力劳动者则较少发生。因疾病行双侧卵巢切除或因放化疗使双侧卵巢功能受损的患者更易发生绝经综合征。

2.临床表现

（1）近期症状

1）月经紊乱：常见症状，可表现为月经稀发，经量逐渐减少，直至绝经。也可表现为月经周期不规则、经期延长、经量增多或者减少。

2）血管舒缩症状：主要表现为潮热、出汗，为血管舒缩不稳定所致，是雌激素降低的特征性症状。反复出现短暂的面部、颈部、胸部皮肤阵阵上涌的热浪，伴皮肤发红、出汗。持续数分钟不等，轻者每日数次，重者达十多次或更多。夜间或应激状态易促发。此症状可持续 1～2 年，有时长达 5 年或更长。潮热严重时可影响妇女的工作、生活和睡眠，是需要性激素治疗的主要原因。

3）自主神经失调症状：常出现心悸、眩晕、头痛、失眠、耳鸣等症状。

4）精神神经症状：常表现为注意力不易集中，并且情绪波动大，如激动易怒、焦虑不安或情绪低落、抑郁、不能自我控制等，记忆力减退也较常见。

（2）远期症状

1）泌尿生殖道症状：主要表现为泌尿生殖道萎缩症状，如阴道干燥、性交困难及反复阴道感染、子宫脱垂、膀胱或直肠膨出、压力性尿失禁、反复发生的尿路感染。

2）骨质疏松：绝经后妇女缺乏雌激素，使骨质吸收增加，导致骨量快速丢失而出现骨质疏松。50 岁以上妇女半数以上会发生绝经后骨质疏松，一般发生在绝经后 5～10 年内，最常发生在椎体。

3）阿尔茨海默病（Alzheimer's disease）：绝经后期妇女比老年男性患病风险高，可能与绝经后内源性雌激素水平降低有关。

4）心血管疾病：绝经后妇女糖、脂代谢异常增加，动脉硬化、冠心病的发病风险较绝经前明显增加，这可能与雌激素水平低落有关。

3.治疗原则　缓解近期症状，早期发现并有效预防骨质疏松症、动脉硬化等老年性疾病。

Etiology

The earliest change of perimenopause is the progressive loss of ovarian function. Later, the pituitary and hypothalamus function degenerate.

Clinical Manifestation

- Recent symptoms.

Menstruation irregularity: Anovulation along with wide fluctuations in estrogen levels is a hallmark of the perimenopausal period and often leads to abnormal vaginal bleeding. The most common symptom of perimenopause is a change in menstrual pattern. More than 50% of women will experience alterations in menstrual cycles before menopause. Irregular menstrual cycles, longer duration and heavier bleeding can be seen in the women. Shorter cycles are typical.

Vasomotor symptoms: The most characteristic vasomotor symptoms in the perimenopause period is the "hot flashes"—an uncomfortable subjective sensation of warmth usually arising in the lower trunk, spreading upwards to the neck, face, shoulders and upper limbs and becoming more marked until the patient breaks out in a sweat or cold sensation, and ranges in duration usually 1 – 3 min. The hot flashes may be accompanied by tachycardia. And tend to occur more frequently at night and in the condition of stress.

Symptoms of autonomic nerve disorders: Often appear palpitations, dizziness, headache, insomnia, tinnitus and other symptoms.

Psychological/Cognitive symptoms: Exposure to estrogen decrease results in changes to brain structure and function. Estrogen deficiency may alter the threshold for clinical expression of various mood and cognitive disorders. The symptoms as depression, irritability, anxiety, loss of libido, and aggression have been commonly reported during the perimenopausal years.

- Forward symptoms.

Genitourinary changes: Decreasing estrogen production leads to atrophy of the vagina and produce the distressful symptoms of senile vaginitis or atrophic vaginitis. This type of vaginitis can cause itching, burning, discomfort dysparenunia, and also vaginal bleeding. The vagina may shorten and narrow. The vaginal walls become pale because of diminished vascularity and are less elastic. Estrogen deprivation may also decrease the collagen content of the structures that support the uterine ligaments causing the uterine prolapse, urine frequency and urine incontinence.

Osteoporosis: Change in the bony skeleton is one of the most profound risks menopausal woman face. About 25% women have osteroporosis during perimenopausal years related to estrogen deficiency. Due to an increase in bone destruction relative to bone formation, bone mass normally declines with age. Osteoporosis is characterized by low bone mass and microarchitectural deterioration, with a consequent increase in fragility and susceptibility to fracture. While there is a reduction in the quantity of bone, there is no alteration in its chemical composition.

Alzheimer's disease: Late postmenopausal women are at higher risk than older men and may be associated with reduced endogenous estrogen levels after menopause.

Cardiovascular disease (CVD): Cardiovascular disease is the leading cause of death among women, over 50% of postmenopausal women will succumb to CVD. Because of the estrogen deficiency after menopause, the total serum cholesterol, low-density lipoprotein (LDL) cholesterol, and high-density lipoprotein (HDL) cholesterol levels increased. The ration of HDL/LDL decreases. The oxidized form of LDL cholesterol damages the vascular endothelium and the risk of CVD increases. Myocardial infarction incidence increases in women after age 50 than in men.

Management

Relieve the recent symptoms, detect the symptom early and prevent osteoporosis, arteriosclerosis and other senile diseases effectively.

【护理评估】

1. 健康史　了解患者年龄、职业、文化水平及性格特征,询问月经史和生育史,有无卵巢切除或盆腔肿瘤放疗史,有无高血压及其他内分泌疾病史等。

2. 身心评估　评估患者因卵巢功能减退及雌激素不足引起的相关症状。对患者进行全身体格检查,排除明显的器质性病变。进入围绝经期后,工作、家庭、社会环境变化加重身体和心理负担,可能诱发和加重绝经综合征的症状。评估近期出现的影响患者情绪的生活事件,应注意排除精神疾病。

3. 辅助检查

(1)卵巢激素测定　检测 FSH 和 E_2 了解卵巢功能。绝经过渡期血清 FSH>10 U/L,提示卵巢储备功能下降。闭经、FSH>40 U/L 且 E_2<20 ng/L,提示卵巢功能衰竭。

(2)抗米勒管激素(AMH)测定　AMH 低至 1.1 μg/L 提示卵巢储备下降;若低于 0.2 μg/L 提示即将绝经。

(3)超声检查　基础状态卵巢的窦状卵泡数减少、卵巢容积缩小、子宫内膜变薄。

【护理诊断】

1. 焦虑　与绝经过渡期内分泌改变,或个性特点、精神因素等有关。

2. 知识缺乏　缺乏绝经期生理心理变化知识及应对技巧。

【护理措施】

1. 一般护理　嘱患者合理饮食,进食高蛋白、高维生素、高钙、高铁、低盐、低脂食物,饮食多样化,多吃新鲜绿色蔬菜和水果,忌食刺激性强的食物,如酒、浓茶、咖啡等。规律运动,刺激成骨细胞、促进血液循环,有利于延缓衰老和骨质疏松症的发生。

2. 用药指导　指导患者正确进行激素替代治疗,可有效缓解绝经相关症状,从而提高生活质量。向患者介绍用药目的、用药途径及方案、用药时间及剂量、适应证、禁忌证、可能出现的不良反应等。首选天然雌激素,剂量应个体化,以最小有效量为佳。嘱患者严格按医嘱用药,不可自行停药和随意更改用药,用药期间如出现子宫不规则出血应及时就诊。长期用药者应定期随访。

3. 心理护理　让患者及家属理解围绝经期是正常生理过程,使患者掌握必要的保健知识,积极参加社会活动,消除恐惧和焦虑。使家属了解围绝经期妇女可能出现的症状,给予理解、同情、安慰和鼓励,帮助患者顺利度过围绝经期。

Nursing Interventions

• General nursing：Perimenopausal women should stop smoking, take healthy diet, and do regular aerobic exercises and deep breathing exercises.

• Medication nursing：Because of the symptoms and serious disease processes that are clearly associated with estrogen deficiency and the onset of menopause, therapy with exogenous estrogen to replace physiologic levels of circulation estrogen has been advocated, with the clear intention of preventing symptoms of the deficiency syndrome rather than treating them after they occur.

Because of the risks associated with HRT(hormone replacement therapy), it is recommended that all women using HRT as prescribed and be seen on an annual basis. They may be instructed to stop hormones for the week before the appointment so that an assessment of the severity of current symptoms can be made. Women who choose to stop HRT may require a slow tapering off for successful cessation.

• Psychological counseling：A psychological counseling can be helpful in helping the patient discover the underlying causes since the symptoms and signs vary greatly in perimenopausal women. The nurse tries to create an equal atmosphere that encourages the patient to ask questions or express her feelings and encourages the patient to use her prior successful skills to cope with stress. Significant others are included in if it is possible.

【健康教育】

介绍绝经前后减轻症状的方法,以及预防绝经综合征的措施,如注意个人卫生,保持外阴清洁,避免尿路感染和阴道炎的发生,加强盆底肌肉锻炼。记录月经卡,以及时发现月经异常。定期健康检查,重点检查生殖系统和乳腺肿瘤。

微课　　　　　　　　课件　　　　　　　练习题及参考答案

（任　美　李文勤）

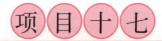

项目十七

妇科其他疾病患者的护理（Nursing of Patients with Other Gynecological Diseases）

◤ 项目描述

本项目主要介绍 3 种妇科疾病，包括子宫内膜异位症、子宫脱垂和不孕症。

This project mainly introduces three gynecological diseases, including endometriosis, uterine prolapse, and infertility.

任务一　子宫内膜异位症（Endometriosis）

■工作情景■

　　患者，31 岁，平时月经规律，既往有痛经史。2 年前曾行足月剖宫产术，术后恢复较好。3 个月前体检时，做 B 型超声发现卵巢处有 3.7 cm 的囊性包块。于 1 周前复查 B 型超声，包块增大，遂入院治疗。

　　①请考虑该患者应进一步做何检查以明确诊断。②请明确该患者主要的护理问题。③根据目前的情况对患者进行正确的护理。

■任务内容■

　　子宫内膜异位症是指具有生长功能的内膜组织出现在子宫腔被覆黏膜以外的身体部位，简称内异症。异位内膜可侵犯全身任何部位，多数位于盆腔内，故又称为盆腔子宫内膜异位症。其中以侵犯卵巢及子宫骶韧带者最常见，其次是子宫浆膜、直肠子宫陷凹、子宫后壁下段等，异位内膜也可出现在手术切口、脐、外阴、肺等部位。子宫内膜异位症一般发生于育龄期妇女，以 25～45 岁多见，发病率为 10%～15%。妇科手术中发现有 5%～15% 患者存在子宫内膜异位症；25%～35% 的不孕患者与子宫内膜异位症有关。绝经后或双侧卵巢切除后异位内膜组织可逐渐萎缩吸收；妊娠或使用性激素抑制卵巢功能，可暂时阻止病情发展，故子宫内膜异位症是激素依赖性疾病。子宫内膜异位症虽为良性病变，但却具有类似恶性肿瘤的远处转移和种植、浸润生长及复发等恶性行为，但极少恶变。

任务目标

◆ 能叙述子宫内膜异位症的定义、病因、临床表现及处理原则。
◆ 能综合评估子宫内膜异位症患者情况,提供相应的护理及健康教育。

【概要】

1. 病因　子宫内膜异位症的病因及发病机制至今尚未完全阐明,目前主要有下列学说:①子宫内膜种植学说;②体腔上皮化生学说;③诱导学说。

2. 病理　子宫内膜异位症的基本病理变化为异位种植的子宫内膜在卵巢激素作用下发生周期性出血,病灶局部反复出血和缓慢吸收导致周围组织增生、粘连,在病变部位形成紫褐色斑点或小泡,最后发展成为大小不等的实质性瘢痕结节或形成囊肿。

子宫内膜异位症发病机制

卵巢最易被异位内膜侵犯,约80%病变累及一侧卵巢,50%双侧卵巢均受累。病变可以是位于卵巢表面的紫褐色斑点或小囊,也可随病情发展,形成单个或多个大小不一的囊肿型的典型病变,称为卵巢子宫内膜异位囊肿。囊肿的直径一般为5~6 cm;大者直径可达25 cm左右。囊肿内含暗褐色黏稠的陈旧血性液体,似巧克力样糊状,故又称卵巢巧克力囊肿,常需手术治疗。子宫颈韧带、直肠子宫陷凹和子宫后壁下段也是子宫内膜异位症的好发部位,可能因处于盆腔后部较低处,与经血中的内膜碎屑接触较多有关。

3. 临床表现　子宫内膜异位症患者的临床表现因病变部位不同而多种多样,症状特征与月经周期密切相关。约25%的患者无任何症状。

(1)症状

1)痛经和下腹痛:约半数以上患者以痛经为主要症状,其特点为继发性痛经且进行性加重;典型的痛经常于经前1~2 d开始,经期第一日最重,以后逐渐减轻并持续整个月经期。疼痛的部位多为下腹深部和腰骶部,并可向会阴、肛门、大腿放射。疼痛严重程度与病灶大小不平行,粘连严重的卵巢异位囊肿可能并无任何疼痛,而盆腔内单个微小病灶也可引起难以忍受的疼痛。也有腹痛时间与月经期不同步者。直肠子宫陷凹处的子宫内膜异位症者,可因出血致纤维增生,使子宫与周围器官发生粘连,表现为性交不适、性交痛、腰骶部疼痛或肛门坠痛。少数患者长期下腹痛,形成慢性盆腔痛,至经期加剧。但也有27%~40%的患者无痛经。

2)不孕:子宫内膜异位症患者中不孕率可高达40%。引起不孕的原因复杂,可以是盆腔粘连、子宫后倾、输卵管粘连闭锁或蠕动减弱等机械性因素,也可能是盆腔微环境改变、卵巢功能异常等内分泌原因。

3)月经失调:15%~30%的患者有经量增多、经期延长、月经淋漓不尽或经前期点滴出血。可能与病灶破坏卵巢组织、影响卵巢的内分泌功能导致排卵障碍和黄体功能不良等有关。

4)其他:①盆腔外任何部分(如肠道、膀胱、腹壁切口瘢痕等处)有异位内膜种植生长时,均可在局部出现周期性疼痛、出血和肿块,并出现相应的症状。②较大的卵巢子宫内膜异位囊肿发生破裂时囊内液流入盆腹腔,患者可出现突发性剧烈腹痛,伴恶心、呕吐和肛门坠胀,引起急腹症。

(2)体征　典型的盆腔子宫内膜异位症患者在进行妇科检查时,可发现子宫粘连,致使后倾、活动受限甚至固定。子宫正常大小或略大,饱满并有轻压痛;一侧或双侧附件区可扪及与子宫相连的不活动囊性包块,囊肿一般<10 cm,有轻压痛;子宫骶韧带、子宫后壁或直肠子宫陷凹可触及不规则的硬结节,触痛明显。若阴道直肠受累,可在阴道后穹隆扪及甚至看到突出的紫蓝色结节。

4.处理原则　治疗子宫内膜异位症的根本目的在于减灭病灶、缓解症状、改善生育功能、减少和避免复发,因此治疗以手术为主,药物为重要的辅助治疗手段。治疗时应依据患者年龄、症状、病变部位及范围、对生育的要求等加以全面考虑,制订个体化治疗方案。原则上症状轻微者采用非手术治疗,可定期随访;症状和病变严重且无生育要求者可考虑根治性手术。

Etiology

Endometriosis is a benign disease. The cause of endometriosis is still uncertain. Various theories have been put forth to explain the mechanisms for the development of this disease: implantation of viable endo-metrial cells theory; coelomic metaplasia theory.

Pathology

The presence of endometriosis is characterized by blue – gray lesion with cycle bleeding on the peritoneal surface over the pelvic peritoneum or pelvic structures accompanied by the ovarian cycle.

The most common site of endometriosis is the ovary, about 80% of patients in one ovary, and in about 50% of patients both ovaries are involved. Early endometriosis may occur either as small, bluish or hemorrhagic areas on the surface of ovary or as small cysts of foci of pink tissue lying beneath the surface epithelium or within the ovarian cortical stroma. The cysts may be multiple in the early stages but subsequently coalesce into a single large cyst. The benign endometrial cyst of the ovary varies from microscopic size to a mass 5–6 cm in diameter. The biggest one can be 25 cm in diameter. These cystic structures have a fibrotic wall with a brown to yellow lining. Endometriomas (ovarian chocolate cysts) are usually small in size and usually contain thick brownish fluid caused by altered blood in the cavity. When the cysts enlarge, the whole ovaries appear grey–bluish.

Clinical Signs and Symptoms

The clinical presentation and symptoms of the disease are frequently related to the anatomical site of the disease. About 25% of patients have no obvious symptoms.

• Pain: Progressive pelvic pain associated with or occurring just prior to menstruation are among 75% of patients. The localization of the pelvic pain is often related to the site involved in the endometriotic lesion. Usually, the pain is most marked just 1–2 d prior to the start of the menstrual flow and extends into the first few days of the menstrual cycle, often the pain in the first day of menstruation is intense. The pain may be acute or chronic. In about half of the patients with severe or extensive endometriosis, the pain is chronic all through the cycle which gets worse right before and during menstruation, and during or shortly after intercourse.

• Infertility: The infertility incidence is about 40% in endometriosis. In patients with severe endometriosis, the extent of the pelvic adhesions, the distortions of the tubes and ovaries, and occasionally because of the destruction of the ovarian tissue, may explain the infertility. However, the cause or relationship of endometriosis in the minimal stage on infertility is not clear.

• Dysfimctional menstruation: 15% – 30% of patients manifest as excessive menstruation, premenstrual spotting, or prolonged menses. The dysfunctional menstruation is possibly related to the anovulation, luteal–phase defects, or incorporated with adenomyosis or leiomyoma of the uterus.

• Other special symptoms: Endometrial implants on the colon or the bladder in more advanced stages may cause pain with bowel movements or urination. When the endometriosis invades fallopian tube, lateral lumbago and urine blood appear, but they are infrequent.

• Signs: Classically, pelvic examination reveals tender nodules in the posterior vaginal fornix and pain upon uterine motion. The uterus may be fixed upon and retroverted due to cul – de – sac adhesions, and tender adnexal masses may be felt because of the presence of endometriosis.

Principle of Management

Management focuses on arresting the progression of the disease, symptom control, and preservation of fertility (if desired).

【护理评估】

1. 健康史　除收集一般健康史外,重点询问患者的月经史、孕产史,应注意询问不孕症患者有无多次人流、引产、手术分娩史,有无多次输卵管通液、碘油造影等宫腔操作史。

2. 身心状况　注意评估患者发生痛经的起始时间、疼痛程度和持续时间,有无性交痛和肛门坠胀感等;了解疼痛是否明显发生于某次盆腔手术或宫腔手术之后。还应判断子宫的位置、活动度、有无触痛,附件区有无肿块及肿块的大小、性质;阴道后穹隆可否扪及包块或结节,是否能见到紫蓝色斑点。

子宫内膜异位症可能使患者产生对疼痛的恐惧和对不孕的担忧,要注意了解患者月经前和经期的心理变化,解答疑虑及提供心理疏导。

3. 辅助检查

(1)B 型超声检查　阴道和腹部 B 型超声检查可以确定卵巢子宫内膜异位囊肿的位置、大小和形状,并可发现盆腔检查时未能扪及的包块。

(2)CA125 测定　CA125 水平可用于动态监测异位内膜病变活动情况。

(3)腹腔镜检查　是目前国际公认的诊断子宫内膜异位症的最佳方法。

【护理诊断】

1. 疼痛　与病灶反复出血刺激周围组织中的神经末梢有关。

2. 恐惧　与经期剧烈的、进行性加重的疼痛有关。

3. 自尊紊乱　与不孕有关。

【护理措施】

1. 一般护理　为患者提供舒适的住院环境,给予患者适当的经期指导,帮助其缓解经期疼痛,加强经期卫生,促进舒适。

2. 提供治疗选择

(1)期待疗法　对于症状轻微者或无症状者,可指导其每 3 ~ 6 个月随访 1 次。有生育要求者,鼓励其尽早妊娠。随访期间症状加重者,可根据情况选择药物或手术治疗。

(2)药物治疗　适用于盆腔疼痛症状较明显、暂时无生育要求、无内膜异位囊肿者。根据经血逆流学说得知,妊娠和闭经可避免月经的来潮,月经停闭可使得异位内膜萎缩退化,故临床上可采用性激素类药物引起患者较长时间的闭经,促使异位内膜的萎缩退化。遵医嘱指导患者选用口服避孕药、达那唑、孕三烯酮、促性腺激素释放激素激动剂等。要特别注意性激素类药物的使用注意事项。

(3)手术治疗　针对药物治疗后症状无缓解、病情进一步加重或迫切希望生育、卵巢囊肿超过 5 ~ 6 cm 者,可选择手术治疗。根据不同的预后要求选择适合的手术方式,包括保留生育功能、保留卵巢功能和根治性手术 3 类。

(4)手术与药物联合治疗　纯手术或单纯药物治疗均有局限性,故而采用联合治疗。术前给药可使异位病灶缩小、软化,利于缩小手术范围、便于手术操作;术后加用药物治疗,有利于巩固手术的疗效。

3.心理护理　鼓励患者倾诉自己的不适和对疾病的认识,了解患者的真实感受、想法,缓解和消除患者的焦虑和担心,争取得到患者及家属对治疗的配合和支持。

Nursing Interventions

● Medication nursing: The nurse should instruct the patients to administer the medication as prescribed, help them to observe the side effects correctly and give them appropriate interventions.

● Pain controlling: In nursing interventions, visual analog pain scores are frequently used. The health-related quality of life may be quantified by the short form−36. The overall individual impressions of satisfaction should also be assessed.

● Surgery nursing: The role of surgery in the management of endometriosis is important especially for those with severe disease or adhesions. Explain the surgery and the process to the patient to relieve her anxiety or fear related to the surgery.

● Psychological counseling: The nurse provides emotional support and encourages the patient to ask questions or express her fears.

【健康教育】

1.防止经血逆流　经期注意休息,避免吃生冷食物,对无孔处女膜、阴道闭锁、子宫颈管粘连及闭锁、残角子宫等先天或后天容易引起经血逆流的疾病,应及早发现及早治疗。

2.药物避孕　避孕药物可抑制排卵,促使子宫内膜萎缩,使经血逆流的机会相对减少。对有家族史或严重痛经患者可考虑以此方法进行避孕。

3.防止医源性子宫内膜种植　经期避免性交和阴道检查及阴道手术操作,凡是进入子宫腔的手术,均应用纱布垫保护好子宫切口的周围术野,以防子宫腔内容物溢入腹腔;缝合子宫壁时,注意缝针不要穿透子宫内膜层。子宫颈治疗应选择在月经干净后 3～7 d 进行,以免子宫内膜进入尚未愈合的手术创面。

4.其他　鼓励母乳喂养,在政策范围内,鼓励重复妊娠,可以预防此病的复发。对于有生育要求的患者,鼓励尽早妊娠,可以对此病起到一定的治疗作用。

任务二　子宫脱垂(Uterine Prolapse)

工作情景

患者,60 岁,G_6P_5,患慢性支气管炎 20 年,经常咳嗽。近 10 年来感觉下身有块状物脱出,开始时卧床休息后块状物可消失,近 5 年来块状物逐渐增大,平卧后也不消失,并伴尿频、尿失禁。妇科检查:阴道前后壁重度膨出,子宫颈及全部宫体脱出在阴道口外。

①请明确该患者发生此病的主要原因。②请明确该患者主要的护理问题及相应护理措施。

任务内容

子宫脱垂是指子宫从正常位置沿阴道下降,子宫颈外口达坐骨棘水平以下,甚至子宫全部脱出阴道口外,常伴有阴道前后壁膨出。

任务目标

◆ 能叙述子宫脱垂的定义、病因、临床表现及处理原则。
◆ 能向患者讲解子宫托的放取方法和注意事项。

【概要】

1. 病因　①分娩损伤；②长期腹压增加；③盆底组织发育不良或退行性变。

2. 临床分度　按患者平卧用力向下屏气时子宫下降程度，将子宫脱垂分为3度（图17-1）。

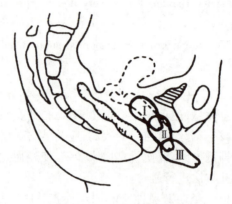

图 17-1　子宫脱垂分度

（1）Ⅰ度　轻型为子宫颈外口距离处女膜缘<4 cm，但未达处女膜缘；重型为子宫颈外口已达处女膜缘，在阴道口可见到子宫颈。

（2）Ⅱ度　轻型为子宫颈已脱出阴道口外，宫体仍在阴道内；重型为子宫颈及部分宫体已脱出阴道口外。

（3）Ⅲ度　子宫颈及宫体全部脱出至阴道口外。

3. 临床表现　Ⅰ度患者多无自觉症状，Ⅱ、Ⅲ度患者主要有如下表现。

（1）腰骶部酸痛及下坠感　由下垂子宫对韧带的牵拉，盆腔充血所致。站立过久或劳累后症状明显，卧床休息以后症状减轻。

（2）肿物自阴道脱出　常在腹压增加时，阴道口有一肿物脱出。开始时肿物在平卧休息时可变小或消失，严重者休息后亦不能回缩，需用手还纳至阴道内。若脱出的子宫及阴道黏膜水肿，用手还纳也有困难，子宫长期脱出在阴道口外，患者行动极为不便，长期摩擦可出现子宫颈溃疡，甚至出血，若继发感染则有脓性分泌物。

（3）排便异常　伴膀胱、尿道膨出的患者易出现排尿困难、尿潴留或压力性尿失禁等症状。若继发尿路感染，患者可出现尿频、尿急、尿痛等。若合并直肠膨出，患者可有便秘、排便困难。

4. 处理原则　除非合并压力性尿失禁，无症状的患者不需治疗。有症状者可采用保守或手术治疗，治疗以安全简单和有效为原则。

（1）非手术治疗　包括支持疗法、盆底肌肉锻炼、放置子宫托、中药和针灸等。

（2）手术治疗　凡非手术治疗无效或Ⅱ、Ⅲ度子宫脱垂者均可根据患者的年龄、全身状况及生育要求等采取个体化治疗。常选择以下手术方法：阴道前后壁修补术加子宫主韧带缩短及子宫颈部分切除术（曼氏手术）、经阴道子宫全切术及阴道前后壁修补术、阴道封闭术及盆底重建手术等。

Etiology

Laceration in delivery；long – term increased abdominal pressure；congenital weakness of supporting tissues in pelvic tissue.

Classification

First degree prolapse is often called vault prolapse，the uterus lies below its normal level but the cervix does not protrude from the vulva. If the distance between external cervix orifice and vaginal membrane minors 4 cm，not reaching to the edge of vaginal membrane is a light one and if the external cervix orifice reaches the edge of vaginal membrane but not beyond the edge is a heavy one. Cervix can be seen at the vaginal orifice in examination.

Second degree uterine prolapse is characterized by protrusion of the cervix from the vulva. If the cervix protrudes the vulva，while the uterus body is still in the vagina，it is called a light one. The heavy one is the cervix and partial uterus protrude the vagina.

Third degree prolapse the cervix and entire uterus is protruded from the vagina and the entire vagina is inverted as a consequence.

Clinical Manifestation

The patients of first degree of prolapse do not cause symptoms. The condition gradually tends to become more severe.

The patient of second degree has a sense of dragging discomfort or an aching or pulling sensation in the lower pelvis is particularly evident after she has been in the erect position for sometime. At the beginning，the masses disappear after relaxation or become smaller. For the third degree patients，even after relaxation，the masses could not be returned. The symptoms of uterine prolapse are those of protrusion of the cervix or uterus through the introitus. They include heaviness，fullness，falling out in the perineal area，feeling of bulging in the vagina or dragging.

Backache that is most painful on arising and abates during the day is likely to be orthopedic in origin. In major degrees of prolapse，the protruding cervix and vagina may ulcerate，with consequent bleeding and discharge or pain. Purulent secretion is often discharged from the cervix and vagina when secondary infection occurs.

Principle of Management

Management depends upon the age of the patient，whether she is in her childbearing years or desirous of having more children. The principle is that the treatment should be safe，simple and effective.

【护理评估】

1. 健康史　了解患者有无产程过长、阴道助产及盆底组织撕伤等病史。同时评估患者有无长期腹压增高情况，如慢性咳嗽、盆腹腔肿瘤、便秘等。

2. 身心状况　了解患者有无腰背酸痛、下腹坠胀感，有无大、小便困难及阴道肿物脱出，是否在用力下蹲、增加腹压时加重上述症状，甚至出现尿失禁，经卧床休息后症状减轻。注意评估患者是否因子宫脱出行动不便，影响生活而出现焦虑、低落、悲观失望等情绪。

3. 妇科检查　在患者增加腹压的情况下重点评估子宫脱垂的程度，子宫颈、阴道壁有无溃疡及溃疡面的大小、深浅等。同时，还应注意有无阴道前后壁膨出和陈旧性会阴裂伤及程度，有无张力性尿失禁等。

【护理诊断】

1. 焦虑　与长期的子宫脱出影响正常生活有关。

2.慢性疼痛　与子宫下垂牵拉韧带、子宫颈,阴道壁溃疡有关。

【护理措施】

1.一般护理　改善患者一般情况,加强患者营养,卧床休息。积极治疗原发疾病,指导患者进行盆底肌肉锻炼,行缩肛运动,用力使盆底肌肉收缩3 s以上后放松,10～15 min/次,2～3次/d。

2.教会患者子宫托的放取方法　以喇叭形子宫托为例。选择大小适宜的子宫托,放置前让患者排尽大小便,洗净双手,蹲下并两腿分开,一只手持托柄,使托盘呈倾斜位进入阴道口,将托柄边向内推边向阴道顶端旋转,直至托盘达子宫颈,然后屏气,使子宫下降,同时用手指将托柄向上推,使托盘牢牢地吸附在子宫颈上(图17-2)。放妥后,将托柄弯朝前,正对耻骨弓后面便可。取子宫托时,手指捏住子宫托柄,上、下、左、右轻轻摇动,等负压消失后向后外方牵拉,即可自阴道滑出。在使用子宫托时应注意:放置前阴道应有一定水平的雌激素作用;子宫托应每日早上放入阴道,睡前取出消毒后备用,避免放置过久压迫生殖器而致糜烂、溃疡;保持阴道清洁;上托以后,分别于第1、3、6个月时到医院检查1次,以后每3～6个月到医院检查1次。

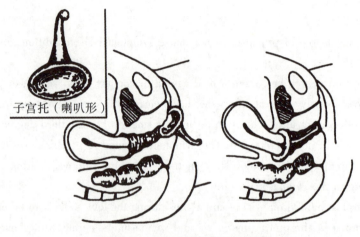

图17-2　喇叭形子宫托及其放置

3.做好术前准备　术前5 d开始进行阴道准备,Ⅰ度子宫脱垂患者应每日坐浴2次,坐浴液一般采取1∶5 000的高锰酸钾或0.2‰的碘伏溶液;对Ⅱ/Ⅲ度子宫脱垂的患者,特别是有溃疡者,行阴道冲洗后局部涂含抗生素的软膏,并勤换内裤。注意冲洗液的温度,一般在41～43 ℃为宜,冲洗后戴无菌手套将脱垂的子宫还纳于阴道内,让患者平卧于床上半小时。用清洁的卫生带或丁字带支托下移的子宫,避免子宫与内裤摩擦。积极治疗局部炎症,按医嘱使用抗生素及局部涂含雌激素的软膏。

4.术后护理　术后应卧床休息7～10 d;留置导尿管10～14 d;避免增加腹压的动作;术后用缓泻剂预防便秘;每日行外阴擦洗,注意观察阴道分泌物的特点;应用抗生素预防感染。

5.心理护理　子宫脱垂患者由于长期受疾病折磨,往往有烦躁情绪,护士应为其讲解子宫脱垂的疾病知识和预后;做好家属的工作,让家属理解患者,协助患者早日康复。

6.出院指导　术后一般休息3个月,禁止盆浴及性生活,半年内避免重体力劳动。术后2个月到医院复查伤口愈合情况;3个月后再到门诊复查,医生确认完全恢复以后方可有性生活。

Nursing Interventions

● Help the patients to use pessaries correctly:Pessaries need periodic attention by the patient and the health provider. The pessary must be removed, cleaned, and replaced at regular intervals. At the same intervals the vaginal walls must be inspected. If any evidence of inflammation or ulceration appears in the vaginal walls, the instrument cannot be worn. A properly fitted pessary should make the patient be unconscious of its presence while it is in the vagina. The patient wearing a pessary should be instructed to return to her physician's office once each 3–6 months for pelvic examination. The choice of pessary for the support of uterine prolapse must be guided by individual circumstances in a particular patient.

● Perioperative nursing: Information is provided about the surgical procedure and consequences, particularly on sexuality and reproductive function. Anesthesia risk, postoperative and recovery processes, and return to normal function are discussed. Following surgery, vital signs are monitored frequently. Bleeding and pain are assessed. Apply antibiotics to prevent infection. Early ambulation is promoted, and diet is progressed as tolerated. The patient needs to relax for 3 months, avoid heavy work in 6 months, check at 2 months after operation.

【健康教育】

①提倡计划生育,防止生育过多、过密。②加强营养,增强体质。积极防治慢性咳嗽、习惯性便秘等。③注意产褥期保健,避免产后过早参加重体力劳动或需增加腹压的劳动;鼓励产后做保健操。④医务人员应正确处理产程,提高助产技术:避免产程延长;正确指导产妇使用腹压;保护好会阴,及时行会阴切开术;会阴撕裂应仔细缝合;有指征者应及时行剖宫产术。

任务三　不孕症(Infertility)

工作情景

患者,27岁,结婚2年不孕。丈夫28岁,检查结果无异常。患者到不孕症门诊就诊。

①请明确患者将进行的不孕特殊检查。②针对检查可能造成的不适,提供相应的护理措施。

任务内容

女性无避孕性生活至少12个月而未受孕,称为不孕症。在男性则称为不育症。不孕症可分为原发性和继发性两类,其中从未妊娠者称为原发不孕,有过妊娠而后不孕者称为继发不孕。夫妇一方有先天或后天解剖生理方面的缺陷,无法纠正而不能妊娠者称为绝对不孕;夫妇一方因某种因素阻碍受孕,导致暂时不孕,一旦得到纠正仍能受孕者称为相对不孕。不孕症发病率因国家、种族和地区不同存在差别,我国不孕症发病率为7%~10%。

任务目标

◆能叙述不孕症的定义、分类及主要检查方法。

◆能综合评估不孕症患者情况,提供相应的护理及健康教育。

【概要】

1. 病因　阻碍受孕的因素包括女方、男方、男女双方因素和不明原因。其中女方因素占 40% ~ 55%，男方因素占 25% ~ 40%，男女双方共同因素占 20% ~ 30%，不明原因约占 10%。

2. 临床表现　不孕症夫妇常有不同程度的全身性疾病，如营养不良、甲状腺功能亢进症等。内、外生殖器官发育及第二性征的发育也可出现异常，如外生殖器畸形或病变；女性处女膜过厚或比较坚韧，阴道有纵隔、瘢痕或狭窄，子宫颈或子宫异常，子宫附件压痛或肿块等。

3. 处理原则　应针对病因进行治疗；改变不良生活习惯，加强锻炼，增强体质；掌握性知识，学会预测排卵，性交次数应适当；积极治疗生殖系统器质性疾病，特别是输卵管炎症及阻塞的治疗，也可采用内分泌疗法，以支持黄体功能和改善子宫颈黏液的性状；根据具体情况采用恰当的辅助生殖技术。

Etiology

Problems related to the female partner, the male partner, and the both female and male partner can result in infertility.

Principle of Management

Identification of appropriate infertility therapy must consider many factors, including the couple's history, medical evaluations, financial resources, ages and other time constraints, and religious and cultural values. Some therapy is simple, such as timing intercourse to better coincide with ovulation. Other procedures may involve considerable expense, discomfort, or unpleasant side effects. Many infertile couples need a combination of treatments to improve their chances of conception.

【护理评估】

1. 健康史　应从家庭、社会、性生殖等方面，全面评估男女双方的健康史。女方重点询问年龄、不孕年限、月经史，是否有生殖器官炎症及慢性疾病史。男性还需询问有无影响生育的疾病史、生殖器官外伤史和手术史。

2. 身心状况　夫妇双方应进行包括第二性征发育情况在内的全身检查，并注意排除全身性疾病；男方应重点检查外生殖器有无畸形或病变；女方应重点检查有无处女膜过厚或坚韧，有无阴道痉挛或横隔、纵隔、瘢痕或狭窄，子宫或子宫颈有无异常，子宫附件有无压痛、增厚或肿块等。不孕症的诊治过程可能是长期且令人心力交瘁的过程，个人在生理、心理、社会和经济方面都可能遭受压力，需要酌情同时对夫妇双方或分别评估其心理反应。

3. 辅助检查　男方检查除全身检查，重点应检查阴茎、阴囊、前列腺的大小、形状等；初诊时男方要进行 2~3 次精液检查，以获取基线数据。女方检查包括卵巢功能检查、输卵管通畅试验、性交后精子穿透力试验、子宫颈黏液、精液相合试验、腹腔镜检查及宫腔镜检查。

【护理诊断】

1. 知识缺乏　缺乏解剖知识和性生殖知识；缺乏性技巧。

2. 自尊紊乱　与不孕症诊治过程中繁杂的检查、无效的治疗效果有关。

【护理措施】

1. 检查护理　向女方解释诊断性检查可能引起的不适。子宫输卵管碘油造影可能引起腹部痉挛感，在术后持续 1~2 h，可以在当日或第 2 天返回工作岗位而不留后遗症。腹腔镜术后 1~2 h 可能感到一侧或双侧肩部疼痛，可遵医嘱给予可待因或可待因类的药物以镇痛。子宫内膜活检后可能引起下腹部的不适感如痉挛、阴道流血。若子宫颈管有炎症,黏液黏稠并有白细胞时会影响性交后试验的效果。

2. 指导女方服药 ①教会女方在月经周期遵医嘱正确按时服药;②说明药物的作用及不良反应;③提醒女方及时报告药物的不良反应如潮热、恶心、呕吐、头痛;④指导女方在发生妊娠后立即停药。

3. 注重心理护理 不孕症对于不孕夫妇来说可能导致系列的心理反应(震惊、否认、悲伤、孤独),护理人员应提供对夫妇双方的护理。当多种治疗措施的效果不佳时,护理人员帮助夫妇正视治疗结果,帮助他们选择是否继续治疗,和不孕夫妇探讨人工辅助生殖技术。

4. 教会女方提高妊娠率的技巧 鼓励女方治疗合并症,保持身心健康状态。在性交前、中、后勿使用阴道润滑剂或进行阴道灌洗,不要在性交后立即如厕,而应该卧床,并抬高臀部,持续 20 ～ 30 min,以使精子进入子宫颈。选择适当的日期性交,可在排卵期增加性交次数。

5. 帮助女方分析和比较几种人工辅助生殖技术 配子输卵管内移植(GIFT)、体外受精(IVF)都具有较高的妊娠率,但 GIFT 可以导致异位妊娠的发生率升高,并且几乎所有的辅助生殖技术都可能引起多胎妊娠。在治疗不孕症的过程中应该考虑到经济因素,一些辅助生殖技术昂贵而成功率并不高。

6. 正视不孕症治疗的结局 不孕症治疗可能的 3 个结局:①治疗失败,妊娠丧失;②治疗成功,发生妊娠;③治疗失败,停止治疗。

Nursing Interventions

- Direct woman to take medicine: Nursing implications include teaching woman to begin taking medication of fifth day of cycle and to take drug at the same time each day; teaching about drug and potential risks and benefits; teaching woman to report symptoms of hot flashes, nausea, vomiting, headache, visual symptoms; instructing woman to stop taking drug if pregnancy is suspected.

- Pay attention to psychologic aspects of infertility: Infertility is a major life crisis for many couples. Nurses and other health care team members often can provide the support necessary for the couple to resolve the crisis of infertility in a positive manner.

- Educate woman to increase fertility: There are several simple things the nurse can educate infertile woman to increase the chances of becoming pregnant. ①To stay healthy. ②To encourage communication with your partner. ③Do not stress conception as the product of sexual relations. ④Do not rise to urinate immediately after intercourse. ⑤Maximize your chances of pregnancy by timing intercourse around the time of ovulation.

- Analyze and compare characterize of the ART: The primary advantage of GIFT and TET over IVF is a higher pregnancy rate. With IVF and TET, evidence of fertilization exists before placement in the uterus or tubes. Either GIFT or TET may result in a tubal pregnancy if the embryo cannot reach the uterine cavity to implant.

- Remind outcomes after infertility therapy: After infertility therapy, three outcomes are possible. Pregnancy loss after infertility therapy; parenthood after infertility; infertility-therapy may be unsuccessful and the couple must decide whether to pursue adoption.

【健康教育】

护理人员应向夫妇宣讲不孕症相关知识,帮助不孕妇女和她的家人进行沟通,提高自我评价,正确应对不孕现实。在治疗过程中保持正常心态,积极配合各种诊断、检查。在妊娠过程中,通过饮食、适量活动等方法保持良好的身体状况,有异常反应立即就诊。

辅助生殖技术

微课

课件

练习题及参考答案

(张艳亭)

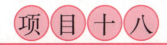

项目十八
计划生育妇女的护理
(Nuring of Family Planning Women)

▶ 项目描述

　　计划生育是妇女生殖健康的重要内容。计划生育措施主要包括避孕、绝育及避孕失败补救措施。避孕方法知情选择是计划生育优质服务的重要内容,实行计划生育应充分尊重夫妻双方的意愿。护士通过宣传、教育、培训、指导等途径,使育龄妇女了解常用避孕方法的相关知识,并协助育龄妇女根据自身特点选择适宜、安全、有效的避孕方法。

　　Family planning is an important part of women's reproductive health. Family planning measures mainly include contraception, sterilization, and contraceptive failure remedies. Assisting the couple to select and use an effective contraceptive method is an important nursing function. The nurse must understand couple's philosophy and beliefs about contraception and avoid presenting biased information. Highly effective contraceptives are available. However, all involve some risk, and their effectiveness may be lowered by inappropriate use.

任务一　避孕方法及护理(Common Methods of Contraception and Nursing Care)

▶ 工作情景

　　小张,25岁,结婚1个月,暂时不想要孩子,口服妈富隆避孕,但担心药物对身体及以后怀孕有影响,故今日来医院咨询,以便选择更为安全的避孕方法。

　　作为护士,请指导小张选择适合她的避孕措施,并对其采取的避孕措施进行相应的健康教育。

▶ 任务内容

　　避孕是计划生育的重要组成部分,是采用科学手段使妇女暂时不受孕。目前常用的女性避孕方法有宫内节育器避孕、药物避孕及外用避孕等。

任务目标

◆ 能叙述女性常用的避孕方法及其作用机制。

◆ 能指导女性选择适合的避孕措施。

◆ 能配合医生完成放、取宫内节育器手术。

避孕主要控制生殖过程中 3 个关键环节：①抑制精子与卵子产生；②阻止精子与卵子结合；③使子宫环境不利于精子获能、生存，或不适宜受精卵着床和发育。理想的避孕方法，应符合安全、有效、简便、实用、经济的原则，对性生活及性生理无不良影响，为男女双方均能接受并乐意持久使用。

一 宫内节育器避孕

宫内节育器(intrauterine device,IUD)避孕是将避孕器具放置于子宫腔内，通过局部组织对它的各种反应而达到避孕效果，是一种安全、有效、简便、经济、可逆的避孕方法，为我国育龄妇女所接受并广泛使用。

1. 种类

(1)惰性 IUD(第一代 IUD)　由金属、硅胶、塑料或尼龙等惰性材料制成。由于金属单环带器妊娠和脱落率较高，已于 1993 年停止生产使用。

(2)活性 IUD(第二代 IUD)　内含活性物质，如铜离子、激素、药物或磁性物质等，可以提高避孕效果，减少副作用。分为含铜 IUD 和含药 IUD 两大类。含铜 IUD 是目前我国临床常用的，含药 IUD 主要有含孕激素的 IUD 和含吲哚美辛的 IUD。

2. 避孕原理　有阻碍受精卵着床、使子宫内膜产生前列腺素、杀精毒胚的作用。

3. 宫内节育器放置术

(1)适应证　凡育龄妇女无禁忌证、要求放置宫内节育器者。

(2)禁忌证　①妊娠或妊娠可疑；②生殖道急性炎症；③人工流产出血多，怀疑有妊娠组织物残留或感染可能；中期妊娠引产、分娩或剖宫产胎盘娩出后，子宫收缩不良，有出血或潜在感染可能；④生殖器肿瘤；⑤生殖器畸形；⑥子宫颈内口过松、重度陈旧性子宫颈裂伤或子宫脱垂；⑦严重的全身性疾病；⑧宫腔<5.5 cm 或>9.0 cm（除外足月分娩后、大月份引产后或放置含铜无支架宫内节育器）；⑨近 3 个月内有月经失调、阴道不规则流血；⑩有铜过敏史。

(3)放置时间　①月经干净 3~7 d 无性交；②人工流产后立即放置；③产后 42 d 恶露已净，会阴伤口愈合，子宫恢复正常；④剖宫产术后半年；⑤含孕激素宫内节育器在月经第 4~7 天放置；⑥自然流产于转经后放置，药物流产 2 次正常月经后放置；⑦哺乳期放置应先排除早孕；⑧性交后 5 d 内放置为紧急避孕方法之一。

(4)放置方法　双合诊检查子宫大小、位置及附件情况。外阴阴道部常规消毒铺巾，阴道扩张器暴露子宫颈后消毒子宫颈与子宫颈管，以子宫颈钳夹持子宫颈前唇，用子宫探针顺子宫位置探测宫腔深度。用放置器将节育器推送入宫腔，宫内节育器上缘必须抵达宫底部，带有尾丝的宫内节育器在距宫口 2 cm 处剪断尾丝。观察无出血即可取出子宫颈钳和阴道扩张器。

(5)术后护理　①术后休息 3 d，1 周内忌重体力劳动，2 周内忌性生活及盆浴，保持外阴清洁。②术后第一年 1、3、6、12 个月进行随访，以后每年随访 1 次直至停用，有特殊情况随时就诊。随访宫内节育器在宫腔内情况，发现问题应及时处理，以保证宫内节育器避孕的有效性。

4.宫内节育器取出术

（1）适应证

1）生理情况：①计划再生育或已无性生活不再需要避孕者；②放置期限已满需更换者；③绝经过渡期停经1年内；④拟改用其他避孕措施或绝育者。

2）病理情况：①有并发症及副作用，经治疗无效；②带器妊娠，包括宫内和宫外妊娠。

（2）禁忌证　①并发生殖系统炎症时，先给予抗感染治疗，治愈后再取出宫内节育器；②全身情况不良或在疾病的急性期，应待病情好转后再取出。

（3）取器时间　①月经干净后3～7 d为宜；②带器早期妊娠行人工流产同时取器；③带器异位妊娠术前行诊断性刮宫时，或在术后出院前取出IUD；④子宫不规则出血者，随时可取，取IUD同时需行诊断性刮宫，刮出组织送病理检查，排除子宫内膜病变。

（4）取器方法　常规消毒后，有尾丝者，用血管钳夹住尾丝轻轻牵引取出。无尾丝者，需在手术室进行，按进宫腔操作程序操作，用取环钩或取环钳将宫内节育器取出。取器困难可在超声下进行操作，必要时在宫腔镜下取出。

（5）护理要点　取器时间以月经干净后3～7 d为宜，出血多者随时可取。带器早期宫内妊娠于人工流产同时取器。带器异位妊娠于术前诊断性刮宫时或术中、术后取器。术后休息1 d，术后2周内禁止性生活和盆浴，并保持外阴清洁。

5.宫内节育器的副作用及护理

（1）不规则阴道流血　是放置宫内节育器常见的副作用，主要表现为经量增多、经期延长或少量点滴出血，一般不需处理，3～6个月后逐渐恢复。若需药物治疗，可按医嘱给予前列腺素合成酶抑制剂。出血时间长者，应补充铁剂。若经上述处理无效，应考虑取出IUD，改用其他避孕方法。

（2）腰腹酸胀感　IUD与宫腔大小、形态不符时，可引起子宫频繁收缩而出现腰腹酸胀感。轻者无须处理，重者应考虑更换合适的节育器。

6.宫内节育器的并发症及处理

（1）节育器异位　操作不当将节育器放到宫腔外；节育器过大、过硬或子宫壁薄而软，子宫收缩造成节育器逐渐移位至宫腔外。确诊节育器异位后，应在腹腔镜下或经腹将节育器取出。

（2）节育器嵌顿或断裂　由于节育器放置时损伤子宫壁或带器时间过长，致部分嵌入子宫肌壁或发生断裂，应及时取出。若取出困难，应在超声或宫腔镜下取出。

（3）节育器下移或脱落　操作不规范，节育器放置未达宫底部；节育器与宫腔大小、形态不符；月经量过多；子宫颈内口过松及子宫过度敏感。常见于放置宫内节育器后1年之内。

（4）带器妊娠　多见于节育器下移、脱落或异位。一经确诊，行人工流产同时取出宫内节育器。

（5）感染　术中无菌操作不严、生殖器本身有炎症、术后过早盆浴或性交均可引起感染，表现为下腹疼痛、白带增多等。一旦发生感染，应给予广谱抗生素，并取出宫内节育器。

为减少并发症的发生，应定期随访。一旦发生IUD并发症，护士需向患者及其家属解释病情，告知正确处理方法，取得配合；严格按医嘱用药，做好术前准备工作。

Intrauterine devices(IUDs) are inserted into the uterus to provide continuous pregnancy prevention. The high-dose copper IUD provides safe, long-term contraception with effective equivalent to tubal sterilization.

Types of Intrauterine Devices

In general, devices are one of two varieties. There are chemically inert and chemically active IUD.

Mechanism of Action

The exact mechanism of action is unknown, but IUDs appear to affect sperm, ova, and the endometrium to prevent fertilization.

Complications of IUDs

● Infection：Pelvic infections have developed with a variety of intrauterine devices. They occur most often in the first few weeks after insertion. Tubal–ovarian abscesses, which may be unilateral, have been described. The major risk of infection is due to insertion and does not increase with long–term use. With suspected infection, the device should be removed, and the woman treated with effective antibiotics.

● Pregnancy：A device within the pregnant uterus may be dangerous for the woman and her fetus. Appropriate steps should be removal of the device.

● Ectopic：If pregnancy occurs in an IUD wearer, it will be ectopic in about 5% of cases. The studies have reported that the IUD did not increase the rates of ectopic pregnancy.

● Uterine perforation：The earliest adverse effects are those associated with insertion. They include clinically apparent or silent uterine perforation, either while sounding the uterus or during insertion of the device. The frequency of this complication depends on operator skill.

● Uterine cramping and bleeding：Uterine cramping and some bleeding are likely to develop soon after insertion, and they persist for variable periods. Cramping can be minimized by administering a nonsteroidal anti–inflammatory agent approximately 1 h, prior to insertion.

● Menorrhagia：Increased menstruation is common problem with the use of IUD and it may be so great as to cause iron–deficiency anemia. This is a troubling side effect, and 10% –15% of women using the copper device have it removed for this problem.

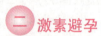 **激素避孕**

激素避孕是指女性应用甾体激素达到避孕效果。目前国内主要为人工合成的甾体激素避孕药,由雌激素和孕激素配伍组成。

1.作用机制　抑制排卵,改变子宫颈黏液性状,改变子宫内膜形态与功能,改变输卵管的功能。

2.适应证　健康育龄妇女均可采用甾体激素避孕药。

3.禁忌证　严重心血管疾病,急、慢性肝炎或肾炎,血液病或血栓性疾病,内分泌疾病,恶性肿瘤、癌前病变、子宫或乳房肿块,哺乳期,月经稀少或年龄大于 45 岁,原因不明的阴道异常流血,精神病生活不能自理。

4.种类

(1)口服避孕药

1)复方短效口服避孕药:雌激素、孕激素组成的复合制剂。根据整个周期中雌激素、孕激素的剂量和比例变化而分为单相片、双相片和三相片 3 种。复方短效口服避孕药的主要作用为抑制排卵,正确使用避孕药的有效率接近100% 。注意事项:若漏服必须于次晨补服。若停药 7 d 尚无阴道出血,于当晚或第 2 天开始第 2 周期服药。若服用 2 个周期仍无月经来潮,则应该停药,考虑更换避孕药物种类或就医诊治。

2)复方长效口服避孕药:由长效雌激素和人工合成孕激素配伍制成,服药 1 次可避孕 1 个月。避孕有效率达96% ~98% 。复方长效口服避孕药激素含量大,副作用较多,市场上已经很少见。

(2)长效避孕针　目前的长效避孕针,有单孕激素制剂和雌激素、孕激素复合制剂两种,有效率达98% 以上。尤其适用于对口服避孕药有明显胃肠道反应者。长效避孕针有月经紊乱、点滴出血或闭经等副作用。由于单孕激素制剂对乳汁的质和量影响小,较适用于哺乳期妇女。复合制剂,由于激素剂量大,副作用大,很少用。

（3）探亲避孕药　适用于短期探亲夫妇。有抑制排卵、改变子宫内膜形态与功能、使子宫颈黏液变稠等作用。探亲避孕药的避孕效果可靠,但是由于探亲避孕药的剂量大,现已经很少使用。

（4）缓释避孕药　又称缓释避孕系统。缓释避孕药是以具备缓慢释放性能的高分子化合物为载体,1 次给药后在体内通过持续、恒定、微量释放甾体激素,主要是孕激素,达到长效避孕目的。目前常用的有皮下埋植剂、阴道药环、避孕贴片及含药的宫内节育器。

5.药物的副作用及处理

（1）类早孕反应　是口服避孕药最常见的副作用,是雌激素刺激胃黏膜引起的。妇女服药后多有食欲减退、恶心、呕吐、困倦、头晕、乳房胀痛、白带增多等类似早孕反应,坚持服药数日后常可自行缓解。症状严重者需考虑更换制剂或停药改用其他措施。

（2）不规则阴道流血　服药期间阴道流血又称突破性出血。多数发生在漏服避孕药后,少数未漏服避孕药也会发生。轻者点滴出血,不用处理,随着服药时间延长而逐渐减少直至停止。流血偏多者,每晚在服用避孕药同时加服雌激素直至停药。流血似月经量或流血时间已近月经期,则停止服药,作为 1 次月经来潮,于下一周期再开始服用药物,或更换避孕药。

（3）闭经　1% ~2% 妇女发生闭经,常发生于月经不规则妇女。对原有月经不规则妇女,使用避孕药应谨慎。停药后月经不来潮,需除外妊娠,停药 7 d 后可继续服药,若连续停经 3 个月,需停药观察。

（4）体重及皮肤变化　早期研制的避孕药中雄激素活性强,个别妇女服药后食欲亢进,体内合成代谢增加,体重增加;极少数妇女面部出现淡褐色色素沉着。近年来随着口服避孕药不断发展,雄激素活性降低,孕激素活性增强,用药量小,副作用也明显降低,而且能改善皮肤痤疮等。新一代口服避孕药屈螺酮炔雌醇片有抗盐皮质激素的作用,可减少雌激素引起的水钠潴留。

（5）其他　个别妇女服药后出现头痛、复视、乳房胀痛等,可对症处理,必要时停药做进一步检查。

Hormonal contraceptives are methods that alter the normal hormone fluctuations of the menstrual cycle. They may be given by implant, by injection, or orally. Oral contraceptives are a combination of estrogen and progestin. Injectable or implantable contraceptives contain progestins alone or a combination of estrogen and progestin.

Oral Contraceptives（OCs）

OCs are the most widely used reversible contraceptive method. Combination OCs contain both estrogen and progestin. Oral contraceptives have a nearly 100% typical effectiveness rate if they are used correctly.

Mechanisms of Action

Preventing ovulation is the mainly mechanism of OCs.

Contraindications

Oral contraceptives should not be used by women with a history of any of the following: Thrombophlebitis or thromboembolic disorders; cerebrovascular or cardiovascular disease; any estrogen-dependent cancer or breast cancer; benign or malignant liver tumors; impaired liver function; suspected or known pregnancy; undiagnosed vaginal bleeding; heavy cigarette smoking.

Side Effects

The side effects are due to estrogen and progestin. Most side effects are minor and include signs and symptoms often seen in pregnancy. Decreasing the amount of estrogen helps relieve nausea, headaches, and breast tenderness, whereas increasing the estrogen content prevents breakthrough bleeding. Other side effects include weight gain or loss, fluid retention, amenorrhea, and chloasma. Side effects often decrease after the first few months of use and are less frequent in low-dose OCs.

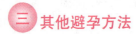 其他避孕方法

1.紧急避孕　无保护性生活后或避孕失败后几小时或几日内,妇女为防止非意愿性妊娠的发生而采用的补救避孕法,称为紧急避孕。紧急避孕仅对1次无保护性生活有效,避孕有效率明显低于常规避孕方法,且紧急避孕药激素剂量大,副作用亦大,不能替代常规避孕。方法包括放置含铜宫内节育器和口服紧急避孕药。

（1）适应证　避孕失败、性生活未采用任何避孕措施、遭受性暴力。

（2）方法

1）放置宫内节育器:采用含铜IUD,在无保护性生活后5 d（120 h）内放置,避孕有效率达99%以上。适合希望长期避孕且无放置IUD禁忌证的妇女。

2）口服紧急避孕药:①激素类,如左炔诺孕酮片,在无保护性性交后3 d（72 h）内首剂1片,12 h后再服1片。②抗孕激素制剂,如米非司酮,在无保护性生活后120 h内服用,单次口服25 mg。

2.外用避孕

（1）阴茎套　也称避孕套,为男性避孕工具。作为屏障阻止精子进入阴道而达到避孕目的,还有防止性传播疾病的作用。

（2）阴道套　也称女用避孕套,既能避孕,又能防止性传播疾病。目前我国尚无供应。

（3）外用杀精剂　外用杀精剂是性交前置入阴道,具有灭活精子作用的一类化学避孕制剂。目前临床常用有避孕栓剂、片剂、胶冻剂、凝胶剂及避孕薄膜等,由活性成分壬苯醇醚与基质制成。壬苯醇具有强烈杀精作用,正确使用外用杀精剂,有效率达95%以上。使用失误,失败率在20%以上,不作为避孕首选药。

（4）安全期避孕　又称自然避孕,是根据女性生殖生理的知识推测排卵日期,在判断周期中的易受孕期进行禁欲而达到避孕目的。安全期避孕法并不可靠。

此外,还有黄体生成激素释放激素类似物避孕、免疫避孕法的导向药物避孕和抗生育疫苗等,目前正在研究中。

Other Contraceptive Methods

• Postcoital emergency contraception: Postcoital contraception is a method to prevent pregnancy after unprotected intercourse. It may be used after contraceptive failure, such as a condom breaking or diaphragm dislodging during intercourse. It also may be used after rape or in other situations. The high hormone levels prevent or delay ovulation to prevent fertilization and may have some effect on endometrial development. The treatment is ineffective if pregnancy has already occurred and does not harm a developing fetus. The most common method involves taking a larger-than-usual dose of a combined OCs as soon as possible and no later than 72 h after unprotected intercourse. A second dose is taken 12 h after the first. Treatment reduces the risk of pregnancy by 75%.

• Male condom: Condoms, the only male contraceptive device currently available, are one of the most popular contraceptive methods in China. They cover the penis to prevent sperm from entering the vagina. Condoms are most often made of latex and may be coated with spermicide. Some condoms are made from polyurethane. Polyurethane condoms are thinner than latex and can be used by people who are allergic to latex. Unfortunately, the polyurethane condom has a significantly higher breakage rate than latex condoms.

Both of latex and polyurethane condoms are effective against sexually transmitted diseases, including HIV.

● Female condom (vaginal pouch): The female condom is made of the polyurethane material with 2 flexible rings at each side. Open ring remains outside the vagina and closed internal ring is fitted under the symphysis like a diaphragm.

四　各时期避孕措施的选择

避孕方法知情选择是计划生育优质服务的重要内容,指通过广泛深入宣传、教育、培训和咨询,帮助育龄妇女根据自身特点(包括家庭、身体、婚姻状况等),选择合适的、安全有效的避孕方法。以下介绍生育年龄各期避孕方法的选择。

1.新婚期

(1)原则　新婚夫妇年轻,尚未生育,应选择使用方便、不影响生育的避孕方法。

(2)选用方法　复方短效口服避孕药使用方便,避孕效果好,不影响性生活,列为首选。男用阴茎套也是较理想的避孕方法,性生活适应后可选用阴茎套,还可选用外用避孕栓、薄膜等。尚未生育或未曾有人工流产手术者,宫内节育器不作为首选。不适宜用安全期避孕、体外排精及长效避孕药。

2.哺乳期

(1)原则　不影响乳汁质量及婴儿健康。

(2)选用方法　阴茎套是哺乳期选用的最佳避孕方式。也可选用单孕激素制剂长效避孕针或皮下埋植剂,使用方便,不影响乳汁质量。哺乳期放置宫内节育器,操作要轻柔,防止子宫损伤。由于哺乳期阴道较干燥,不适用避孕药膜。哺乳期不宜使用雌激素、孕激素复合避孕药或避孕针及安全期避孕。

3.生育后期

(1)原则　选择长效、可逆、安全、可靠的避孕方法,减少非意愿妊娠进行手术带来的痛苦及并发症。

(2)选用方法　各种避孕方法(宫内节育器、皮下埋植剂、复方口服避孕药、避孕针、阴茎套等)均适用,根据个人身体状况进行选择。对某种避孕方法有禁忌证者,则不宜使用此种方法。

4.绝经过渡期

(1)原则　此期仍有排卵可能,应坚持避孕,选择以外用避孕为主的避孕方法。

(2)选用方法　可采用阴茎套。原来使用宫内节育器无不良反应者可继续使用,至绝经后半年内取出。绝经过渡期阴道分泌物较少,不宜选择避孕药膜避孕,可选用避孕栓、凝胶剂。不宜选用复方避孕药及安全期避孕。

Special Consideration for Contraception

● Adolescent: Concerns about confidentiality and lack of money deter teenagers from seeking and obtaining contraception. Combined oral contraceptives are excellent choice for this age group because they provide effective contraception, increase bone density and can be used to improve acne and regulate menstrual cycle. The only disadvantage is daily requirement of pill taking.

● Barrier method: Provide protection against STDs but they are not good choices for adolescent as they require preplanning and motivation for proper use. Barrier method should be considered primarily as backup method and protective method for STDs.

● Contraception for older than 35 years: Though fertility begins to decline at 35-40 years old, there is still the risk for unwanted pregnancy and STDs. The choice for them are as follows：combined oral contraceptive，injectable depot medroxyprogesterone acetate，intrauterine device，barrier method.

- Lactating mothers：Breastfeeding is important to infant health and to child spacing. Lactating in itself is not a reliable method of family planning. Waiting for first menses involves a risk of pregnancy because ovulation usually antedates menstruation. Progestogen only contraception is a preferred choice in most case. If infant is on partial breastfeeding，IUD can also be recommended.

任务实施

宫内节育器放置术操作步骤见表18-1。

表18-1　宫内节育器放置术操作步骤

项目	内容
术前准备	1. 评估：评估受术者一般情况，有无异常阴道流液症状，意识状态，生命体征，术前3 d禁止性生活；签署知情同意书。适应证：育龄女性自愿要求放置而无禁忌者；某些疾病的辅助治疗，如宫腔粘连、异常子宫出血及子宫腺肌病等的保守治疗。禁忌证：严重的全身性疾病；急慢性生殖系统炎症，如盆腔炎；妊娠及可疑妊娠；生殖器官肿瘤；产后42 d恶露未干净或会阴伤口未愈；严重痛经者
	2. 准备用物：治疗托盘、消毒上环包、碘伏、棉签、手套、合适型号和类型的宫内节育器、抢救用药（阿托品注射液）
	3. 仪表端庄，着装整洁，洗手
手术步骤	1. 核对，解释取得合作，嘱排空小便，将受术者带入手术操作间
	2. 打开上环包：助手核对刮宫包使用期限，用手打开外层包布，再用持物钳打开内层包布。操作者正确戴手套后亦可打开内层包布
	3. 体位及铺巾：受术者取膀胱截石位，常规消毒外阴、阴道。铺无菌巾：①垫治疗巾；②套腿套；③铺无菌孔巾。进行手术器械整理（子宫颈扩张器按从小到大排序）。行双合诊检查了解子宫及双侧附件情况。更换手套（或右手戴2只手套，检查后脱掉1只）
	4. 扩开阴道及消毒处理 （1）手术阴道扩张器暴露子宫颈 （2）消毒子宫颈和子宫颈管口 （3）更换阴道扩张器，暴露子宫颈，子宫颈钳钳夹子宫颈前唇，轻轻向外牵拉
	5. 扩张子宫颈及放置节育器 （1）探查宫腔深度、方向并告知助手记录 （2）子宫颈扩张器逐一扩开子宫颈至适当大小（一般由4号扩至6号即可） （3）宫内节育器种类繁多各有特点：环形或宫形节育器、V形宫内节育器、T形节育器、母体乐、Y形节育器等；注意节育器上缘要达到宫腔底部；带尾丝节育器放置成功后，子宫颈管外尾丝要保留1.5~2.0 cm长度 （4）再次消毒子宫颈及阴道
	6. 术后处理 （1）观察有无活动性出血 （2）取下子宫颈钳，撤出阴道扩张器 （3）向受术者交代注意事项（禁同房2周）

续表 18-1

项目	内容
注意事项	1. 严格无菌操作
	2. 动作稳、准、轻、细

任务二　避孕失败的补救措施（Remedies for Contraceptive Failure）

工作情景

王女士，26岁，已婚。平素身体健康，月经规律，现在月经推迟半个月未来潮，自测尿妊娠试验阳性。因个人身体原因要求流产，但惧怕做人工流产手术，故来院咨询终止妊娠的其他方法及流产的注意事项。

①王女士目前的主要护理诊断是什么？②在终止妊娠前必须做哪项辅助检查？③确诊宫内妊娠后，建议贺女士采取什么方法终止妊娠？

任务内容

因意外妊娠、疾病等原因而采用人工方法终止妊娠称为人工流产，是避孕失败的补救方法。人工流产对妇女的生殖健康有一定的影响，做好避孕工作，避免或减少意外妊娠是计划生育工作的真正目的。终止早期妊娠的人工流产方法包括手术流产和药物流产。

任务目标

◆能叙述手术流产和药物流产的适应证。
◆能根据患者的情况指导其选择适宜的终止早期妊娠的方法。
◆能协助医生完成手术流产。

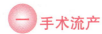 手术流产

【操作方法】

手术流产包括负压吸引术和钳刮术。

1. 负压吸引术　利用负压吸引原理，将妊娠物从宫腔内吸出，称为负压吸引术。适用于妊娠10周内要求终止妊娠而无禁忌证，或因某种疾病（包括遗传性疾病）不宜继续妊娠者。禁忌证包括各种疾病的急性阶段、生殖器炎症、术前两次体温在 37.5 ℃ 以上及全身健康状况不良，不能承受手术者。

（1）体位　受术者排空膀胱，取膀胱截石位。常规消毒外阴、阴道，铺盖无菌洞巾。作双合诊复查子宫位置、大小及附件情况，用阴道扩张器暴露子宫颈并消毒。

（2）探测宫腔　子宫颈钳夹持子宫颈前唇，用子宫探针探测子宫屈向和深度。

（3）扩张子宫颈　子宫颈扩张器扩张子宫颈管,一般扩张至大于所用吸管半号或 1 号。

（4）吸管负压吸引　吸引前,需进行负压吸引试验。无误后,按孕周选择吸管粗细及负压大小,负压不宜超过 600 mmHg。一般按顺时针方向吸引宫腔 1~2 周,即可将妊娠物吸引干净。当感觉宫腔缩小,宫壁粗糙,吸头紧贴宫壁,移动受阻时,表示已吸净,然后慢慢取出吸管。

（5）检查宫腔是否吸净　用小号刮匙轻刮宫腔,尤其要注意宫底及两侧宫角部。全部吸出物用纱布过滤,检查有无绒毛、胚胎或胎儿组织,有无水泡状物。肉眼观察发现异常者,即送病理检查。

2. 钳刮术　适用于妊娠 10~14 周以内自愿要求终止妊娠而无禁忌证,或因某种疾病(包括遗传性疾病)不宜继续妊娠或其他流产方法失败者。禁忌证同负压吸引术。近年来由于米非司酮、前列腺素等药物的应用,钳刮术将逐渐被药物引产取代。为保证钳刮术顺利进行,应先作扩张子宫颈准备。术中应充分扩张子宫颈管,先夹破胎膜流尽羊水再酌情用子宫收缩药;钳夹胎盘与胎儿组织;必要时搔刮宫腔一周,观察有无出血,若有出血加用宫缩剂;术后注意预防宫腔积血和感染。

【并发症及防治】

1. 人工流产综合征　是指部分受术者在术中或手术刚结束时出现恶心呕吐、心动过缓、心律失常、血压下降、面色苍白、头晕、胸闷、大汗淋漓,甚至出现昏厥和抽搐等迷走神经兴奋症状,也称人工流产综合征。一旦出现应立即停止手术,安慰受术者,给予吸氧,一般可自行恢复。一旦出现心率减慢,静脉注射阿托品 0.5~1.0 mg,即可迅速缓解症状。

2. 子宫穿孔　是手术流产的严重并发症,但发生率低。多见于哺乳期子宫、瘢痕子宫、子宫过度倾屈或畸形者,术者未查清子宫位置或技术不熟练,手术器械如探针、吸管、刮匙、子宫颈扩张器及胎盘钳等均可造成子宫穿孔。一旦出现应立即停止手术,应用子宫收缩剂和抗生素,密切观察受术者生命体征,必要性时行剖腹探查术。

3. 吸宫不全　是指手术流产后宫腔内有部分妊娠产物残留,是手术流产常见并发症。术后阴道流血超过 10 d,血量过多,或流血停止后再现多量流血,均应考虑为吸宫不全。B 型超声检查有助于诊断。若无明显感染征象,应尽早行刮宫术,刮出物送病理检查,术后用抗生素预防感染。若同时伴有感染,应在控制感染后再行刮宫术,术后继续抗感染治疗。

4. 漏吸或空吸　已确诊为宫内妊娠,术时未能吸出胚胎或胎盘绒毛称为漏吸。主要与孕周过小、子宫畸形、子宫过度屈曲及术者技术不熟练等有关。一旦发现漏吸,应复查子宫位置、大小及形状,并重新探查宫腔,再行吸宫术。必须将吸刮的组织全部送病理检查,警惕异位妊娠。

5. 术中出血　多发生在妊娠月份较大、吸管过小时,妊娠产物不能迅速排出而影响子宫收缩所致。可在扩张子宫颈管后注射缩宫素,并尽快钳取或吸出妊娠产物。

6. 术后感染　多因吸宫不全、术后过早性交、敷料和器械消毒不严及术中无菌观念不强所致。初起为急性子宫内膜炎,若治疗不及时,可扩散至子宫肌层、附件及盆腔腹膜,严重时可导致败血症。主要表现为发热、下腹痛、白带混浊和不规则阴道流血。妇科检查时子宫或附件区有压痛。治疗原则为半卧位休息、全身支持疗法、应用广谱抗生素。

7. 羊水栓塞　少见,偶发于钳刮术,往往由于子宫颈损伤和胎盘剥离使血窦开放,此时应用缩宫素促使了羊水进入母体血液循环而发生羊水栓塞。妊娠早、中期时羊水中有形成分极少,即使发生羊水栓塞,其症状和严重性也不如晚期妊娠发病凶猛。

【护理要点】

（1）术前应详细询问停经时间、生育史及既往病史,测量体温、脉搏和血压,根据双合诊检查、尿

hCG 检查和 B 型超声检查进一步明确早期宫内妊娠诊断,并进行血常规、出凝血时间及白带常规等检查。协助医生严格核对手术适应证和禁忌证,签署知情同意书。

（2）术前告知受术者手术过程及可能出现的情况,解除其思想顾虑,取得更好的配合。

（3）术中陪伴受术者身边,指导其运用深呼吸减轻不适。

（4）术后受术者应在观察室卧床休息 1 h,注意观察腹痛及阴道流血情况。

（5）遵医嘱给予药物治疗。

（6）嘱受术者保持外阴清洁,1 个月内禁止性生活及盆浴,预防感染。

（7）吸宫术后休息 3 周,钳刮术后休息 4 周。若有腹痛及阴道流血增多,随时就诊。

二　药物流产

药物流产是指用药物终止妊娠的方法,又称药物抗早孕。具有安全、简单、不需宫腔内操作、痛苦小等优点。目前临床常用的药物为米非司酮配伍米索前列醇,完全流产率达 90% 以上。

【适应证】

妊娠 7 周内的宫内妊娠,本人自愿、年龄<40 岁的健康妇女;人工流产术的高危人群,如瘢痕子宫人群、哺乳期人群等;有多次人工流产术史,对手术流产有顾虑和恐惧心理者。

【禁忌证】

使用米非司酮的禁忌证:肾上腺疾病及其他内分泌疾病、血液疾病、血栓性疾病、妊娠期皮肤瘙痒等。使用米索前列醇的禁忌证:心血管疾病、青光眼、癫痫、哮喘、结肠炎等。其他:过敏体质、带器妊娠、异位妊娠、妊娠剧吐等。

【用药方法】

米非司酮有顿服法和分服法。顿服法:于用药第 1 天顿服 200 mg,在服药第 3 天早晨口服米索前列醇 0.6 mg。分服法:米非司酮 150 mg 分次口服,用药第 1 天早晨服 50 mg,8 ~ 12 h 再服 25 mg,第 2 天米非司酮早、晚各服 25 mg,第 3 天早晨 7 时再服 25 mg,1 h 后加服米索前列醇 0.6 mg。每次服药前后至少空腹 1 h。

【不良反应】

1. 下腹痛　由米索前列醇所致的子宫收缩引起,排出妊娠物过程中出现,一般可以忍受,严重者可用药物镇痛。

2. 出血　出血量多于月经量或阴道流血持续 2 周以上,应行清宫术,如果出血过多发生失血性休克,应抗休克同时尽早行刮宫术或吸宫术。药物流产必须在有正规抢救条件的医疗机构进行。出血时间长、出血量多是药物流产的主要副作用。

3. 胃肠道反应　部分患者服药后可出现恶心、呕吐、腹痛、腹泻等,一般不需处理。

4. 感染　与出血时间长及流产后不注意外阴清洁或过早性生活有关,一旦出现应使用抗生素治疗。

【健康教育】

加强休息,保持外阴清洁,禁止性生活和盆浴 1 个月。服用米索前列醇后应留院观察 6 h,注意观察有无用药副作用及胚囊是否排出。出现阴道流血后应用便盆接阴道排出物,医护人员认真检查排出的绒毛情况,判断流产是否完全。嘱患者密切观察阴道流血情况,如果流血量大、时间长或出现异味、腹痛等情况应及时就诊。指导患者正确避孕,再次妊娠应安排在月经复潮 6 个月后。

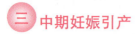

三 中期妊娠引产

终止中期妊娠的方法多采用依沙吖啶(利凡诺)和水囊引产。依沙吖啶是一种强力杀菌剂,将其经腹壁注入羊膜腔内,具有较强的杀菌和刺激子宫收缩的作用。水囊引产是将水囊置于子宫壁与胎膜之间,向囊内注入适量0.9%氯化钠注射液,刺激宫缩,促使胎儿及其附属物排出。

【适应证】

妊娠13~27周,本人自愿要求终止妊娠而无禁忌证者。因患某种疾病,不宜继续妊娠者。

【禁忌证】

严重全身性疾病。各种疾病的急性期(如急性传染病)、慢性疾病急性发作期。生殖器官急性炎症。术前24 h内两次体温≥37.5 ℃。对依沙吖啶有过敏史者不宜用依沙吖啶引产。妊娠期反复阴道流血者不宜行水囊引产。瘢痕子宫或子宫颈陈旧性裂伤者。

【操作方法】

1. 依沙吖啶引产

(1)经腹羊膜腔内注入法 孕妇排尿后取平卧位,常规消毒铺巾。腰椎穿刺针进入羊膜腔后,拔出针芯有羊水流出后接注射器注入依沙吖啶50~100 mg(用注射用水或羊水溶解,切忌用0.9%氯化钠注射液,以免发生药物沉淀),注药完毕插入针芯,快速拔出穿刺针,用无菌纱布压迫2~3 min,观察无出血,胶布固定。一般在注射后12~24 h开始宫缩,约在用药后48 h内胎儿胎盘娩出。

(2)羊膜腔外给药 孕妇排尿后取膀胱截石位,外阴、阴道常规消毒,铺无菌单。将导尿管经子宫颈插入宫壁与胎膜间,注入依沙吖啶100 mg,扎紧导尿管末端,无菌干纱布包裹,放入阴道。24 h后取出纱布和导尿管。一般注药后3~7 d内可见妊娠组织流出,流产后应密切观察阴道流血情况,检查胎盘、胎膜是否完整,疑有残留时需清理宫腔。

(3)依沙吖啶引产的注意事项 用药剂量要准确,一般用量为100 mg。穿刺成功拔出针芯后,如从穿刺针向外溢血或注射器回抽有血液时(可能是刺入胎盘)应向深部进针或向后退针稍改变方向后进针,若仍有血,应更换穿刺点,但不能超过3次。用药后24 h仍无宫缩,可加用缩宫素缓慢静脉滴注。羊膜腔内注药者,如第一次失败,可在72 h后行第二次操作。严格无菌操作。用药5 d后仍未出现宫缩者即为引产失败,应告知家属,并协商再次给药时间或改用其他引产方法。

2. 水囊引产 孕妇排空膀胱,取膀胱截石位。常规消毒铺巾,暴露子宫颈,用长镊或卵圆钳夹持水囊导尿管,经子宫颈送入宫腔,使其置于子宫壁和胎囊之间。向囊内注入无菌0.9%氯化钠注射液,注液量以每孕月100 mL计算,最多不超过500 mL。注液完毕,将导尿管末端折叠、扎紧,用无菌干纱布包裹置于阴道后穹隆部,24 h后取出水囊。

【护理要点】

1. 术前准备 ①询问病史、全面体格检查,协助医生严格掌握适应证与禁忌证。②指导受术者行B型超声检查,进行胎盘定位及穿刺点定位,并了解羊水量。③嘱受术者术前3 d禁止性生活,并且每天冲洗阴道1次。④局部常规皮肤准备。⑤了解受术者中期妊娠引产的原因,耐心答疑,为其提供情感表达的机会,并介绍手术经过、注意事项,解除其顾虑,利于术中配合。⑥准备好穿刺包、水囊和消毒手套等用物。

2. 术中配合 ①为受术者提供安静舒适的环境,术中陪伴,提供心理支持,使其积极配合。②协助医生抽取药物。③密切观察受术者有无呼吸困难、胸痛、发绀等症状,发现异常报告医生。

3. 术后护理 ①留受术者在观察室休息12 h,观察受术者生命体征、宫缩、破膜时间、阴道流血、宫底高度等情况。②产后仔细检查软产道有无裂伤及胎盘、胎膜的完整性。

【健康教育】

①注意休息，加强营养。②及时退奶。③保持外阴清洁，术后 6 周内禁止性交及盆浴。④提供可靠的避孕措施。

Causes of Abortion

Abortion is done for a number of reasons to end a pregnancy which threatens a woman's life (e. g. ,pregnancy in a woman with heart disease) or which involves a fetus found on amniocentesis to have a chromosomal defect;to end a pregnancy that is unwanted because it is the result of rape or incest;or to terminate the pregnancy of a woman who chooses not to have a child at this time in her life.

Methods for Induced Abortion

- Surgically induced abortion：① Vacuum extraction. Vacuum extraction is the simplest type of abortion procedure. It may be performed on an out-patient basis under 10 weeks after the last menstrual period. ②Dilatation and curettage. If the gestation age of the pregnancy is 11 – 14 weeks, the dilatation and curettage may be performed as the procedure.

- Medically induced abortion：RU 486 (mifepristone) is a compound that blocks the effect of progesterone and is currently used as a commonly prescribed drug for abortions. The compound has a 95% effectiveness rate when it is administered with a prostaglandin within 49 d of the last menstrual period, 90% if it is used without a prostaglandin.

Advantages are the decreased risk of damage to the uterus and use of anesthesia necessary for surgically performed abortions.

Complications of Abortion

The surgically induced abortion methods share common hazards：failure of the primary procedure to produce abortion within a reasonable time, incomplete abortion, hemorrhage and infection.

Psychological Aspects of Abortion

Women of all ages, married or unmarried, with or without children, request induced abortions. The usual profile of a woman who is having an abortion is young, unmarried, no previous live births and undergoing the procedure for the first time. Most women feel anxious when they appear at the hospital or clinic for an abortion. Some of the anxiety comes from having made a difficult decision to reach this step;some may come from feelings of loss or shame and sadness that they had to make a decision with which they are not totally comfortable.

Nursing Considerations

Women having surgically induced abortions have laboratory studies performed before the procedure, including a pregnancy test, complete blood count, blood typing, gonococcal smear, a serologic test for syphilis, urinalysis, and a Pap smear. Women with medically induced abortion are tested the type "B" ultrasonic to make sure the embryo size.

The woman void and her perineum is washed with an antiseptic at preoperation. The anesthetic block, the cervix is dilated by graduated dilators until a uterine sound and a curette can be inserted through the cervical os. The women may be educated an oral medicine to ensure full uterine contraction following the procedure. Following the procedure, the woman should remain in the rest room for 2 h. She is given the same careful assessment of vital sighs and perineal care as a women following childbirth receives. If there are no complications, she may return home after approximately 2 h and after being told of the danger signs of abortion and pertinent contraceptive counseling. The danger signs should be reported or visit to clinic.

The perineum area should keep cleaning. She should not douche, use tampons, or resume coitus until 2 weeks after the procedure. She should return in 2 weeks for a pelvic examination and pregnancy test to be certain that the procedure was successful and her pregnancy was effectively terminated.

任务实施

人工流产术操作步骤见表18-2。

表18-2　人工流产术操作步骤

项目	内容
术前准备	1. 与受术者沟通,简单询问病史,缓解受术者紧张情绪,解除受术者思想顾虑
	2. 测体温、血压,进行全身检查、妇科检查,完善病历书写
	3. 对精神紧张者,适当给予镇静药物
手术步骤	1. 术者穿清洁工作服,戴帽子、口罩,肥皂洗手,戴无菌手套
	2. 受术者体位:排空膀胱,取膀胱截石位,常规清洁外阴、阴道
	3. 将手术器械依次放妥,铺无菌巾,妇科检查行双合诊,再次确定子宫大小、倾曲度
	4. 以阴道扩张器暴露子宫颈,消毒阴道(碘伏)、子宫颈(碘伏)
	5. 以子宫颈钳钳夹子宫颈前唇中部,稍向外牵拉,使子宫呈水平位
	6. 探测宫腔深度、曲度(探针顺宫腔方向)
	7. 扩张子宫颈:由小到大扩至大于吸管半号至1号(执笔式,稳、准、轻,禁止跳号)
	8. 吸管选择:根据宫腔大小选择吸管(<10 cm 选6号,10~12 cm 选7号,12 cm 选8号)
	9. 连接宫腔吸管:一端连接吸管末端,另一端由助手接在负压吸引瓶上
	10. 送入吸管,开动负压:负压400~500 mmHg,孕9周以上用7~8号,负压450~550 mmHg,不宜超过600 mmHg。顺时针方向或逆时针方向吸引宫腔1~2周,紧贴子宫壁上下移动,至宫壁粗糙、宫腔缩小、仅见少量血性泡沫表示吸净宫腔,停止操作
	11. 取出吸管:夹毕吸管、关闭负压,取出吸管、释放压力
	12. 检查宫腔是否吸净:以小号刮匙轻刮宫角,测量宫腔深度可缩小1~3 cm
	13. 擦净阴道血性物,取下子宫颈钳及阴道扩张器
	14. 检查吸出物,有无绒毛膜胚胎组织,与妊娠月份是否相符,如有异常,送病理科。估计失血量,写手术记录
	15. 写术后医嘱:①休息2 h,注意阴道流血情况;②1个月内禁房事、盆浴;③发生腹痛、发热、阴道流血多或持续2周以上应随诊;④指导避孕;⑤1个月后随访

续表 18-2

项目	内容
注意事项	1. 严格无菌操作
	2. 动作稳、准、轻、细

女性绝育方法及护理

微课

课件

练习题及参考答案

（刘淑霞）

参考文献

[1] 安利彬,陆虹. 妇产科护理学[M]. 7 版. 北京:人民卫生出版社,2022.

[2] 谢幸,孔北华,段涛. 妇产科学[M]. 9 版. 北京:人民卫生出版社,2018.

[3] 狄文,曹云霞. 妇产科学[M]. 北京:人民卫生出版社,2019.

[4] 魏碧蓉. 助产学[M]. 北京:人民卫生出版社,2019.

[5] 余艳红,陈叙. 助产学[M]. 北京:人民卫生出版社,2017.

[6] 张欣,胡向莲. 妇产科护理学[M]. 3 版. 西安:第四军医大学出版社,2015.

[7] 何俐. 妇产科护理[M]. 郑州:河南科学技术出版社,2015.

[8] 谢幸,苟文丽. 妇产科学[M]. 8 版. 北京:人民卫生出版社,2013.

[9] 郑修霞. 妇产科护理学[M]. 5 版. 北京:人民卫生出版社,2012.

[10] 沈铿,马丁. 妇产科学[M]. 3 版. 北京:人民卫生出版社,2015.

[11] 何俐,赵远芳. 妇科护理学[M]. 北京:人民卫生出版社,2016.

[12] 夏海鸥. 妇产科护理学[M]. 3 版. 北京:人民卫生出版社,2014.